INTERPROFESSIONAL APPROACH TO

REFUGEE HEALTH

Interprofessional Approach to Refugee Health

A Practical Guide for Interdisciplinary Health and Social Care Teams

Edited by Emer McGowan, Djenana Jalovcic and Sarah Quinn

OpenBook Publishers

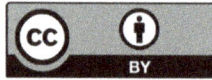

https://www.openbookpublishers.com

All external links were active at the time of publication unless otherwise stated and have been archived via the Internet Archive Wayback Machine at https://archive.org/web

Digital material and resources associated with this volume are available at
https://doi.org/10.11647/OBP.0479#resources

Information about any revised edition of this work will be provided at
https://doi.org/10.11647/OBP.0479

ISBN Paperback: 978-1-80511-658-5
ISBN Hardback: 978-1-80511-659-2
ISBN PDF: 978-1-80511-660-8
ISBN HTML: 978-1-80511-662-2
ISBN EPUB: 978-1-80511-661-5
DOI: https://doi.org/10.11647/OBP.0479

Cover image: Photo by Annalisa Overgaard, a shadow of a tree on a wall, November 7, 2024, https://unsplash.com/photos/a-shadow-of-a-tree-on-a-wall-CiymNBWclhE
Cover design: Jeevanjot Kaur Nagpal

Contents

V. SOCIAL AND OCCUPATIONAL DETERMINANTS OF MENTAL HEALTH FOR REFUGEES

The book is part of the Persons with Refugee Experience Education - Interprofessional project (https://prosjekt.hvl.no/prep/) implemented with support from the European Commission. Views and opinions expressed are those of the authors only and do not necessarily reflect those of the European Union or the European Education and Culture Executive Agency (EACEA). Neither the European Union nor EACEA can be held responsible for them.

Co-funded by
the European Union

Notes on Contributors

Hassan Alipanahzadeh, M.Sc. Lecturer, Department of Health and Functioning, Western Norway University of Applied Sciences, HVL.

Amira* (name changed) Freelance Journalist, Damascus, Syria.

Kerstin Berr, M.Sc. Occupational therapist, Project Manager, Robert Bosch Center for Innovative Health, Stuttgart, Germany.

Méabh Bonham Corcoran Occupational Therapist, PhD Candidate, Discipline of Occupational Therapy, School of Medicine, Trinity College Dublin, The University of Dublin.

Ousman Drammeh Occupational Therapist, Bremen, Germany.

Huseyin Emlik, PhD Candidate M.Sc. Sociologist, Advisor, Center for Migration Health (CMH), Bergen, Norway. PhD Candidate, Department of Health and Functioning, Western Norway University of Applied Sciences.

Mohammad Ali Farhat, M.R.S. M.Sc (rehebilitation science), B.A (psychology).

Franziska Grünberg-Lemli, M.Sc. Physiotherapist, Center for Social Paediatrics, Celle, Germany.

Dr Aisling Hearns, PhD, MA (Addiction Studies), MA (Cognitive Science), MA (Psychotherapy), BA (Psychology).

Dr Rachel Hoare, PhD, Assistant Professor, School of Languages, Literatures and Cultures, Trinity College Dublin, The University of Dublin. Director of The Centre for Forced Migration Studies, Trinity College Dublin.

Dr Djenana Jalovcic, EdD, MPA, MSc (ed.) Associate Professor, Department of Health and Functioning, Western Norway University of Applied Sciences.

Kass Kasadi, Founder of baobab – zusammensein e.V.; Project manager for Elikia.

Dr Emer McGowan, PhD (ed.), Assistant Professor in Interprofessional Learning, Discipline of Medical Education, School of Medicine, Trinity College Dublin, The University of Dublin.

Sarah Quinn (ed.), Assistant Professor, Discipline of Occupational Therapy, School of Medicine, Trinity College Dublin, The University of Dublin.

Angelika Roschka, M.Sc. Occupational Therapist, Lecturer, Researcher, Trainer and Coach for Anti Bias, Democracy and Transculture, Ernst-Abbe-Hochschule Jena, University of Applied Sciences and Hochschule Fulda, Fulda Graduate Centre of Social Sciences.

Dr Sandra Schiller, PhD, M.Sc., Dipl.-Bibl., Honorary Professor, Lecturer, HAWK University of Applied Sciences and Arts Hildesheim/Holzminden/Göttingen, Faculty of Social Work and Health, Hildesheim, Germany.

Dr Fintan Sheerin, PhD, Associate Professor in Intellectual Disability Nursing, School if Nursing and Midwifery, Trinity College Dublin, The University of Dublin.

Christine Spevak-Grossi, M.Sc., Occupational Therapist, Lecturer, Researcher, IMC Krems University of Applied Sciences, Piaristengasse, Krems, Austria.

Rolf Vardal, Physiotherapist, Center for Migration Health (CM), Bergen, Norway.

Dr Frédérique Vallières, PhD, Associate Professor in Global Health and Psychology, Director of the Trinity Centre for Global Health, Trinity College Dublin, The University of Dublin.

Kathrin Weiß, M.Sc., Occupational Therapist, Lecturer, HAWK University of Applied Sciences and Arts Hildesheim/Holzminden/Göttingen, Faculty of Social Work and Health, Hildesheim, Germany.

Andreas Wolfs, M.A., Lecturer, HAWK University of Applied Sciences and Arts Hildesheim/Holzminden/Göttingen, Faculty of Social Work and Health, Hildesheim, Germany.

Dr Ganzamungu Zihindula, PhD, Centre for Global Health, Trinity College Dublin, Ireland. Global Atlantic Fellow for Health Equity, Oxford University, UK. Institut Superieur pour le Development Rural (ISDR-Kaziba).

List of Illustrations and Tables

Illustrations

Tables

Foreword

Aisling Hearns

As a mental health professional who has spent most of my career working with refugees—many of whom have endured unimaginable suffering before finding refuge in Ireland—I have witnessed first-hand the profound and lasting impact of displacement. These experiences have deeply influenced my approach to providing care, emphasizing the need for a compassionate, holistic, and culturally sensitive approach. This holistic model of care was a key finding in my doctoral research, which focused on working with torture survivors seeking international protection in Ireland. I found that providing certainty, a sense of control, and empowerment in healthcare settings is essential for facilitating healing.

Understanding the global context in which refugees live is crucial to delivering effective care. Section 1 of this book provides an essential overview of global migrations, the reasons behind forced migration, and the impact these experiences have on health. This broader context is critical for health professionals who seek to offer care that is both informed and empathetic, recognizing the complex realities that refugees face.

One of the most important lessons I have learned is the value of creating a therapeutic space where refugees feel safe, respected, and heard. Many individuals I have worked with carry deep emotional and psychological scars from their experiences of war, torture, and persecution. Section 2 delves into how healthcare professionals can provide person-centred care by creating such therapeutic environments. Building trust is key, and this often means taking the time to listen to

     https://doi.org/10.11647/OBP.0479.15

experiences, active involvement in care, and addressing not just physical symptoms but the whole person.

Interprofessional collaboration is another cornerstone of effective refugee healthcare. The complex needs of this population require the coordinated efforts of various professionals. In my practice, I have seen how integrated teamwork can significantly enhance the care provided to refugees. Section 3 explores the importance of professional identity, critical reflection and effective collaboration between professionals in ensuring that refugees receive comprehensive, high-quality care.

Cultural competence is an ongoing process of learning and reflection, rather than a skill to be simply acquired. Refugees come from diverse backgrounds, with unique beliefs, values, and practices that influence their perceptions of illness and healthcare. Section 4 emphasizes the need for healthcare providers to develop a deep understanding of these cultural dimensions. In my experience, the most effective care comes from professionals who approach their work with humility and a willingness to learn from the people they serve.

Finally, I have been deeply inspired by the resilience and strength of the refugees I have worked with. Despite immense suffering, many find ways to rebuild their lives, regain their sense of purpose, and contribute to their new communities. Providing opportunities for social connections, empowerment, and meaningful engagement is crucial to this healing process. Section 5 discusses the social and occupational determinants of mental health, highlighting how these factors can support refugees in regaining control over their lives and finding a sense of belonging.

Throughout my career, I have been continually inspired by the stories of survival, resilience, and hope shared by those I have been fortunate enough to have worked with. This book offers a comprehensive guide to improving refugee healthcare, drawing on both practical strategies and personal narratives. *Interprofessional Approach to Refugee Health* is a call to action for healthcare professionals to deepen their understanding, enhance their skills, and approach their work with empathy and respect. By doing so, we can make a meaningful difference in the lives of refugees, helping them to heal, rebuild, and thrive in their new communities.

0. Introduction

Emer McGowan, Djenana Jalovcic, and
Sarah Quinn

Global displacement of populations continues to rise, with millions of individuals and families forced to move by conflict, persecution, climate change, environmental degradation and socioeconomic instability. As displaced populations seek safety and refuge in host countries, they frequently encounter complex challenges that can have profound implications on their physical health, mental wellbeing, and social integration. People with refugee experience can face significant barriers to accessing appropriate health and social care, including linguistic and cultural differences, legal and administrative challenges, trauma-related mental health conditions, and socioeconomic exclusion. Overcoming these barriers requires not only compassionate care but also a coordinated, interprofessional response. This book explores the complex intersection of health and social care in the context of forced migration. It aims to illuminate the health-related challenges that refugees can face, and the strategies and approaches that health and social care providers can implement to support these vulnerable populations.

This book aims to be a resource and practical guide for health and social care professionals to prepare them to work with, and provide services for, people with refugee experience. It is targeted at health and social care professionals who are new to working with people who have been forcibly displaced. As the number of people with refugee experience continues to increase, health and social care professionals in a range of contexts will be tasked with providing effective, equitable, and culturally responsive health and social care to refugee populations whose needs are complex and often unmet. Research has demonstrated

    https://doi.org/10.11647/OBP.0479.00

that refugees can present with complex and unmet healthcare needs, and that health professionals can feel underprepared to adequately meet these needs. The intention of this book is to provide practical suggestions and evidence-based approaches to assist health and social care professionals to improve the services they provide to people with refugee experience. It is not only for health and social care professionals, but also policymakers, educators, students, and anyone committed to building more inclusive and equitable healthcare systems.

Drawing on current evidence, global best practice, and frontline experiences, this book features contributions from authors with backgrounds in a range of different health and social care professions including nursing, occupational therapy, psychology, psychotherapy, physiotherapy, and speech and language therapy. The heterogeneity of the contributors and range of professional practices presented mean that this book will be relevant and useful to a variety of health and social care professionals. Factors including mental health challenges, trauma, chronic illness, housing insecurity, and language barriers contribute to a complex picture that demands a holistic and person-centred approach. No single profession can fully meet the diverse needs of people with refugee experience. Effective care delivery relies on the collaborative efforts and effective teamwork of professionals across health and social care. Given the diversity of the contributing authors' backgrounds, it is not possible to give a list of definitions used in the book. Where applicable, the authors have included definitions of key terms within the text of their chapter. The reader should take these into account, along with the professional and geographic background of each contributing author, when reading their contributions.

The book is primarily focused on providing care for people who have been forcibly displaced and as such encompasses people with refugee experience and asylum seekers. While much of the content will be relevant to other types of migrants, the text has been written with those who have been forcibly displaced across countries in mind. Throughout this book, readers will find analysis of key themes such as health equity, mental health and psychosocial support, person-centred care, cultural competence, interprofessional collaboration, and integration. Real-world case studies and reflective practice prompts are presented to support both academic inquiry and practical application.

Across the globe, the number of people forcibly displaced continues to rise as people flee war, persecution, poverty, environmental catastrophe, and the effects of climate. Behind each statistic is a person with a story, a family, and a way of life that they have had to leave behind. The need for compassionate, culturally competent, and accessible health and social care has never been greater. The lived experiences of people with refugee experience are of central importance in this book. No two refugees will have the same experiences.

To bring lived experiences to the centre of our attention and to illustrate the far-reaching impact of forced migration in a person's life, personal stories from three people with refugee experience are included in this introduction. These writings demonstrate the importance of listening to someone's history and experience when working with them in a health and social care context. Each person is very different, but each conveys the trauma of leaving their country of origin and being forcibly displaced, and how their experience of being a refugee continues to influence many aspects of their life.

Personal Narratives

Personal Narrative 1: Before and After

There is a deep scar that divides my life into before and after the war. Everything else is in between.

Before

Peace, prosperity, freedom, growth, care, love, brotherhood and unity, fun, travel, education, work, joy... My life was no different from the lives of my peers in any other part of Europe. And then the unimaginable happened.

In Between

The war swept my homeland, catching us unprepared for all the horrors that it brought. Some saw it coming, but for the majority of us it was inconceivable to think that it could happen to us. We lived and loved together, shared values, respected each other, and built the country and our future together. The country in which I was born fell apart. Our friends became enemies. "Our army" with its heavy artillery besieged the city with tanks and cannons targeting the city. We demonstrated for peace. We took over the streets that were blocked by masked gunmen. Until they started killing us. Every day, every moment from every weapon they had. In disbelief that the war was happening to us, we started to gather the pieces of our destroyed lives, homes, families, friendships, libraries, schools, hospitals... like *kintsugi,* the Japanese art of repairing broken pottery by connecting it with gold... we started putting our lives together, connected by the only gold we had, our unbreakable bonds of love, respect, solidarity, and friendship.

In my head I rewound millions of times the memories from the beginning of the war. The scenes I had watched from the window of my office: the enemy tank just two blocks away firing at the municipal building. In black and white. Sounds of the shells being launched. Sounds of the shells coming towards you. Sounds of explosions. The thick unbreathable air filled with the dust of destroyed buildings and smell of gunpowder mixed with burned lives and livelihoods.

The bread-line massacre. The first of many massacres of people trying to live.

No water. No electricity. No food. No windows. No fuel. No communication. No transportation. No...

Destroyed libraries, research institutes, educational institutions, health facilities... A gaping hole in the ceiling of my brother's room. My cousin killed while collecting water. Her two small children survived. The entrance to my building blown up. My little cousin killed while playing with his brother in front of their building, his brother severely wounded.

People killed and wounded in their homes, offices, streets, shelters, while collecting water, waiting in the bread lines, attending the funerals. Children killed and wounded everywhere, while they were playing inside and outside. On their way to and from schools and during their classes. Health workers killed while saving lives. News of family members, friends, neighbours who had been killed, wounded.

Dead bodies lined up in front of the hospital morgue. Washing the office floor in the hospital, the blood, flesh, and brain of an unknown person killed in front of it. Cleaning the debris of what was left of our sitting room after being directly hit by a shell. Hoping for this nightmare to end.

Peacekeepers. International humanitarian agencies. Incredible humanitarians of all professions who left the comfort and safety of their homes to support us, defend our collective humanity, experience the horror, help, witness, and share.

The power of life. Finding energy to survive from precious moments we shared with others. Joy of seeing loved ones alive. Long and strong hugs we gave each other every time we met, like it was the last time. Warm, irresistible scent of the tasty pie that mama magically made of rice and flour, the only staples we had. Being fit from always running to avoid snipers and carrying dozens of litres of water to the top floor of the building on the top of the hill where we lived. Listening to the music on a crackling radio connected to the car battery. Celebrating when the rabbit-shaped thermometer showed the room temperature of eight degrees next to the woodstove in the middle of the long and cold winter.

We carried on. Fought back by being dignified in life and death. By going to work, distributing medicines and medical supplies, helping others, sharing, partying, grieving and hoping together, by organizing make-shift shelters, health facilities, support centres, radio programs, exhibitions, performances, concerts, book readings, festivals...

Every day every citizen of this besieged city was going towards her or his shell or bullet, or away from it.

No past. No future. Present, in between.

No safe place. Fear for my family, fear for my friends, fear for my life. Will this bloody war ever finish?

Walking through the vibrant streets of a European metropolis filled with happy, worriless people. Lost in a new and beautiful place. Not belonging. Crying uncontrollably. Waiting for any piece of news from my home and fearing that it would be devastating. Crying uncontrollably. Fainting. Attending language classes with other refugees from other parts of the world who understood. Attending rallies to stop racism. Crying uncontrollably. Waiting for resettlement. Living in uncertainty. Crying uncontrollably. Checking newspapers for any photos from the besieged city. Recognizing people. Violently shaking. Crying uncontrollably. I survived. Feeling guilty because I survived. Crying uncontrollably. It never occurred to me to seek professional help.

News from home. Genocide.

Resettlement.

Military intervention.

Crying uncontrollably.

Recurring nightmare: endless columns of the enemy soldiers and tanks are advancing towards my home city.

Peace.

After

Starting a new life from scratch as who I was did not count. Working hard to be able to support rehabilitation and recovery efforts back home. Being positive and hopeful. Healing through the war stories told over, and over again. Making new friends. Finding spaces to grow and develop in a new country. Going back to school. Finding a new home. And homeland. Nurturing friendships. Feeling safe and free. Making life choices to enable me to give back. Feeling the pain of intergenerational trauma of First Nations and Indigenous People on whose land I settled uninvited. Feeling responsible for supporting others who have been experiencing war, genocide and displacement. Solidarity. Finding peace with my own multiple identities. Loving my new home country. Her vast land, beautiful lakes and magnificent autumns, her diverse people, and all those working on truth and reconciliation.

Through work witnessing peace negotiated in two countries after decades of war. Hearing a helicopter triggers the memory. Violently shaking.

Keeping positive and hopeful. My tears dried out but the excruciating pain of seeing other people suffering remains.

Returning to my country of origin and being there for its rebuilding and fragile recovery.

I remember. Walking through the streets of a once-besieged city that looks like any other European city. Beautiful and vibrant. As I walk her streets, I remember people killed and wounded in this street, at that corner. I can still clearly see where once the sign "be aware of sniper" was placed. I can still hear sniper bullets around my head. As I cross this bridge, I see my cousin crawling over it from the occupied part of the city while they were shooting at her. When I climb the mountains around the city, I realize what easy targets we were. I hate fireworks.

Recurring nightmare: endless columns of the enemy soldiers and tanks are advancing towards my home city.

Somehow, 29 years later still feeling vulnerable.

I am not safe and free until everyone is safe and free.

Personal Narrative 2: A Son of a Stateless Society

Telling or writing your own story might seem like an easy task, but it is far more challenging than it appears. To narrate a life spent in continuous struggle, fighting just to declare "I am alive", this is no simple feat. I ask myself, was this struggle my choice? Or did I fight because there was no other option but to resist the darkness that sought to consume me, to annihilate me?

Imagine the worst atrocities that a hegemonic structure bent on annihilating an entire people could commit: civil wars, massacres, deaths, the stench of blood, tortures. Envision babies, children, the elderly, women, pregnant women, and helpless people being brutally burned alive. Is it possible to stay silent in the face of such horrors? To remain indifferent? I couldn't stay silent. To be silent, I would either have to kill myself or be killed.

I wanted to describe myself this way: I am a son of a stateless society. To know this, to be aware of it and to live with this awareness, and either to be totally silent in the face of a system that is so thoroughly assimilationist, or to fight against it. This is my reality. I had no other choice. The poverty that enveloped me and my family, and all the negative conditions it caused, stemmed from the colonisation of my country. It took me a few years to understand and recognize this.

Colonialism is like a dark hole. I am not talking here about the Western kind of colonialism but instead about settler colonialism, which denies your existence and builds its own state on your land. If you want to live here, you must exist within the homogeneous national identity they desire. This is why I compare settler colonialism to a dark hole. This dark hole tries to pull you in no matter what. If you resist assimilation, this system will resort to all sorts of brutal policies to subdue you. It sees itself above the people and all social values, organized and constructed on a single national identity, and it employs every fascist practice to melt all different ethnic identities living within the borders of its constructed nation-state into the same homogeneous national identity.

In this system, being Kurdish is enough to be killed, imprisoned, tortured, or impoverished. This is the oppression my people have been subjected to for a century. For a hundred years, the Kurdish people, who have endured numerous genocidal attempts and hundreds of massacres, have tried to survive in this vortex of oppression. The oppression has not ended; it continues. Despite this brutal oppression, the Kurdish people, one of the ancient nations of the fertile Mesopotamian geography between the Tigris and Euphrates rivers, do not give up their language, culture, and identity.

I wanted to describe myself as an individual who is part of such a social identity. All the uniqueness that makes me who I am emerged under these social conditions. In primary school, when I told my teacher that I wanted to be educated in my native language, Kurdish, I was subjected to physical and psychological violence and eventually expelled from school. This experience shaped my consciousness, leading me to become a human rights activist in my high school years. I witnessed a major civil war following a period of armed internal conflicts. During my university years, as an activist fighting for our most natural human rights, many of my friends who fought alongside me were arrested and imprisoned. Balancing the fight for justice and my academic studies, I evolved my struggle into the academic field and continued the intellectual fight for Kurdish rights at an intellectual level as an activist.

The state declared curfews, and explosions and gunfire were heard everywhere. The sound of a bomb explosion, the screams of fear from the crowd, the smell of blood... The sound of bullets hitting walls, war helicopters and planes, and fear... Living during all this had become shameful for me. Yes, living can sometimes be a heavy burden. Innocent people were being killed, and I was alive. It is impossible to describe in words how heavy this burden is. Having narrowly escaped death a few times did not make me happy because I lost many friends and human rights defenders in these terrorist acts.

During all this turmoil, I continued my master's education and began conducting professional academic research. In my master's thesis, I wanted to investigate the sociological manifestations of this century-long oppression the Kurds have faced. I aimed to research the societal trauma caused by war and genocidal policies inflicted on the Kurdish people, particularly focusing on recent social memory. Through intellectual activism, I wanted to pay a small part of my debt to my people. However, as in all other areas, the field of academic research had come under heavy pressure from the ruling powers. Academic freedom had almost vanished, and conducting critical and objective academic research on the Kurdish question had become forbidden. People were being killed, unjustly imprisoned, exiled, and subjected to demographic cleansing in the Kurdish region. Any critical voice or study of these oppressive policies was also banned. Researchers who wanted to advocate for the Kurds and to document history through academic work were being expelled from universities one by one, in an attempt to render them passive individuals.

During such a period, my master's thesis was also obstructed, and the institute where I was to conduct my research threatened me, saying, "We cannot accept this work; if you insist, we will expel you from school." However, I did not want to give up, and I completed my research and wrote my thesis. Unfortunately, as expected, my thesis was not accepted by the institute, and I was forced to find a new thesis topic. However, I did not abandon my research field. This entire process made life increasingly unbearable for me. I had to either remain silent, becoming a mute devil, because, for me, remaining silent in the face of oppression is also supporting it, or find a new alternative to continue my activism. These harsh conditions led me to emigrate from the country because I needed to feel free to say that I was truly living.

In Exile

Exile is the common destiny of the children of Kurdistan and I have become a subject of this common destiny. The fascist state policies that intensify every day, the government's increasing repression in all areas, and the growing pressure on dissenters compelled me to emigrate to a northern European country to continue my academic education, marking the beginning of my exile.

Experiencing exile first-hand led me to question this phenomenon and how I should navigate this process from my perspective. For me, exile is not the imprisonment of the "cursed identities" (Fanon, 2023) that I carry, but rather a space where an intellectual reclaims and asserts their power. Thus, exile can be seen not as a well of suffering or the depths of despair romanticized by others, but as a site heralding a new rebellion.

The state of exile or the garden of sorrow that comes with separation, in my view, is not just about being far from home or longing for a lost home. It is also about re-engaging with one's personal political history. Being exiled, especially coming from the Kurdish area ingrained with memories of war and violence, means embarking on this journey with a certain memory and engaging in new intellectual activities within this new homeland. For the oppressed, exile can signify a colonial history in their memory and simultaneously a rebirth in the present. Exile serves as a space of protest, a place where the body can find new freedom, and where a wounded language and fragile identity can emerge as new political subjects.

Exile is a space where the fragile, the overlooked, tries to define itself between existence and non-existence. Edward Said (1996), while discussing exile from Palestine, does not describe it as a pit of destiny. Instead, he views this traumatic space as an area of liberation. He describes it as an opportunity for the intellectual, encountering new narratives and witnessing new geographies, to facilitate the reformation of their distant homeland here. When we speak of the Kurdish area, we see that the issue of Kurds and Kurdistan, from the moment it began to emerge on the 20th-century stage, particularly affected the Kurdish intelligentsia with significant experiences of exile. Drawing inspiration from this historical legacy, I find myself closely aligning with Edward Said's definition of the intellectual in exile. I do not want to view exile merely as an area of suffering or nostalgia. Instead, following Said's perspective, I want to contemplate how an intellectual in exile can transform exile into an intellectual capacity, a field of knowledge, and even a celebration.

Exile should be read as a place of escape, a refuge for dissenters, not only from a totalitarian regime, war, and violence but also from a society steeped in hatred. Hence, although I may be in exile out of necessity, this necessity also presents itself as a desire. For me, this situation is not merely a trap or a pit of nostalgia. When I came into exile, I asked myself how I could turn the political consequences of this into a new living space. How can we resist fascism? How have those who have been unable to see their families and loved ones for years endured exile? Imagine coming from a deranged social realm and experience of political power, and, for you, exile is both a refuge and a place where you can consciously shape your daily existence into a form of personal political resistance.

While exile often leads to some becoming pathologically introverted, it functions exactly as the veil Said mentions. For Kurds and other stateless peoples, it becomes a space to meet, encounter, and dialogue with transnational values. Exile is a form of neighbourliness; it is a place where you recreate and share certain values through your own agency. In this sense, exile has been for me an area where I established my dark memory with an anti-colonial consciousness and viewed it as a place to liberate that memory.

With such an understanding, I reconstructed the reality that made me a subject in the diaspora. I completed my master's degree with a thesis focusing on Kurdistan's century-long colonization in a northern European country where I have lived for about seven years without ever falling into despair. I strive to strengthen and transform the struggle I maintain for my people using the advantages my current circumstances provide. For me, the diaspora has been a space where I develop new perspectives and strategies, meet people from different nations who share common concerns that strengthen my struggle, and nurture my hope further. This struggle and hope have allowed me to work in a field today where I can create solutions for the challenges of people from various nations and serve them.

The French philosopher Voltaire (2004) said, "We only have two days to live, it is not worth spending them kneeling in front of scoundrels!" I did not kneel in front of fascism for my own individual interests and chose the struggle. Life has been a field of struggle for me since I was born and will remain so until there is not a single oppressed person left on earth. I would like to conclude my personal story with a verse from poet Adnan Yücel (2013): "that fight has not finished yet and it will continue until the earth's surface will be the surface of love."

Personal Narrative 3: My Only Sorrow

Hassan Alipanahzadeh

Writing this text wasn't easy for me. I opened my laptop several times and sat down to write, each time starting with a thought that would take me on a journey, dragging me down like a terrifying nightmare. Along with the fear, anxiety, and worry that tormented me, I would close my laptop again, with a heart full of sorrow, without having written anything. I sought help from my friends who were writing about their own experiences. It was effective; I felt that I wasn't alone, that all of us were going through similar pain, and that this shared feeling was a source of comfort and healing for our wounds.

The story of my fate is a strange one—unbelievable to some, a tragedy to others. It's the story of someone who was born into displacement and migration from the very beginning, the story of an ethnic group that has always suffered, that has never had an identity or a place and has always experienced bitter genocide and forced migration, even within their own country (Raza, 2018).

Amir Abdur Rahman Khan, who spared no effort to exile and massacre my people, even forcing religious clerics to issue a Fatwa to justify his actions, began the slaughter and exile of the Hazara people. Many still believe in that Fatwa today, and it has been the ideological basis for terrorist groups in Afghanistan for the genocide of the Hazara people (Hakimi, 2023).

When the Soviet war and the civil wars intensified, the fear of war, the killing of innocent people, and famine forced my father, a poor, illiterate villager who was opposed to migration, to leave his homeland. The only seemingly better destination was Iran, due to the linguistic and religious similarities and our limited financial means, given the young age of his children.

I was born in Iran in a state hospital. My mother said that Iran was at war with Iraq at the time, but it was still better than Afghanistan. While I was in the hospital due to some medical problem in the neonatal ward, a rocket hit nearby. My family thought I might not survive, but the part of the hospital where I was remained undamaged. Many times, in my life, I have wished that the rocket had hit the part where I was; maybe it would have been easier, simpler for me. But fate seemed to have another plan for me—to survive and fight for my life.

We lived in Iran for years with a special ID card for Afghan refugees, labelled with large red letters. Without any human or civil rights, my only chance was being able to go to school. Despite the relative calm during that time, even with that ID, my father was arrested and humiliated several times under the pretext of not being allowed to work or to be in Iran, before being released. But even that seemed better than being in Afghanistan, especially during the initial period when the Taliban were taking over. Every day, we were tormented by distressing news of Hazara massacres, hoping that the Iranian government wouldn't force us to return.

In 2002, Tabriz, the border city where we were living, was declared a restricted area for Afghans. We had to leave the city and everything that we had made from scratch—our home and friends that we had grown accustomed to and found some solace in. This time, my father was no longer young; the wrinkles on his forehead testified to his tiredness and inability to endure more humiliation, relocation, and confusion. After discussing with friends and relatives, and with the relative calm created by the presence of the United States and its allies, and the fall of the Taliban regime, hopes were higher, and my father was determined to go back to Afghanistan. Despite all the challenges, I had just been accepted into university and wanted to celebrate this, but I knew I would be alone and had to continue the journey on my own. My father, who had always been my support during tough times, squeezed my arms and said, "You have grown up now. Stay and finish your studies so that you don't end up like me—displaced. Have a better fate." I found strength and tried to continue.

After completing my bachelor's and master's degrees at the University of Tehran, while the light of hope was still shining in Afghanistan, I decided to go back to my homeland, both to share the little knowledge I had gained with my people and to perhaps find my lost identity. I will never forget when I said goodbye to my closest friend; his eyes were filled with sorrow as he told me, "You're lucky you studied." He had decided to go to Germany via Turkey and the illegal routes. He even suggested that we go together, but I was tired of migration and determined to go to Afghanistan. I firmly declined and went back. I started working at a private medical university and, a year later, joined Kabul Medical University as a faculty member in the Anatomy Department. It was fulfilling for nearly a decade that I was in Afghanistan. Despite the insecurity, explosions, pressures, and ethnic discriminations, I felt good in my homeland. I felt useful and had become a positive role model for the younger generation of my relatives, especially those in Iran. I always encouraged them that education was the only way out of this tough situation.

In Afghanistan, I was intensely involved in my work, focused only on my goals—improving the department and teaching. During my lectures, I had found a unique opportunity to not only teach anatomy and share my experiences but also to speak about enlightenment and resistance against Taliban brutality and dictatorial ideologies. Many welcomed this, although some gave me hostile looks and whispered among themselves.

In the department, my colleagues and I (as the first anatomist of anatomy department) managed to obtain religious and court permissions for cadaver dissection for the first time in years. With the help of the International Organization for Migration (IOM), we acquired a cadaver, and I became responsible for the dissection. Despite the fears and threats from religious extremists who opposed the dissection, we began our work. Establishing the first dissection centre after so many years was truly gratifying.

I was full of energy, feeling like I was making a difference, and I was happy that I no longer had to hide my identity as a Hazara. I felt obligated to raise my voice for justice, against ethnic discrimination, and against the prejudice towards Hazara people that even extends, in many cases, to support for their enslavement. In this way, I actively participated in demonstrations such as the Enlightenment Movement and the Tabassum movement (Hugueley, 2019). During the Enlightenment Movement demonstration, I even witnessed a suicide bombing near Deh Mazang Square in Kabul, where about one hundred people lost their lives, just 500 meters away from me (Jawad, 2014).

I always encouraged my students to raise their voices against discrimination and to actively participate in the political and social struggles of our country as educated individuals. My emotions had overcome my fears; despite the threats, I was not particularly afraid and kept moving forward. I had like-minded friends who were close to me, and they often advised me, for the sake of my safety and that of my family, to temper my criticisms, especially against religious extremism. I had transitioned from poverty to the middle class due to my job, leading a relatively comfortable life, and I felt good about my progress. I was proud of my journey—sometimes slow, sometimes quick, but always moving forward.

But even this period of relative peace didn't last. Once again, there were whispers of the Taliban regaining control, and the sounds of displacement echoed in my ears. I had students with Taliban-like mindsets; their glances grew more intense, their voices louder. Yet many of us still didn't believe that the Taliban would actually return to power. Unfortunately, that day came. I turned to my father for guidance, drawing from his experiences of migration and displacement, as I had no other support besides him and he was aware of every aspect of my life and problems. Although disheartened, my father had no intention of leaving our homeland.

However, he strongly advised me to leave Afghanistan and not return as long as this regime remains in power. He urged me to fulfil my duty as a father to my family, especially to my two young daughters, and to at least provide them with some semblance of peace. Once again, that familiar, painful lump formed in my throat, and, once again, displacement and forced migration led me back to Iran, as it was the most practical option. My daughter, separated from her kindergarten friends, was deeply upset, but there was no other choice, and I didn't have the heart to explain it to her. My entire time in Iran felt like living in a bitter nightmare, one I wished I could wake up from and end.

I had lost everything—my home, my life, and the friends whose departures left me even more saddened and isolated. But what hurt me the most was seeing the younger members of my extended family, whom I had always encouraged to study for a better future, possibly losing their faith in education and that brighter future when they looked at me. Sometimes, I thought of my friend who had gone west when I returned to Afghanistan; now he had a Western passport, a job, and peace. I wondered if, instead of pursuing my studies, I should have made the same decision he did.

I became determined to do something for the sake of my family, my daughters, the younger members of my extended family who looked up to me, and for all the years of hard work I had invested. I knocked on every door until, finally, one opened, and an opportunity to go to Norway as a researcher presented itself. It felt as if I had been reborn after all the despair, and I felt closer to my friends. I was happy, though my daughter was upset at the thought of losing her school friends again. All I could offer was a fatherly promise that this might be the last move.

This was now my new home. I began to enjoy going to university again and the smiles I received from people as I was walking the streets and starting everything from scratch—something I had learned to do several times before. But it wasn't long into my stay that I received the heart-breaking news of my father's death. It was unbelievable; I could never see him again, nor could I be by his side or attend his funeral in Afghanistan. I had lost the pillar of my support, the one whose prayers had sustained me through the hardest days of my life. It was tough, but I endured it, just as I had endured all the hardships in my life, like so many other Afghans. At least I find some comfort in knowing that my father saw my progress and knew I had reached a safe country with my family. My only sorrow is for my fellow countrymen who are left behind, stranded in Afghanistan, and whom I can't help.

References

Fanon, Frantz. 2023. 'Black skin, white masks', in *Social Theory Re-Wired*, 3rd edn., ed. by Longhofer, Wesley, and Daniel Winchester (Routledge), pp. 364–371, https://doi.org/10.4324/9781003320609

Hakimi, Mehdi J. 2023. 'The Afghan state and the Hazara genocide', *Harvard Human Rights Journal*, 37: 81–116.

Hugueley, Savannah. 2019. 'The Enlightenment Movement', *Radicle: Reed Anthropology Review*, 4.1.

Jawad, Ali Aqa Mohammad. 2014. 'Dynamics of Protest Mobilization and Rapid Demobilization in Post-2001 Afghanistan: Facing Enlightening Movement', *International Journal of Humanities and Social Sciences*, 14.8: 564–577.

OHCHR. 2017. *Report on the Human Rights Situation in South-East Turkey*, https://www.ohchr.org/sites/default/files/Documents/Countries/TR/OHCHR_South-East_TurkeyReport_10March2017.pdf

Raza, Ali. 2018. 'Identity crisis in the wake of mass migration: A study of identity crisis and acculturation strategies of Hazara diaspora living in Arendal' (Universitetet i Agder: University of Agder).

Said, Edward W. 1996. *Representations of the Intellectual* (New York: Vintage).

Voltaire, Francois. 2004. *Philosophical dictionary* (Penguin: UK).

Yücel, Adnan. 2013. *Yeryüzü Aşkın Yüzü Oluncaya Dek* (Yurt Kitap Yayın).

I. Global Migrations

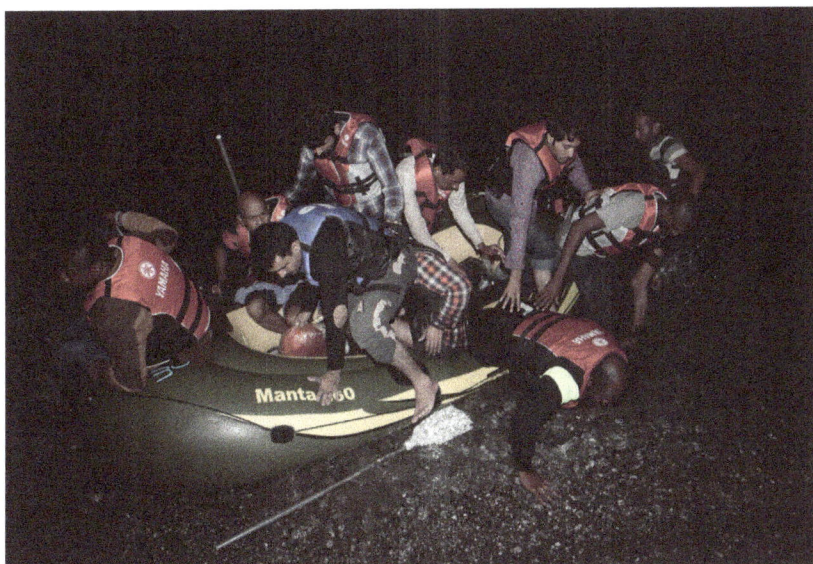

1. Global Migrations and Persons with Refugee Experiences

Huseyin Emlik

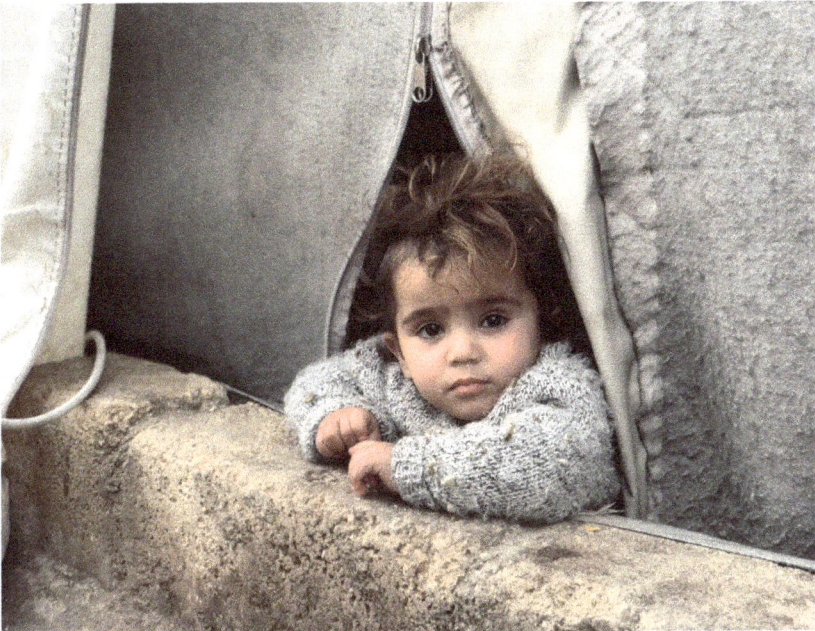

Refugees are neither seen nor heard, but they are everywhere. They are witnesses to the most awful things that people can do to each other, and they become storytellers simply by existing. Refugees embody misery and suffering, and they force us to confront terrible chaos and evil. (Helton 2002).

 https://doi.org/10.11647/OBP.0479.01

Introduction

The issue of forced migration has gained considerable attention in global discussions, highlighting significant humanitarian, legal, and socio-economic difficulties. The term "persons with refugee experiences" refers to individuals who have been compelled to leave their countries of origin due to a legitimate fear of persecution, armed conflict, or other forms of violence and have sought shelter in another country (Helton 2002). This group includes those who have been officially recognized as refugees under international law, as well as asylum seekers who are in the process of having their claims assessed. Comprehending the experiences and obstacles faced by these individuals is essential for creating effective policies and interventions aimed at their protection and integration.

In an era marked by unprecedented levels of forced displacement, comprehending the experiences of persons with refugee backgrounds is more critical than ever. This chapter delves into the complexities of global migration, focusing on individuals compelled to leave their home countries due to conflict, persecution, and other crises. By examining the legal, social, economic, and health-related aspects of refugee experiences, this chapter aims to illuminate the challenges and opportunities faced by displaced populations.

The chapter is structured to provide a comprehensive analysis of migration trends, the legal frameworks governing refugee protection, and the lived realities of those navigating forced migration. It begins with an overview of global migration patterns and the factors driving displacement, including geopolitical instability, climate change, and economic disparities. Following this, it examines the legal definitions of refugees, asylum seekers, and internally displaced persons (IDPs), as well as the challenges in accessing protection under international law.

A central focus of this chapter is the multi-stage refugee experience, encompassing pre-migration trauma, the dangers of migration journeys, and the complex process of integration into host societies. The mental and physical health implications of forced migration are highlighted, along with a discussion of the policies and interventions that can support successful resettlement. Furthermore, the role of host countries in providing humanitarian assistance and fostering social inclusion is explored, while also addressing barriers such as discrimination, legal restrictions, and economic challenges faced by many refugees.

This chapter is intended for a broad audience, including policymakers, researchers, practitioners in migration and refugee studies, humanitarian workers, and students in the fields of sociology, international relations, and public health. By integrating empirical research, case studies, and theoretical perspectives, it aims to provide a nuanced understanding of the refugee experience and the broader implications of global migration trends. Whether engaged in academic research, policy development, or frontline humanitarian work, this chapter offers readers valuable insights into the realities of displacement and the pathways toward effective refugee support and integration.

Global Migration Trends and Context

International migration has remained a persistent feature of globalization. As of 2020, nearly 280 million people were living outside their country of birth, constituting approximately 3.6% of the world's population (IOM 2024). While this figure may appear significant, it is essential to contextualize it.[1] Over the past three decades, the proportion of international migrants in relation to the global population has remained relatively stable, fluctuating between 2.8% and 3.6%. However, due to overall population growth, the absolute number of migrants has steadily increased (See Table 1.1: Overview of migrants between 1990 and 2020). In 1990, there were approximately 153 million international migrants, but by 2020, this number had grown by nearly 85%, reflecting broader demographic trends and intensified migration drivers.

---

1   Since some organization and countries may have different definition of migrants, and different criteria, their numbers may vary.

Year	Number of migrants	Migrants as a % of the world's population
1990	152,986,157	2.9 %
1995	161,289,976	2.8 %
2000	173,230,585	2.8 %
2005	191,446,828	2.9 %
2010	220,983,187	3.2 %
2015	247,958,644	3.4 %
2020	280,598,105	3.6 %

Table 1.1. Overview of migrants between 1990 and 2020 (IOM 2024).

Among these 280 million migrants, labour migration remains the dominant form, as the vast majority of people relocate for work, education, or family reunification. However, a growing subset of international migrants consists of forcibly displaced persons—those who have fled their homes due to persecution, armed conflict, or environmental disasters. By the end of 2023, the United Nations High Commissioner for Refugees (UNHCR) reported that 117.2 million individuals were forcibly displaced worldwide, meaning that roughly 42% of all international migrants fall into this category.

Major Migration Corridors and Forced Displacement

Migration corridors offer valuable insights into the ways historical, economic, and geopolitical relationships influence mobility. The Mexico–United States corridor remains the largest globally, with nearly 11 million migrants (IOM 2024). Conversely, the Syria-Türkiye corridor has emerged as the largest refugee movement worldwide, with Türkiye hosting over 3.6 million Syrian refugees following the protracted Syrian civil war (see Figure 1.1). These corridors underscore distinct migration dynamics: economic migration versus forced displacement due to conflict. Notably, these migrants represent only a small fraction of those who express a desire to migrate (World Bank 2018). The Gallup World Poll indicates that 13% of the global population would like to migrate.

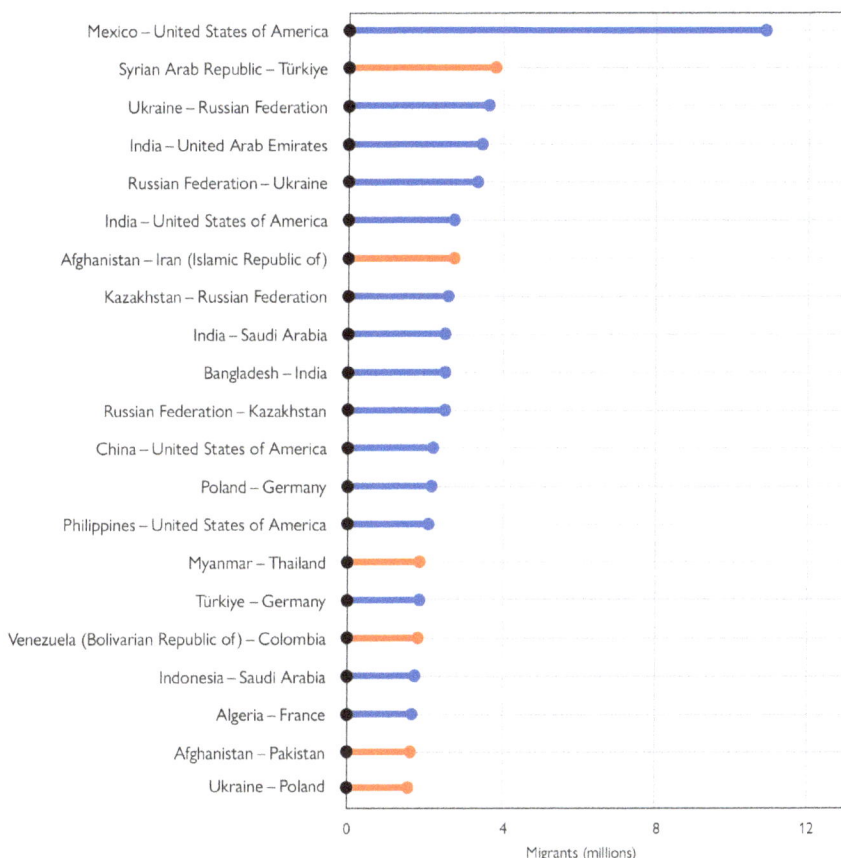

Notes: The corridors represent the number of international migrants (millions) born in the first-mentioned country and residing in the second. Corridors represent an accumulation of migratory movements over time and provide a snapshot of how migration patterns have evolved into significant foreign-born populations in specific destination countries.

Those corridors comprising mainly displaced persons are coloured orange. Revisions have been made based on large-scale displacement from Ukraine to neighbouring countries (as at end October 2023).

Fig. 1.1 Top international country-to-country migration corridors, 2024 (IOM 2024).

The sharp increase in forced displacement is alarming, as the number of forcibly displaced persons has nearly doubled in just a decade. In contrast, the overall international migrant population has not grown at a comparable rate, suggesting an increasing proportion of individuals moving out of necessity rather than choice. According to the United Nations High Commissioner for Refugees (UNHCR), the number of forcibly displaced persons has reached unprecedented levels, with over 117.2 million individuals projected to be displaced or stateless in 2023 (UNHCR 2023). Of these 117.2 million forcibly displaced individuals in 2023, nearly 62 million were internally displaced persons (IDPs), indicating displacement within their own countries. This distinction is significant: while international migration garners global attention, most displacement occurs within national borders.

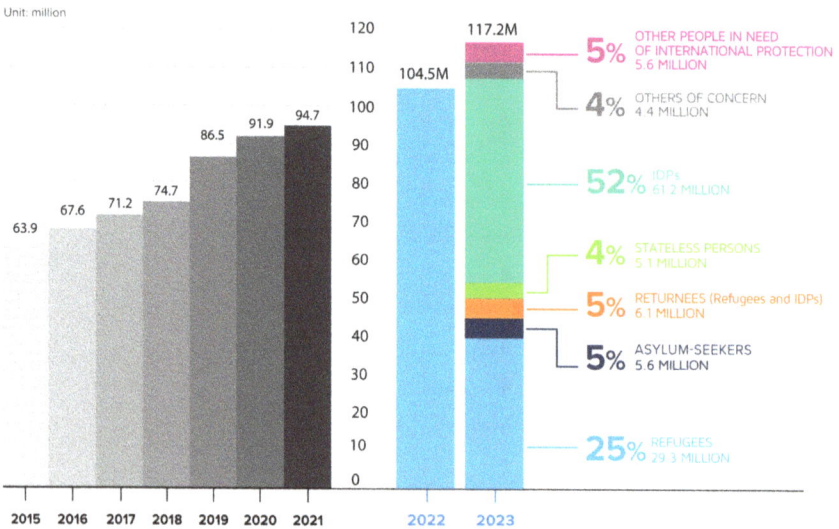

Fig. 1.2 117.2 million forcibly displaced and stateless people in 2023 (UNHCR 2023).

The rise in IDPs suggests that addressing displacement requires both national and international efforts, focusing not only on cross-border refugees but also on the millions forced to relocate within their own countries due to violence, persecution, or climate change.

Migration Risks and Humanitarian Concerns

Migration, particularly forced migration, frequently entails life-threatening risks. A significant humanitarian challenge is presented by the perilous routes migrants undertake in their quest for safety. The Missing Migrants Project (IOM 2024) has documented over 63,000 deaths and disappearances along migration routes between 2014 and the end of 2023, with numerous fatalities occurring in the Mediterranean Sea, at the US-Mexico border, and in the Sahara Desert (IOM 2024) (see Figure 1.3). However, there are substantial challenges in data collection, suggesting that this number may be higher.

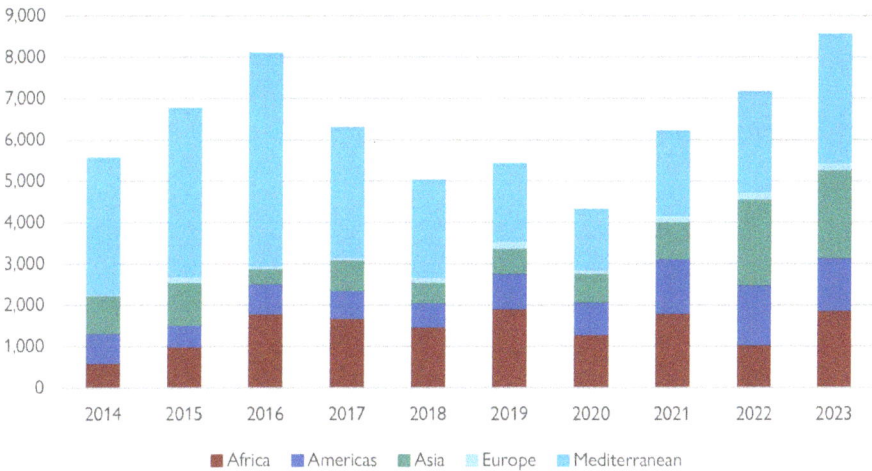

Note: Data include recorded deaths as well as those reported as missing. See the Missing Migrants Project webpage for details of methodology and geographic regions.

Fig. 1.3 Migrant deaths by region between 2014 and 2023 (IOM 2024).

The data on migrant fatalities underscores the severe consequences of irregular migration. Numerous individuals risk their lives attempting to traverse seas, deserts, and conflict zones due to the absence of legal and safe migration pathways. These fatalities highlight the urgent need for enhanced humanitarian interventions, search and rescue missions, and international cooperation to address the structural causes of forced migration and to improve protection mechanisms for vulnerable populations.

The 1951 Convention relating to the Status of Refugees, along with its 1967 Protocol, serve as the foundation of international refugee protection. These documents establish a comprehensive framework for the rights and obligations of refugees, as well as the responsibilities of host states (UNHCR 2011; UNHCR 2023). The Convention defines a refugee as an individual who, due to a legitimate fear of persecution based on factors such as race, religion, nationality, social group membership, or political opinion, is outside their country of origin and unable or unwilling to seek protection from that country (UNHCR 2011; UNHCR 2023). This definition has had a significant impact on shaping both national and international policies related to refugee protection and asylum procedures (Goodwin-Gill & McAdam 2007).

Despite the legal protections provided by international agreements, refugees often encounter formidable obstacles in integrating into host countries. These obstacles include legal and bureaucratic challenges, discrimination, and limited access to essential services such as healthcare, education, and employment (Bozorgmehr, Schneider & Joos 2015). The integration of refugees is further complicated by socio-economic disparities and cultural differences, which can impede their ability to adapt to new environments and achieve self-sufficiency (Ager & Strang 2008).

Contemporary integration frameworks emphasize that integration is a dynamic and bidirectional process necessitating adjustments from both refugees and host communities. Strang and Ager (2010) underscore the imperative for host societies to modify institutional structures, policies, and attitudes to facilitate successful integration, while also recognizing the role of refugees in actively engaging with their new environment. This reciprocal perspective ensures that integration transcends mere assimilation, fostering mutual adaptation and co-existence (Strang & Ager 2010). Ager and Strang's (2008) framework delineates four key domains essential to integration: achievements in employment, education, housing, and health; social connections through bonds, bridges, and links; facilitators such as language and cultural knowledge; and a foundation of rights and citizenship. These interconnected elements shape the integration trajectory, highlighting that legal recognition alone is insufficient without access to resources that enable participation in society (Strang & Ager 2010). Furthermore, integration is not a linear process but a fluid and context-dependent experience that varies based on local policies, societal attitudes, and individual aspirations (Phillimore & Goodson 2008). Refugees often navigate barriers related to discrimination, economic disparities, and policy restrictions, underscoring the critical role of host society adaptation in shaping successful integration experiences (Ager & Strang 2008). Thus, fostering inclusive environments, equitable opportunities, and policies that promote long-term social cohesion is essential to achieving meaningful refugee integration. Recognizing refugees as active contributors rather than passive recipients reshapes the discourse around migration and integration, reinforcing the importance of reciprocal engagement between newcomers and host communities.

The experiences of refugees are profoundly shaped by the circumstances surrounding their migration, encompassing pre-migration, migration, and post-migration phases. Research by Steel et al (2009) indicates that pre-migration experiences often involve exposure to traumatic events, such as torture, violence, and the loss of loved ones. During migration, refugees may encounter perilous journeys, exploitation, and separation from family members (UNHCR 2023). Post-migration, they may grapple with physical and mental health issues stemming from the challenges of adapting to a new country, navigating legal systems, and overcoming social marginalization (Helton 2002). Schweitzer et al (2011) argue that these incidents underscore the necessity of a comprehensive approach to refugee protection that addresses both immediate humanitarian needs and long-term integration and well-being. Recent research emphasizes the importance of adopting a multidisciplinary approach to investigating refugee experiences, incorporating perspectives from law, social sciences, public health, and human rights (Betts & Collier 2017). By integrating multiple viewpoints, this approach facilitates a more thorough understanding of the various factors that shape refugee experiences and their outcomes. Moreover, it highlights the necessity of implementing policies and practices guided by empirical evidence and rooted in principles of fairness and social justice (Fazel, Wheeler & Danesh 2005). This chapter explores the complexities of refugee experiences, analysing the legal, socio-economic, and personal dimensions that shape the trajectories of refugees in host societies. Rather than focusing solely on the challenges they face, it also examines the reciprocal nature of integration, considering how both refugees and host communities contribute to successful adaptation. By viewing integration as a shared process, this chapter seeks to provide insights into policies and strategies that promote inclusion, resilience, and long-term societal cohesion for displaced populations.

Reasons for Migration

The process of international migration is influenced by various macro, meso, and micro-level factors. In this chapter, we focus on the combination of "push" and "pull" factors to simplify the complex motivations behind migration.

Push factors are conditions in the migrant's home country that drive them to leave (Wickramasinghe & Wimalaratana 2018; Urbański 2022). These factors include high unemployment rates, political instability, or limited educational opportunities, compelling individuals to seek better prospects elsewhere. Conversely, pull factors are attractions associated with the destination country, such as higher wages, better living conditions, or greater access to quality healthcare and education. For example, a software engineer from a developing country may be driven to migrate to a tech hub like Silicon Valley due to limited job opportunities (push factor) in their home country and the potential for better career growth and compensation in the United States (pull factor). Here are some examples of push and pull factors.

Push factors:

- Wars, Conflicts, and Political Instability: These can create unsafe living conditions, prompting people to seek safety and stability elsewhere.

- Ethnic and Religious Persecution: Discrimination and persecution based on ethnicity or religion can force individuals to flee their home countries.

- Natural and Man-Made Disasters: Events such as earthquakes, floods, or industrial accidents can devastate communities and livelihoods.

- Poverty: Lack of financial resources and economic opportunities can drive people to look for better living conditions abroad.

- Unemployment, Low Wages, and Poor Working Conditions: The absence of job opportunities or decent working conditions can push individuals to migrate.

- Shortages of Food, Water, or Healthcare: Basic needs are critical, and shortages can force people to seek environments where these needs can be met.

- Limited Opportunities: Whether in education, career growth, or personal development, limited opportunities can push individuals to seek greener pastures.

Pull factors:

- Better Quality of Life and Standard of Living: Countries offering higher living standards and quality of life attract migrants.

- Varied Employment Opportunities and Higher Wages: Better job prospects and the potential for higher earnings are significant pull factors.

- Better Healthcare and Access to Educational Services: Quality healthcare and educational opportunities are strong attractions for migrants.

- Political Stability and More Freedom: Stable political environments and greater personal freedoms draw individuals seeking a safer and freer life.

- Better Life Prospects: Overall, better prospects for personal and professional growth are strong incentives.

- Services for Retirees and Environmental Characteristics: For retirees, specific services and desirable environmental features, such as coastal areas, can be attractive.

The research conducted by Urbański (2022) comparing Poland and Romania highlights that pull factors generally have a greater influence on migration than push factors. In Poland, significant pull factors include economic opportunities, political stability, and social benefits such as better healthcare and education. Conversely, push factors like political instability and poor governance have a notable impact in Romania. Urbański's (2022) findings demonstrate that pull factors significantly contribute to migration, even in peaceful democratic regimes like Poland and Romania. It is natural to assume that individuals in undemocratic or war-torn countries have an even stronger incentive to take risks for a brighter future.

From Migration Motivations to Forced Displacement

While economic opportunities and improved living standards are significant drivers of migration, not all movement is voluntary. For many individuals, migration is not a matter of choice but one of survival. Forced migration occurs when individuals and families flee their countries due to war, persecution, natural disasters, or human rights violations. Unlike those driven by economic incentives, refugees and asylum seekers do not migrate for better opportunities but rather to escape conditions that threaten their lives and freedoms.

The distinction between voluntary migration and forced displacement is crucial for understanding global migration patterns. Economic migrants typically retain some level of agency in their decision-making process, evaluating risks and rewards before relocating. Refugees, on the other hand, often leave their homes under duress, with little time for planning or securing resources for their journey. While both groups face significant challenges, refugees frequently experience heightened vulnerability, legal uncertainties, and prolonged periods of liminality in transit or host countries (Bakewell 2021; Mandic 2021).

Recent research has highlighted the complexities surrounding the dichotomy between voluntary and forced migration. Bakewell (2021) critiques the rigid separation between these categories, arguing that migration decisions often involve an intricate interplay of choice and compulsion, making it difficult to define clear boundaries. Similarly, Mandic (2021) emphasizes that forced migration is not only the result of immediate threats but also the product of structural inequalities, protracted insecurity, and systematic exclusion that gradually erode an individual's ability to remain in their home country. These perspectives call for a more nuanced understanding of displacement, recognizing that many migration experiences exist along a spectrum rather than as distinct categories.

Refugee Experiences

Migrants generally exhibit better health than both the population they depart from and the population of the destination country (Wickramage et al. 2018). This phenomenon, often referred to as the Healthy Immigrant Effect (HIE), suggests that migrants, particularly those who migrate voluntarily, tend to have better health outcomes upon arrival than native populations. This is attributed to self-selection biases, where healthier individuals are more likely to undertake migration (Abraído-Lanza et al. 1999; Kennedy et al. 2006). However, for refugees and forcibly displaced populations, the Healthy Immigrant Effect (HIE) is often less pronounced or absent due to the extreme hardship they experience before, during, and after migration (Norredam et al. 2010).

Regardless of the nature of the migration process, fleeing is a significant burden, and settling in a new country constitutes a profound transition. The migration process can be categorized into three stages: pre-migration, migration, and post-migration. Each of these stages features important factors that can have either a positive or negative impact on health. The different phases and critical factors that can influence health in both the short and long term are depicted in Figure 2.4. Additionally, a potential return phase has been incorporated in this representation.

The migration process for individuals with refugee experiences is divided into several key phases. The pre-migration phase involves pre-migratory events such as conflict, human rights violations, and economic disparities, as well as the migrants' epidemiological profiles and the linguistic, cultural, and geographic proximity to their destination. The movement phase covers the journey's duration, conditions, and associated risks, including violence and exploitation, particularly for irregular migration flows. The arrival and integration phase addresses the legal status, access to services, social dynamics such as discrimination and exclusion, and the adaptation to new cultural and linguistic environments. Finally, the return phase considers the duration of absence, the capacity of home community services, remaining social ties, and changes in the behavioural and health profiles of both the returnees and the host community, with cross-cutting aspects like gender, age, socio-economic status, and genetic factors influencing all stages.

Understanding these phases provides a necessary foundation for analysing the broader health implications of migration. However, migration health research has long debated whether migrants maintain better health than host populations upon arrival, as suggested by the HIE phenomenon. Furthermore, while voluntary migrants may initially exhibit superior health outcomes due to self-selection and pre-departure screenings, the extent to which this effect applies to refugees and asylum seekers remains contentious. The following section critically examines the HIE, highlighting its limitations, complexities, and the factors that contribute to the erosion of migrant health over time.

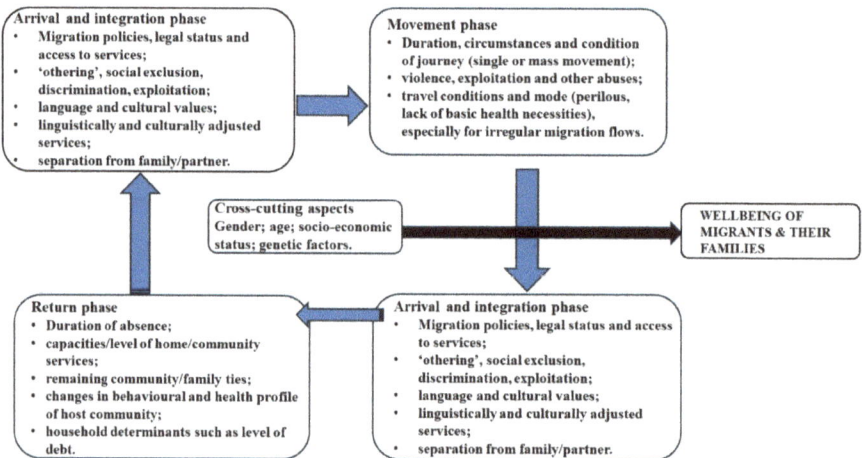

Fig. 1.4 Factors influencing the health and wellbeing of migrants and their families along the phases of migration (Wickramage et al., 2018).

Healthy Immigrant Effect (HIE)

The HIE has long been regarded as a paradox in migration health research. Furthermore, certain migration systems include pre-departure health screenings, which contribute to a temporary advantage in health status (Domnich et al. 2012). Additionally, recent research highlights the role of educational selectivity, where migrants often come from socioeconomic backgrounds that promote healthier lifestyles, reinforcing the perception of superior health outcomes upon arrival (Ichou et al. 2017). However, the assumptions underpinning the HIE warrant critical scholarly investigation, as its applicability is far from universal. Rather than having a protective effect, the migration experience exacerbates pre-existing vulnerabilities, making the very notion of HIE misleading when applied uncritically across all migrant groups (Vang et al. 2015). The lived experiences of refugees illustrate how the challenges of forced migration intersect with the erosion of the HIE.

A compelling example is the case of Tarik, a refugee from Iraq whose journey underscores the systemic barriers that impede professional and social integration.

> In 2018, Tarik arrived in Norway as a refugee from Iraq. He was a trained dentist who had previously operated his own dental practice, employing two additional staff members. A portion of the practice's surplus revenue was allocated to support a local sports club in which his children were actively involved. Additionally, Tarik served as a coach and contributed to the club's activities. He was also engaged in local politics. Tarik arrived in Norway alone and was granted residency relatively quickly on humanitarian grounds. Upon arrival, he commenced an introduction program. Shortly thereafter, his family was able to join him, and over time, they became more familiar with their new country. However, Tarik's dental qualifications were not recognized in Norway. He was offered the opportunity to enrol in an additional education program designed for dentists without approved qualifications. The waiting list for this program was extensive, and he was informed that it would take several years before he could commence his studies. This situation led Tarik to experience a profound sense of helplessness, a stark contrast to the resourceful individual he had been accustomed to being, both for himself, his family, and the community around him.[2]

Tarik's case exemplifies the challenges faced by highly skilled refugees who, despite possessing substantial qualifications and professional experience, encounter systemic barriers in accessing the labour market. These barriers exacerbate stress and diminish well-being, thereby challenging the traditional notion that migrants enjoy superior health

---

2   Tarik's case is drawn from the Center for Migration Health (CMH) data storage, where he was registered as a patient.

outcomes upon arrival. Furthermore, the HIE is increasingly recognized as a temporary phenomenon that deteriorates over time due to the cumulative impact of post-migration stressors. While initial health advantages may be observable among certain migrant groups, long-term studies indicate a decline in migrant health trajectories, a process referred to as the Healthy Migrant Paradox (Hynie 2018). The erosion of the HIE is particularly pronounced among migrants facing legal and economic precarity, as many are compelled into precarious labour markets, unstable housing conditions, and exclusion from essential social services. The accumulation of such disadvantages amplifies stress-related health burdens, especially for asylum seekers and undocumented migrants, who often experience prolonged uncertainty and restricted access to healthcare (Priebe et al. 2016).

Another significant factor contributing to the decline in HIE is acculturation stress and behavioural changes. The process of adapting to a new society involves substantial modifications in diet, physical activity, and exposure to novel health risks, often leading to an increased incidence of non-communicable diseases (NCDs), such as cardiovascular disease and diabetes. Migrants who initially exhibit strong health profiles may adopt unhealthy dietary habits over time due to economic hardship and limited access to fresh, nutritious foods. This transition can exacerbate chronic health conditions and challenge the assumption that migration inherently confers health advantages (Vang et al. 2015). Moreover, structural inequities in healthcare systems pose significant barriers to migrants' sustained health advantages. Barriers related to language, cultural unfamiliarity, discrimination, and limited healthcare accessibility prevent many migrants from seeking timely medical intervention, exacerbating long-term health disparities (Hynie 2018). This is particularly evident among asylum seekers who may experience prolonged waiting periods before gaining legal recognition, during which they may lack healthcare access. Undocumented migrants, fearing deportation, are often reluctant to seek medical assistance, further exacerbating preventable health conditions (Priebe et al. 2016). Mental health constitutes a critical challenge in understanding the decline in the HIE.

Empirical studies have consistently demonstrated that post-traumatic stress disorder (PTSD), depression, and anxiety disorders are disproportionately prevalent among refugees and asylum seekers. This prevalence is largely attributable to pre-migration trauma, exposure to violence, and post-migration social marginalization, which collectively induce distress and significantly impact well-being (Juárez & Hjern 2017). Unlike physical health conditions that may be promptly observed and addressed, psychological distress can remain latent and exacerbate over time if left untreated. For many refugees, the stress associated with legal insecurity, financial instability, and cultural dissonance persists long after resettlement, thereby reinforcing patterns of psychological distress and complicating integration efforts. From a policy perspective, the continued reliance on the HIE as a generalizable principle obscures the profound disparities among different migrant groups. While certain voluntary migrants may indeed arrive healthier, refugees and asylum seekers experience profound vulnerabilities that necessitate targeted intervention. A more nuanced approach to migration health research must recognize that migrant well-being is not a static condition but rather an evolving trajectory shaped by structural determinants, legal status, and integration policies. Failure to acknowledge these intersecting factors perpetuates the misleading assumption that all migrants experience positive health outcomes upon arrival.

Migration health research must adopt a dynamic framework that captures the evolving and intersectional nature of migrant health rather than relying on static models. The deterioration of migrant health over time is inextricably linked to experiences that commence prior to migration. Many refugees and asylum seekers encounter profound physical and psychological stressors in their home countries, which set the stage for challenges that persist throughout their migration trajectories. To fully comprehend the health consequences of displacement, it is essential to consider the pre-migration phase, wherein exposure to violence, economic instability, and a lack of healthcare services shape initial health vulnerabilities. The following section explores refugees' pre-migration experiences and how these factors influence their well-being during transit and upon arrival in host countries.

Pre-Migration Experiences

This phase encompasses the decision to migrate and the preparation for the move. It involves emotional and practical preparations, such as saying goodbye to friends and family, obtaining necessary documents and planning the journey (Vinke et al. 2020). The duration of this phase varies; some individuals spend months or even years making arrangements, while others must flee suddenly due to urgent threats to their safety. Migration preparation can take different forms depending on circumstances. Some migrants meticulously research possible destinations, save money, and arrange housing, employment, and education (ibid). Others may not have the luxury of preparation and instead flee in haste, often in a state of flux, with little to no resources.

Migration is a phenomenon that transcends the traditional notion of family-based movement. Individuals embark on migratory journeys alone, in small groups, or within broader networks of displaced persons, each navigating unique socio-political and economic landscapes. Unaccompanied minors, the elderly, and single adults face distinct vulnerabilities that differ significantly from those of family units. These groups must contend with heightened exposure to exploitation, social isolation, and systemic barriers in access to humanitarian aid and legal protection.

Understanding migration through this broader lens allows for a more nuanced approach to policy development and humanitarian intervention, ensuring that support mechanisms are tailored to the diverse realities of displaced individuals. The motivations for migration are multifaceted, often described through the push-and-pull factors, where economic, social, political, and environmental aspects influence movement decisions. Typical push factors include economic instability, political repression, conflict, and environmental disasters, while pull factors include employment opportunities, political stability, and access to healthcare and education. Prior to fleeing their home countries, many refugees experience significant hardship, including persecution, violence, and human rights violations. These traumatic experiences frequently serve as the primary impetus for their displacement. Many refugees experience extreme adversity before departure, including war, torture, and systematic persecution, which have long-term repercussions on mental health (Steel et al. 2009). Migration may be motivated by positive aspirations, such as improving living conditions, or negative drivers, such as escaping oppression, or a combination of both (Czaika & Reinprecht 2022). However, trauma does not end upon leaving a conflict zone; rather, it accumulates throughout migration and resettlement, shaped by insecurity, exploitation, and structural exclusion at each stage.

Research shows that pre-migration trauma can have enduring consequences on refugees' mental and physical health. For instance, a systematic review by Fazel, Wheeler and Danesh (2005) found that refugees have a higher likelihood of developing serious mental health disorders when compared to the general population. This emphasizes the necessity of providing adequate mental health support to refugees from the moment they arrive in host countries. The primary health concerns experienced by migrants at this stage include mental health issues, poor healthcare, and an increased risk of violence and abuse. Migrants can grapple with stress and anxiety as a result of the uncertainty and unpredictability of their journey and future. Moreover, reasons for migration, such as conflict or economic instability, can lead to prolonged stress and strain, negatively impacting mental health (Kumar & Diaz 2019). Furthermore, some migrants may face poor healthcare due to economic insecurity or limited access to healthcare in their home country, which can result in health problems going untreated and worsening over time (ibid). In addition, migrants may be at a heightened risk of violence and abuse prior to migrating, particularly if they reside in areas with high crime or conflict. This can lead to physical and psychological injuries that can affect health in both the short- and long-term (ibid). These vulnerabilities are especially pronounced for women, unaccompanied minors, and LGBTQ+ individuals, who often face increased risks of exploitation and persecution during this stage.

Many refugees originate from regions affected by conflict, persecution, and human rights abuses. As a result, they frequently encounter significant physical and psychological trauma before leaving their home countries. Pre-migration health issues include injuries sustained from violence, chronic conditions left untreated due to disrupted health services, and psychological disorders such as PTSD, depression, and anxiety (Fazel, Wheeler & Danesh 2005). These conditions can have long-lasting effects on refugees' health and complicate their ability to integrate into new societies. By recognizing the diverse migration constellations beyond family-based migration and addressing the specific challenges faced by individual migrants, unaccompanied minors, and other vulnerable groups, policies and interventions can be better tailored to meet the needs of displaced populations.

During/Under Migration Experiences

The migration journey itself represents one of the most perilous and uncertain phases of displacement. This phase involves the actual physical move to a new location and can involve feelings of excitement, fear, and disorientation. The journey towards safety is often marked by danger and uncertainty. Refugees may encounter hazardous travel routes, fall prey to smugglers, and become separated from their loved ones during migration. The United Nations High Commissioner for Refugees (UNHCR) reports that many refugees risk their lives crossing deserts, seas, and conflict zones in pursuit of safety and protection (UNHCR 2023).

The trauma experienced during migration is often overlooked but remains a critical determinant of mental and physical health. The vulnerability of displaced individuals during this phase is exacerbated by systemic barriers to protection and assistance. Women and children, in particular, face a heightened risk of sexual violence and trafficking. The Women's Refugee Commission (2019) documents extensive cases of gender-based violence throughout displacement journeys, underscoring the need for targeted interventions, including secure transit routes, access to legal protections, and immediate medical support. Additionally, individuals fleeing alone, including unaccompanied minors and elderly refugees, face severe social isolation, increasing their susceptibility to exploitation and harm.

The arduous nature of migration exerts a profound toll on physical and mental health. The imagery of overcrowded boats in the Mediterranean Sea and perilous desert crossings epitomizes the extreme risks associated with forced migration. Refugees frequently endure malnutrition, dehydration, and infectious diseases due to inadequate access to clean water, healthcare, and sanitation. Kumar and Diaz (2019) highlight the particularly dire conditions in transit camps, where makeshift shelters, inadequate medical facilities, and limited access to education and employment compound the hardship of displacement. While some camps offer structured support, many are overcrowded and lack essential services, exposing residents to acute and chronic health risks.

Furthermore, migration is rarely a linear process. For some, displacement is temporary, with the expectation of eventual return; for others, it is the beginning of a protracted limbo, often extending over years or even decades. Social networks forged during migration can offer solidarity and support, yet they can also reinforce patterns of dependency and marginalization. Individuals experience migration in diverse ways— some embark on solitary journeys, while others travel in groups, forming surrogate communities in the absence of familial structures.

The following testimonies illustrate the deeply personal nature of displacement:

> I was very stressed both before and during the journey itself. It was the worst journey I have ever taken. We did not know how we would be treated, or what to expect. We heard stories that we would be stripped naked and body-searched, that we would be put in isolation, and that we would be treated very poorly.
>
> During the escape, there was no time to think about our own health; we had two children to take care of. The only focus was on finding practical solutions so that the children were as safe as possible.

These quotes are taken from interviews with refugees conducted through the Physiotherapy and Refugees Educational Project (HVL 2018-2021). The first quote is from an interview with a man who came on a planned flight to Norway. He came as a quota refugee and had all his papers in order. Nevertheless, he experienced enormous fear and uncertainty about what awaited him in Norway. The second quote is from a man who was fleeing with his family for several years. They lived in several refugee camps before they came to Norway and were granted asylum here.

Post-Migration Experiences

Moving to a new country initiates a phase in which one tries to adapt to the new place, language, culture, and people. Although reaching safety constitutes a significant milestone, it does not signify the cessation of hardship. The initial post-migration period is often characterized by a blend of relief and optimism, tempered by grief, uncertainty, and the challenge of reconstructing one's life in an unfamiliar society. Both refugees and asylum seekers must navigate legal systems, secure housing and employment, learn a new language, and establish social networks, tasks that can be both empowering and overwhelming.

However, asylum seekers often experience a distinct and heightened level of vulnerability due to their precarious legal status and the uncertainty surrounding their future. Unlike recognized refugees who have obtained legal protection, asylum seekers frequently endure prolonged waiting periods, restricted access to healthcare and employment, and the persistent fear of deportation (Lindencrona et al. 2008; Hynie 2018). These structural barriers contribute to prolonged psychological distress, exacerbating the burdens already carried from pre-migration and migration experiences. The insecurity surrounding their status often results in chronic stress, social marginalization, and exclusion from essential public services, further complicating their ability to integrate (Silove et al. 2017).

The Healthy Immigrant Effect (HIE), which suggests that migrants initially exhibit better health outcomes upon arrival, is often diminished or absent among refugees due to pre-migration trauma and migration hardships (Norredam et al. 2010). Even individuals who arrive in relatively good health frequently experience a gradual deterioration of physical and mental well-being as they navigate systemic barriers to healthcare, economic instability, restrictive asylum policies, and acculturative stress (Domnich et al. 2012; Hynie 2018). Studies indicate that prolonged asylum processes, social isolation, and precarious living conditions significantly elevate the risk of PTSD, depression, and anxiety (Silove et al. 2017; Priebe et al. 2016).

The psychological trauma of displacement often resurfaces in post-migration life, compounded by structural and social barriers. Some refugees experience an early phase of overcompensation, wherein they strive intensely to assimilate and conform to their new environment (Sluzki 1979). This period can be stressful, as individuals may struggle to balance personal identity with the expectations of their host society. Over time, some experience cultural dissonance, marked by homesickness, frustration, and disappointment with the realities of life in their new country. Limited employment opportunities, difficulties forming social connections, and the persistent longing for familiarity can contribute to emotional distress.

Legal and bureaucratic barriers further complicate the integration process. Many refugees encounter significant challenges in accessing healthcare, education, and employment due to linguistic and cultural differences, lack of legal documentation, or discriminatory practices (Bozorgmehr, Schneider & Joos 2015). The psychological toll of pre-migration trauma, coupled with the stress of resettlement, often results in heightened rates of PTSD, depression, and anxiety (Steel et al. 2009; Schweitzer et al. 2011).

A case study illustrating these challenges is that of Yana, a 15-year-old refugee who arrived in Norway in 2015:

> Yana is 15 years old and came with her family to Norway in 2015. She and her family have been back to their home country, but for Yana, it is here in Norway that she feels most at home. She speaks fluent Norwegian, has good friends, does well in school, and has leisure activities she enjoys. She sees that there are differences between the rules she has at home and some of what her friends have, which has recently led to some conflicts at home. In a conversation with her mother, the mother expresses the difficult situation where she feels she stands with one foot in Norway and one foot in her home country. Some of the things they do in Norway would have been completely unthinkable in their home country, such as being out with boys, going to a youth club, and the like. On one hand, she actually thinks it is okay, but on the other hand, she feels guilty and feels that she is not a good enough mother for Yana when she lets her do the same as her friends do.

Mental health poses a significant challenge for refugees due to the multiple traumas they endure. Studies have shown that refugees are at a higher risk for mental health disorders compared to the general population (Steel et al. 2009). Common mental health issues among refugees include PTSD, depression, anxiety, and adjustment disorders. The cumulative impact of pre-migration trauma, migration stressors, and post-migration challenges necessitates comprehensive mental health support tailored to the unique needs of refugees (Schweitzer et al. 2011).

The experiences of refugees highlight the complex interplay between adaptation, resilience, and the enduring impact of past traumas. The protracted nature of asylum processes, combined with legal insecurity and exclusion from key social services, underscores the need for comprehensive policies that address the challenges faced by displaced individuals in the post-migration phase (Priebe et al. 2016). Yana's story is a testament to the ongoing challenges and successes that come with resettling in a new country. Addressing the multifaceted needs of refugees requires a holistic approach that encompasses legal, social, economic, and health support systems. Ensuring comprehensive and accessible support is crucial for fostering successful integration and improving the overall well-being of refugee populations.

Conclusion

The global phenomenon of forced migration remains a critical issue. It poses significant humanitarian, legal, socio-economic, and health challenges. This comprehensive review of people with refugee experiences underscores the urgent need for strong international policies and interventions that address both immediate and long-term needs.

Pre-migration trauma, including persecution, violence, and human rights violations, has a significant impact on the mental and physical health of refugees, requiring tailored mental health and psychosocial support upon arrival in host countries. Research shows that refugees have higher rates of PTSD, depression, and anxiety than the general population, highlighting the need for early and sustained mental health interventions (Steel et al. 2009; Schweitzer et al. 2011).

During or under migration, refugees often undertake perilous journeys associated with threats of exploitation, unsafe conditions and separation from family members. The journey itself poses significant health risks, including exposure to infectious diseases, physical injuries, and severe psychological stress. This underscores the need for international cooperation to ensure safe migration routes and provide adequate protection and assistance during transit (UNHCR 2023).

Post-migration, refugees face the challenging task of integrating into new societies, learning new languages, and navigating unfamiliar cultural landscapes. This phase is often marked by a combination of relief and ongoing psychological distress as refugees reconcile their traumatic pasts with the challenges of building new lives. The mismatch between expectations and reality can lead to frustration and homesickness, further complicating the integration process (Sluzki 1979).

Migration can act as a catalyst for innovation and economic growth in host countries. Refugees bring diverse skills, perspectives, and resilience that can contribute to local economies and enrich cultural landscapes. However, this potential is often unrealized due to restrictive policies and social barriers, highlighting the need for more inclusive and forward-thinking approaches to migration management (Papademetriou & Benton 2016). The integration of refugees is further hampered by socio-economic disparities, discrimination, and limited access to basic services such as healthcare, education, and employment. Effective integration requires a comprehensive approach that includes legal protection, social support networks, and economic opportunities. Studies have shown that inclusive policies and community-based support systems significantly improve refugee integration and well-being (Ager & Strang 2008; Bozorgmehr, Schneider & Joos 2015). New research highlights the potential of using technology and digital platforms to support refugees. Applications such as mobile health, virtual learning environments, and online social networks can provide refugees with critical information, facilitate access to services, and foster social connections. These innovative solutions can play a significant role in bridging gaps in service delivery and enhancing the overall integration process (Betts & Collier 2017). In addition, addressing the root causes of forced migration, such as armed conflict, human rights violations, and environmental crises, remains essential. The increasing number of forcibly displaced people, as reported by UNHCR, calls for comprehensive international efforts to promote peace, stability, and sustainable development in the affected regions (Comte 2020; UNHCR 2023).

In conclusion, the complex and multifaceted needs of refugees require a holistic and coordinated global response. The integration of legal protection, socio-economic support, and innovative technological solutions can significantly improve the integration and well-being of refugee populations. Continued research, policy development, and international cooperation are essential to ensure that the rights and dignity of refugees are maintained and that their journeys of hardship are transformed into journeys of resilience and hope.

References

Abraído-Lanza, A. F., Dohrenwend, B. P., Ng-Mak, D. S., & Turner, J. B. 1999. 'The Latino mortality paradox: A test of the "salmon bias" and healthy migrant hypotheses', *American Journal of Public Health*, 89.10: 1543–1548.

Ager, Alastair, and Alison Strang. 2008. 'Understanding Integration: A Conceptual Framework', *Journal of Refugee Studies*, 21.2: 166–191, https://doi.org/10.1093/jrs/fen016

Bakker, L., Dagevos, J., & Engbersen, G. 2014. 'The importance of resources and security in the socio-economic integration of refugees. A study on the impact of length of stay in asylum accommodation and residence status on socio-economic integration for the four largest refugee groups in the Netherlands', *Journal of International Migration and Integration*, 15: 431–448.

Betts, Alexander, and Paul Collier. 2017. *Refuge: Transforming a Broken Refugee System* (UK: Penguin).

Biermann, Frank, and Ingrid Boas. 2008. 'Protecting climate refugees: the case for a global protocol', *Environment: Science and Policy for Sustainable Development*, 50.6: 8–17.

Bozorgmehr, Kayvan, Christine Schneider, and Stefanie Joos. 2015. 'Equity in access to health care among asylum seekers in Germany: Evidence from an exploratory population-based cross-sectional study', *BMC Health Services Research*, 15: 1–12, https://doi.org/10.1186/s12913-015-1156-x

Chiswick, B. R., & Miller, P. W. 2008. 'Why is the payoff to schooling smaller for immigrants?', *Labour Economics*, 15.6: 1317–1340.

Comte, Emmanuel. 2020. *The European Asylum System: A Necessary Case of Differentiation*, No. 3 (European Union), https://www.iai.it/sites/default/files/euidea_pp_3.pdf

Czaika, Mathias, and Constantin Reinprecht. 2022. 'Migration drivers: Why do people migrate', in *Introduction to Migration Studies: An Interactive Guide to the Literatures on Migration and Diversity*, ed. by Scholten, Paul (Springer), pp. 49–82.

Domnich, A., Panatto, D., Gasparini, R., & Amicizia, D. 2012. 'The "healthy immigrant" effect: Does it exist in Europe today?', *Italian Journal of Public Health*, 9.3.

Fazel, Mina, Jeremy Wheeler, and John Danesh. 2005. 'Prevalence of serious mental disorder in 7000 refugees resettled in Western countries: A systematic review', *The Lancet*, 365.9467: 1309–1314, https://doi.org/10.1016/S0140-6736(05)61027-6

Goodwin-Gill, Guy S., Jane McAdam, and Emma Dunlop. 2021. *The Refugee in International Law* (Oxford: Oxford University Press).

Harris, Ricci, et al. 2006. 'Racism and health: The relationship between experience of racial discrimination and health in New Zealand', *Social Science & Medicine*, 63.6: 1428–1441, https://doi.org/10.1016/j.socscimed.2006.04.009

Helton, Arthur C. 2002. *The Price of Indifference: Refugees and Humanitarian Action in the New Century* (Oxford: Oxford University Press).

Hynie, M. 2018. 'The social determinants of refugee mental health in the post-migration context: A critical review', *Canadian Journal of Psychiatry*, 63.5: 297–303, https://doi.org/10.1177/0706743717746666

Ichou, M., & Wallace, M. 2019. 'The healthy immigrant effect', *Demographic Research*, 40: 61–94.

International Organization for Migration (IOM). 2019. *Glossary on Migration*, 34 (Geneva: International Organization for Migration), https://publications.iom.int/system/files/pdf/iml_34_glossary.pdf

Kumar, Bernadette, and Esperanza Diaz (eds). 2019. *Migrant Health: A Primary Care Perspective* (Florida: CRC Press).

Juárez, S. P., & Hjern, A. 2017. 'The weight of inequalities: Duration of residence and offspring's birthweight among migrant mothers in Sweden', *Social Science & Medicine*, 175: 81–90.

Kennedy, S., McDonald, J. T., & Biddle, N. 2006. 'The healthy immigrant effect and immigrant selection: Evidence from four countries', *Social and Economic Dimensions of an Aging Population Research Papers*, 164.

Lindencrona, F., Ekblad, S., & Hauff, E. 2008. 'Mental health of recently resettled refugees from the Middle East in Sweden: The impact of pre-resettlement trauma, resettlement stress and capacity to handle stress', *Social Psychiatry and Psychiatric Epidemiology*, 43: 121–131.

Mandić, D. 2022. 'What is the force of forced migration? Diagnosis and critique of a conceptual relativization', *Theory and Society*, 51.1: 61–90.

Mangrio, Elisabeth, and Katarina Sjögren Forss. 2017. 'Refugees' experiences of healthcare in the host country: A scoping review', *BMC Health Services Research*, 17: 1–16, https://doi.org/10.1186/s12913-017-2731-0

Miller, Kenneth E., and Andrew Rasmussen. 2017. 'The mental health of civilians displaced by armed conflict: An ecological model of refugee distress', *Epidemiology and Psychiatric Sciences* 26.2: 129–138, https://doi.org/10.1017/S2045796016000172

Næss, Anders. 2020. 'Migration, gender roles, and mental illness: The case of Somali immigrants in Norway', *International Migration Review*, 54.3: 740–764, https://doi.org/10.1177/0197918319867381

Norredam, M., Nielsen, S. S., & Krasnik, A. 2010. 'Migrants' utilization of somatic healthcare services in Europe: A systematic review', *European Journal of Public Health*, 20.5: 555–563.

Ortiz-Ospina, Esteban, et al. 2022. 'Migration', *Our World in Data*, https://ourworldindata.org/migration

Papademetriou, D. G., & Benton, M. 2016. 'Towards a global compact for migration: A development perspective', *Migration Policy Institute*. https://www.migrationpolicy.org/programs/international-program/global-compact-migration

Phillimore, J., & Goodson, L. 2008. 'Making a place in the global city: The relevance of indicators of integration', *Journal of Refugee Studies*, 21.3: 305–325, https://doi.org/10.1093/jrs/fen025

Priebe, S., Giacco, D., & El-Nagib, R. 2016. Public health aspects of mental health among migrants and refugees: A review of the evidence on mental health care for refugees, asylum seekers and irregular migrants in the WHO European Region, *WHO Regional Office for Europe,* https://apps.who.int/iris/handle/10665/326308

Schweitzer, Robert D. et al. 2011. 'Mental health of newly arrived Burmese refugees in Australia: Contributions of pre-migration and post-migration experience', *Australian & New Zealand Journal of Psychiatry,* 45.4: 299–307, https://doi.org/10.3109/00048674.2010.543412

Sluzki, Carlos E. 1979. 'Migration and family conflict', *Family process,* 18.4: 379–390, https://doi.org/10.1111/j.1545-5300.1979.00379.x

Steel, Zachary et al. 2009. 'Association of torture and other potentially traumatic events with mental health outcomes among populations exposed to mass conflict and displacement: A systematic review and meta-analysis', *Jama,* 302.5: 537–549.

United Nations. n.d. 'Peace, dignity and equality on a healthy planet', https://www.un.org/en/global-issues/migration

United Nations High Commissioner for Refugees (UNHCR). 2011. *The 1951 Convention and its 1967 Protocol* (Geneva: UNHCR), https://www.unhcr.org/sites/default/files/legacy-pdf/4ec262df9.pdf

United Nations High Commissioner for Refugees (UNHCR). 2023. *Global Trends: Forced in 2022* (Denmark: UNHCR), https://www.unhcr.org/sites/default/files/2023-06/GlobalTrends_2023_v16.pdf

United Nations High Commissioner for Refugees (UNHCR). 2024. *Global Trends: Forced Displacement in 2023* (Denmark: UNHCR), https://www.unhcr.org/sites/default/files/2024-06/global-trends-report-2023.pdf

Urbański, Mariusz. 2022. 'Comparing push and pull factors affecting migration', *Economies,* 10.1: 21, https://doi.org/10.3390/economies10010021

Vinke, Kira, et al. 2020. 'Migration as adaptation?', *Migration Studies,* 8.4: 626–634, https://doi.org/10.1093/migration/mnaa029

Wickramage, Kolitha, et al. 2018. 'Migration and health: a global public health research priority', *BMC Public Health,* 18: 1–9, https://doi.org/10.1186/s12889-018-5932-5

Wickramasinghe, A. A. I. N., and Wijitapure Wimalaratana. 2016. 'International migration and migration theories', *Social Affairs,* 1.5: 13–32.

World Bank. 2018. *Moving for Prosperity: Global Migration and Labor Markets* (Washington, DC: World Bank), https://documents.worldbank.org/en/publication/documents-reports/documentdetail/238411612756666941/overview

2. Refugee Rights Are Human Rights

Sandra Schiller, Mohammad Ali Farhat, and

Djenana Jalovcic

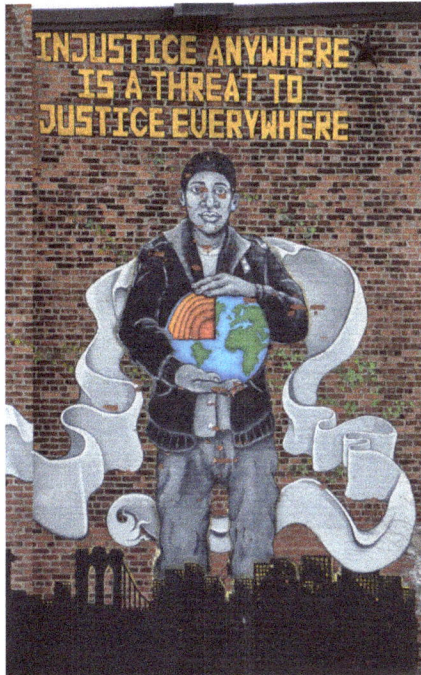

Injustice anywhere is a threat to justice everywhere. We are caught in an inescapable network of mutuality, tied in a single garment of destiny. Whatever affects one directly, affects all indirectly. (Martin Luther King Jr., 16 April 1963). Image: © Sandra Schiller / Groundswell Mural Projects, CC BY.

 https://doi.org/10.11647/OBP.0479.02

Introduction

By focusing on the interconnectedness between the rights of persons with refugee experience and human rights, this chapter emphasizes the relevance of a human-rights-based perspective in the developing field of refugee health. The refugee context is constantly changing; therefore, the frameworks used in refugee health should be frequently reviewed and reflected upon to protect the welfare of persons with refugee experience. In light of this, a fundamental cornerstone in refugee health is the role of health professionals who recognize that patients with refugee experience possess the inherent right for their unique health needs to be addressed in the most effective way.

Clinical settings such as hospitals or rehabilitation centres have often been remote from patients' everyday life experiences. However, health research informed by the humanities and social sciences has increasingly broadened the biomedical focus on the 'universal patient', and highlighted the need for a more nuanced understanding of health and well-being that considers the impact of health inequalities shaped by macro-economic, environmental, social, and political factors. In the context of forced migration, such a shift requires health professionals to understand the key legal frameworks that define and influence the lives of people with refugee experience, and to adopt the principles of universal human rights as their moral guideline. In other words, healthcare professionals need a moral stance that is based on the universality of human experience and the equality of all human beings, and that is characterized by solidarity and empathy. This can be a challenge given geographical distance, media portrayals that tend to show anonymous masses of people, and the frequent stereotyping and dehumanisation of persons with refugee experience.

What does knowing about refugee rights mean for health professionals? We argue that they should not only be aware of the specific rights to which refugees are entitled but they should also understand the underlying justifications for these rights. This is particularly important in relation to the right to reside in a host country and to be treated with fairness and humanity, regardless of their lack of citizenship status. This requires an understanding of the global human rights perspective as advocated by the United Nations (UN), the World Health Organization (WHO) and other relevant international bodies. In addition, health professionals should be able to identify disparities between human rights ideals and the reality in their own country, and be prepared to address these issues.

We begin by examining the concept of international protection for refugees as it emerged from the 1951 Refugee Convention. This is followed by a description of the characteristics of forced migration today, illustrated through the personal example of a healthcare professional who fled from Afghanistan in 2021. The next section outlines the increasing influence of human rights legislation and global human rights scholarship. This influence is particularly relevant to the human right to health, which is then described as a fundamental guideline for quality refugee healthcare. The chapter concludes with links to recent health research that warns of the dangers of violating the human rights of persons with refugee experience.

The International Protection of Persons with Refugee Experience

The protection of citizens' rights is the responsibility of each individual state. However, when a state fails to ensure these rights—whether due to inability or unwillingness to provide protection—and individuals are forced to flee, it becomes the responsibility of another country to step in to ensure these rights are respected. International protection refers to safeguarding individuals who cannot return to their home country due to a risk of persecution or serious harm, and whose own country cannot or will not protect them.

In 1951, the United Nations signed the Convention Relating to the Status of Refugees, commonly known as the Refugee Convention or Geneva Convention (UNHCR 2010). This initiative aimed to protect European refugees in the aftermath of the Second World War, which had displaced millions of people across Europe, including numerous survivors of the Holocaust and other wartime atrocities who were in need of protection and resettlement.

> A refugee used to be a person driven to seek refuge because of some act committed or some political opinion held. Well, it is true we have had to seek refuge; but we committed no acts and most of us never dreamt of having any radical opinion. With us the meaning of the term "refugee" has changed. Now "refugees" are those of us who have been so unfortunate as to arrive in a new country without means and have to be helped by Refugee Committees. (Arendt 1994: 110)

Furthermore, the Cold War, i.e., the ideological battle between the Western bloc (led by the United States) and the Eastern bloc (led by the Soviet Union), was also already underway at the time so that another aim of the Convention was to provide legal protections for individuals fleeing persecution due to political reasons (Gatrell 2016). Two central components primarily determine how protection is ensured: the definition of 'refugee' and the principle of non-refoulement, which prohibits signatory states from returning refugees to territories where their life or freedom would be threatened. This effort to protect the rights and dignity of individuals who have lost the protection of their home countries is part of a broader movement towards establishing international norms and standards for the protection of human rights, as exemplified by the Universal Declaration of Human Rights in 1948. The 1967 Protocol later extended the Refugee Convention's scope in terms of time and geography and to this date, it is still the fundamental basis for the international protection of persons with refugee experience. The Convention clearly defines who a refugee is, their rights, and what kind of legal protection—including the right to protection from persecution and other assistance—refugees should receive from the 149 states around the world who have signed the Refugee Convention and the 1967 Protocol.

However, some countries are avoiding their international obligations by manipulating who, if any, among those forced to flee their countries, will be granted refugee status, i.e., be officially recognized as refugees, and receive protection and support as required under the Geneva Convention (Fiddian-Qasmiyeh 2021). While human rights are universally applicable due to the inherent dignity of every human being, refugee status is conditional upon identifying a specific category of protected persons to which the individual belongs (Chetail 2014). From the beginning, the Refugee Convention was intended as "a compromise between unfettered state sovereignty over the admission of aliens, and an open door for non-citizen victims of serious human rights violation" (Chetail 2014: 24). In fact, the definition of a refugee in Article 1 of the Geneva Convention includes a number of conditions: a person who is outside their country of origin and who has a well-founded fear of being persecuted for reasons of race, religion, nationality, membership of a particular social group, or political opinion, and is unable to avail themselves of the protection of that country or to return to it owing to such fear of persecution (UNHCR 2010). The selective nature of this definition has been increasingly criticized as arbitrarily privileging the rights of some forced migrants over others (McAdam & Wood 2021). On the other hand, the central concept of persecution is not defined by the Refugee Convention, but left to the subsequent interpretation of the individual states. However, human rights treaties and standards adopted since the Geneva Convention provide a universal framework that aids in harmonizing the interpretations of state parties and offers a more predictable basis for determining refugee status. The concept of persecution, central to refugee law, has increasingly been interpreted through the lens of human rights standards, promoting a more principled and less subjective application (Chetail 2014). Considering that the reasons why people in today's world become refugees have also been changing, this is an important development.

Why Is Forced Migration a Global Phenomenon Today?

Why do people leave their home or country? Because they hope for a better life elsewhere for a variety of reasons: e.g., the lifestyle documented by popular reality TV programmes about European expatriates; because they are recruited as workers or encouraged to migrate in order to boost the local economy; or because they have to flee their country due to wars, political persecution, whether as dissidents or as members of ethnic or religious minorities, natural disasters or the effects of climate change. As detailed in Chapter 1, when people flee from their homes due to war, conflict or fear of persecution, and cross international borders, they become refugees in need of protection and assistance as they face inherent dangers and extreme circumstances. Consequently, refugee rights mean first and foremost that people are allowed to leave their country and go to another, and that they enjoy protection from persecution in that country or in another country to which they can go from there.

According to the UN Refugee Agency (UNHCR) the number of people displaced by crises in various regions of the world is growing steadily. In 2024, the UNHCR reported that surpassed 117 million (UNHCR 2024). The majority of those who are forced to flee—currently 68 million—are classified as internally displaced persons within their own countries. Unlike those who cross international borders, these individuals are not considered refugees under international law as defined by the Geneva Refugee Convention. Of those who do flee their country, most (currently 69%) remain in immediate neighbouring countries. Consequently, 75% of all refugees currently reside in low- and middle-income countries, and 20% in the least developed countries (UNHCR 2024). This global context must be understood when discussing those who come to Europe, driven by the geographical proximity of their home countries and/or the aspiration for a better future.

Unfortunately, a greater number of people in need worldwide does not necessarily correspond to a greater willingness to help among those who are in a position to do so. The terms "compassion fatigue" or "collapse of compassion" describes the phenomenon that people feel more empathy and a stronger moral obligation to help when they are presented with individual stories of suffering compared to large-scale statistical data (Jenni & Loewenstein 1997; Small Loewenstein & Slovic 2007; Slovic 2023). At the same time, the difficulty of telling those stories and the emotional burden of listening to them needs to be taken into consideration. The renowned German journalist and writer Carolin Emcke emphasizes that "there are experiences that cannot be described immediately, indeed, there are experiences that cannot even be understood immediately, because they overwhelm us, because they override everything else that applies, because they exceed all expectations of what people can do to each other" (Emcke 2023: 8, own translation). In her work, Emcke frequently addresses questions of witnessing and discursive justice (Emcke 2013). Discursive justice is crucial for amplifying marginalized voices, ensuring that those who are often overlooked or suppressed have the opportunity to share their stories and perspectives. Another significant aspect for Emcke is the promotion of empathy and dialogue. She views witnessing as a means to foster empathetic connections and facilitate dialogue among different individuals and communities. To fully grasp the importance of a human-rights-based perspective in refugee health, people are needed who are able and willing to share their stories and also people who are willing to listen and be empathetic.

Ali's Story: Losing Your Fundamental Human Rights in Your Own Country

Ali joined the Person with Refugee Experience Education Project – Interprofessional (PREP IP) in 2022. He brought to the project his unique and 'real-time' perspective—he had just fled his home in Afghanistan and was living in unsafe environments, experiencing discrimination, losing his human rights as we were implementing the project activities. Ali generously shared the story of his flight in spring 2022 with a group of European health and social care professionals. Two years later, Ali, together with his mother and sister, is safe and settled in a third country. The rest of this section is written by Ali.

First of all, I would like to share my educational level and experience with PREP IP. I received my M.Sc. in Rehabilitation Science from Bangladesh Health Professions Institute in March 2021. Recently, I got a job at an international medical aid organization where I worked as a psychosocial support supervisor on a USAID-funded project.

Everyone knows that the dark days came back for the people of Afghanistan due to the Taliban regime, a group of terrorists, taking power in Afghanistan in August 2021. A majority of the Afghan population live in extremely bad conditions and their lives are in danger in Afghanistan: members of the Hazara nations; members of minority religions; women activists; Afghan soldiers; and whoever worked with NATO, with American people or for any project sponsored by USAID. The Taliban are trying to create an insecure environment for minority religious communities, and in particular they want to expel the Hazara people who are an ethnic and religious minority (Shia) from Afghanistan. For instance, they use violence against women; bombs planted in a mosque, in a place of education, and in a wedding hall full of Hazara people; and they force the Hazaras to leave their homes. I am also Hazara and proud of that because we are honest and have worked very hard to live in peace in Afghanistan. Circumstances rapidly changed in Afghanistan—no one had expected that everything would change so quickly in just one night.

Suddenly the Taliban regime seized the entire country. A majority of men, women, children, and older people had to flee from Afghanistan. On 25 August 2021 we (my mother, my sister and I) also decided to leave our homeland. It was a very difficult decision to leave our own country. But we had no other choice. In 2014, the Taliban regime had killed my father because my older brother had worked with a foreign International Non-Governmental Organisation (INGO). I had also worked with an INGO in Afghanistan and I heard and observed that the Taliban regime killed those who worked for, helped, and supported foreign people. I was concerned about myself and my family, especially about my sister, because we heard from the media and the news that the Taliban forced young girls to marry them and that no one could stop them. Also, when the Taliban took control of the country, girls were banned from participating in the education systems in Afghanistan, which meant that my sister couldn't pursue her education anymore. So we decided to leave for Pakistan.

For ten days, we stayed in a border city trying to cross to Pakistan. For ten days, we tried to cross the border four or five times every day, but we couldn't succeed. Each time we attempted to pass the border we thought that we would die; it was an extremely horrible situation, the worst that I had ever faced in my life. My mother was sick and she had back problems. Every time we used a wheelchair for her because she was not able to walk. Thousands of men, women, children, young people, and older people wanted to leave Afghanistan. The Taliban and the Pakistan militia both said that Hazara people were not allowed to cross the border. Finally, we managed to escape Afghanistan without the Taliban catching us.

I left my suitcase on the way because my heart was racing, and I was scared of the Taliban and the militia of Pakistan. I thought they would shoot or arrest me. On our journey a Pakistan militia arrested us and kept us imprisoned with other Hazara people for one-and-a-half hours, while Pashtun and Tajik people remained free and were laughing and drinking tea with the militia of Pakistan. This was humiliating and an example of the discrimination that I faced during my journey. After this time, when the driver and militiamen reached a deal, we were released from jail and they gave us permission to enter Pakistan. On Pakistani territory, there were ten or more police checkpoints; at each police checkpoint the driver needed to pay some money for the Hazara passengers to receive permission to pass the checkpoint, but not for Tajiks or Pashtuns.

Refugee Rights Are Human Rights: We Are All Born Equal

On 10 December 1948, the United Nations General Assembly proclaimed the Universal Declaration of Human Rights, which consists of 30 articles that present a comprehensive set of civil, political, economic, social, and cultural rights (United Nations 1948). It has served as a foundational text for many of the conventions, laws, and treaties concluded since 1948, e.g., the European Convention on Human Rights. While the Universal Declaration of Human Rights does not have the legally binding force of a treaty that can be ratified by individual states, it carries significant political and moral authority (Rudolf 2023). This importance is underscored by the fact that its provisions have been incorporated into many national constitutions. Some of its provisions now constitute binding customary international law. In some instances, these principles have even attained the status of mandatory international law, which no state may derogate from. Notable examples of such non-derogable norms include the prohibition of slavery, torture, and racial discrimination.

To give the human rights contained in the Universal Declaration a binding form under international law, the United Nations adopted two human rights charters in 1966: the International Covenant on Economic, Social and Cultural Rights (Social Covenant) (United Nations 1966a) and the International Covenant on Civil and Political Rights (Civil Covenant) (United Nations 1966b). Both came into force in 1976. Together with the Universal Declaration of Human Rights and the two additional protocols to the Civil Covenant, they form the so-called International Bill of Human Rights, a term used mainly in English-speaking countries.

Self-reflection exercise:

As a basic introduction to the concept of human rights, watch the following video created by the Raoul Wallenberg Institute of Human Rights and Humanitarian Law: What Are Human Rights, Really? (4 minutes), https://www.youtube.com/watch?v=GDdJ-EI3sVU.

For more information on the Universal Declaration of Human Rights, visit the website of the United Nations: https://www.ohchr.org/en/universal-declaration-of-human-rights

1. How could you incorporate the human-rights-based perspective in your own professional work? Where does this change your perspective?

2. What aspects do you need to learn more about to integrate a human-rights-based perspective into your work?

3. What challenges and what potential does adopting this approach present to you?

In literature across various disciplines, numerous arguments assert that refugee rights are human rights. These arguments are frequently addressed in an interdisciplinary manner, as refugee rights encompass legal, political, ethical, and social dimensions. Consequently, the universal rights of refugees today are not solely based on the Refugee Convention but also derive from the general standards of international human rights law as another primary source:

> General human rights law adds a significant number of rights to the list codified in the Refugee Convention, and is regularly interpreted and applied by supervisory bodies able to refine the application of standards to respond to contemporary realities (Hathaway 2021: 154).

Despite these international laws, the lived experiences of refugees often reflect the gap between the existing laws and the harsh realities on the ground. Ali's story provides a compelling illustration of this disconnect.

For two years, from September 2021 to November 2023, we lived in Quetta, Pakistan, and we didn't have enough money or other facilities to live there like normal people. We didn't have access to our basic necessities and human rights such as: shelter, food, health care services, education, permission to work, and so on. We also went to the UNHCR office to get refugee cards. We had passed many interviews with the UNHCR Office, and then we got our asylum seeker cards, as the UNHCR did not give refugee status to anyone in Pakistan. Unfortunately, we didn't receive any other services from the UNHCR Office located in Quetta.

Theories of global justice argue that injustices experienced by refugees are often a result of global power structures and inequalities, for which wealthier states also bear responsibility (e.g., Farmer 2004; Pogge 2005). Reports on the situation of refugees worldwide (e.g., Bast et al. 2020; O'Flaherty 2023) systematically document the human rights violations that refugees often face, thus underscoring the need to comprehensively understand and protect their rights as human rights. On 19 September 2016, the United Nations General Assembly unanimously adopted the New York Declaration for Refugees and Migrants (United Nations 2016). This declaration reaffirms the importance of the international refugee regime and includes a wide array of commitments by member states to strengthen and enhance mechanisms for the protection of displaced persons.

According to a fact sheet on human rights jointly published by the Office of the High Commissioner for Human Rights (OHCHR) and the WHO (2008), human rights are universal and inalienable. They apply equally, to all people, everywhere, without distinction. Human rights standards—to food; health; education; to be free from torture, inhuman or degrading treatment—are also interrelated. The improvement of one right facilitates advancement of the others. Likewise, the deprivation of one right adversely affects the others.

Ali's experiences in Quetta, Pakistan, underscore the challenges that many refugees face daily, despite the existence of robust international human rights and legal frameworks. His story provides a reminder of the ongoing struggle to bridge the gap between human rights laws, theories, and practice, emphasizing the urgent need to reinforce and implement these rights universally and effectively. By reflecting on Ali's narrative, we are called to consider how we can integrate and uphold a human-rights-based perspective in our own professional and personal lives to ensure that these rights are not only ideals, but lived realities for all.

The Human Right to Health

As described in Chapter 1, current national and international studies show that individuals who have experienced displacement face specific health risks before and during their flight, and that these risks are further influenced by living conditions in the host country. An insecure residence status, limited access to healthcare, experiences of discrimination, and lack of social participation negatively impact the health of those affected. The philosopher Hannah Arendt already described this experience in her 1943 essay 'We Refugees':

> Our optimism, indeed, is admirable, even if we say so ourselves. [...] We lost our home, which means the familiarity of daily life. We lost our occupation, which means the confidence that we are of some use in this world. We lost our language, which means the naturalness of reactions, the simplicity of gestures, the unaffected expression of feelings. We left our relatives in the Polish ghettos and our best friends have been killed in concentration camps, and that means the rupture of our private lives (Arendt 1994: 110).

In such a context, health professionals need to understand the complex nature of refugees' different situations, which are influenced by a wide range of factors, in order to act competently. In particular, it is essential to understand the profound impact that legal status has on an individual's circumstances. Legal status significantly affects access to healthcare services, opportunities for meaningful activities—particularly gainful employment—and the capacity for social and societal participation (Bozorgmehr et al. 2022; Nowak et al. 2023). This includes not only integration into the labour market, but also access to the education system and cultural activities. Furthermore, legal status influences an individual's future prospects, psychosocial stress levels, and housing conditions, including the choice of residence or place of living. Scholars in migration and refugee studies have pointed out that the classification of legal status is a factor in "processes that stratify access to material and symbolic resources" (Menjívar 2023). The treatment of people fleeing the conflict in Ukraine within the European Union has shown that alternative legal frameworks can indeed be established. Following the armed conflicts in the former Yugoslavia during the 1990s, the European Union adopted the Temporary Protection Directive in 2001 to provide immediate and temporary protection in the event of a (potential or actual) mass influx of displaced persons from non-EU countries who are unable to return to their country of origin (European Council 2001). On 4 March 2022, the EU interior ministers adopted a Council decision to implement this directive for the first time, aiming to offer swift and effective assistance to individuals fleeing the Russian invasion and subsequent war in Ukraine (European Commission Directorate-General for Migration and Home Affairs n.d.). This facilitated the granting of humanitarian residence permits to refugees from Ukraine across the European Union without necessitating their participation in an asylum procedure. Consequently, individuals seeking protection from Ukraine are granted access to employment, education, social benefits, and medical care throughout Europe. This example demonstrates the potential for adaptable legal mechanisms to better accommodate displaced populations (European Union Agency for Fundamental Rights 2022).

Article 25 of the Universal Declaration of Human Rights (United Nations 1948: 1) addresses the issue of health as a basic human right:

> Everyone has the right to a standard of living adequate for the health and well-being of himself and of his family, including food, clothing, housing and medical care and necessary social services, and the right to security in the event of unemployment, sickness, disability, widowhood, old age or other lack of livelihood in circumstances beyond his control.

Similarly, the Constitution of the World Health Organization (1948: 1) acknowledges health as a basic human right by stating that:

> The enjoyment of the highest attainable standard of health is one of the fundamental rights of every human being without distinction of "race", religion, political belief, economic or social condition.

The right to the highest attainable standard of physical and mental health is expressed in a number of international legal instruments, including the International Convention on the Elimination of All Forms of Racial Discrimination (United Nations 1965), the International Covenant on Economic, Social and Cultural Rights (United Nations 1966), the International Convention on the Elimination of All Forms of Discrimination Against Women (United Nations 1979), the Convention on the Right of the Child (United Nations 1989), the International Convention on the Protection of the Rights of All Migrant Workers and

Members of Their Families (United Nations 1990), and the Convention on the Rights of Persons with Disabilities (United Nations 2006). All of these international treaties are essential reference points for a human-rights-based approach to health that "provides a set of clear principles for setting and evaluating health policy and service delivery, targeting discriminatory practices and unjust power relations that are at the heart of inequitable health outcomes" (WHO 2023).

The right to the highest attainable standard of physical and mental health encompasses both freedoms and entitlements. Freedoms include the right to control one's health and body and to be free from interference, such as torture and non-consensual medical treatment and experimentation—an aspect particularly pertinent for persons with disabilities (WHO 2023). Entitlements, on the other hand, include the right to access quality health services without discrimination (WHO 2023). As a consequence, the states that have endorsed the right to health in their constitution have legally committed themselves to ensure provision of the determinants of health and to safeguard access to quality healthcare in a "timely, acceptable and affordable" manner. A human-rights-based approach to health "commits countries to develop rights-compliant, effective, gender-transformative, integrated, accountable health systems and implement other public health measures that improve the underlying determinants of health, like access to water and sanitation" (WHO 2023). This approach requires countries to ensure that their legislation, health policies, and health services respect and promote the realisation of human rights.

Self-reflection exercise:

Read the core principles and standards of a human-rights-based approach that are detailed in the WHO (2023) Fact Sheet on Human Rights: https://www.who.int/news-room/fact-sheets/detail/human-rights-and-health

- Core principles: accountability, equality and non-discrimination, and participation.
- Core components of the right to health: availability, accessibility, acceptability, and quality.
- (N.B.: Quality health services should be safe, effective, people-centred, timely, equitable, integrated, and efficient.)

4. What are the current legal and structural foundations in your country e.g., legal framework, government institutions, economic, political and social systems, infrastructure, etc.? Does your health and social care system facilitate the recognition of these fundamental human rights principles in regard to individuals with refugee experience?

5. Does your workplace already incorporate the core principles and standards of a human-rights-based approach to healthcare delivery? If not, what changes are necessary to achieve this? If yes, are further improvements needed? How might these improvements be implemented, and who would be responsible for taking action?

In the 2018 Edinburgh Declaration, participants from over 50 countries at the First World Congress on Migration, Ethnicity, Race, and Health (MERH) made a number of recommendations that are highly relevant for refugee health:

Eliminating barriers to access to healthcare and promoting protection of health of all people on the move, including those in an irregular situation, needs to be prioritised.

The full participation of migrants, ethnic minorities, indigenous populations and Roma in policy development, service planning, healthcare delivery, and research and evaluation is vital.

Relevant and appropriate data are required urgently for policy makers and service providers to tackle inequities.

Harmonization of, and agreement on, definitions and concepts should be sought by building on the consensus achieved at MERH 2018.

Strengthening collaboration between institutions, organizations and countries aimed at improving the health of migrants and ethnic minorities.

A Global Society should integrate academic, professional and community work on health and healthcare in this field (First World Congress on Migration, Ethnicity, Race and Health 2018).

The World Health Organization's *Global Action Plan on Promoting the Health of Refugees and Migrants, 2019–2023* establishes a comprehensive "framework of priorities and guiding principles [...] to promote the health of refugees and migrants" (World Health Organization 2019). It envisions both short-term and long-term public health interventions and strongly advocates for integrating migrant and refugee health into global, regional, and national agendas. By promoting refugee-sensitive and migrant-sensitive health policies, the Action Plan seeks to ensure that the unique health needs of these populations are adequately addressed. Furthermore, it underscores the importance of intersectoral collaboration and the integration of health services to provide holistic care. It also emphasizes the necessity for targeted health strategies that consider the social determinants of health, fostering environments where refugees and migrants can attain the highest standards of health and well-being. This comprehensive approach not only enhances individual health outcomes but also contributes to public health resilience and cohesion within host communities.

Recognizing the Rights of Others

In an examination of human rights, citizenship, and migration, philosopher Seyla Benhabib (2004) explores the principles and practices employed to negotiate between maintaining the boundaries of existing political communities and acknowledging the rights of others, i.e., aliens and strangers, immigrants and newcomers, refugees and asylum seekers, as they seek incorporation into these entities. Ali's personal story embodies this struggle to balance protection and integration.

Our lives were in danger in Pakistan too because circumstances had recently changed there, and the government had revised their policies regarding refugees. These changes were due to more refugees arriving there since the Taliban had come to power in Afghanistan. Most of the refugees were forcibly deported by Pakistani militias to Afghanistan. The cost of food, rent of houses and other basic necessities had doubled there. I didn't have any financial support from anyone. My brother had also been living as a refugee since 2014 in Indonesia and he was not able to support our family. I would have loved to work and support my family, but I didn't have a permission to work in that environment and couldn't find any job in that limbo, and it was really hurting me that I couldn't support my family. We were also hiding from police in Pakistan. If they found us they would send us back to Afghanistan; if we went back to Afghanistan the Taliban regime would kill us as they killed my father.

As persons with refugee experience flee from persecution, war, and human rights violations, there is an ethical imperative (or humanitarian duty) to offer them protection. Nevertheless, in 2011, António Guterres, the United Nations High Commissioner for Refugees at the time, observed:

> In Europe alone, the 1951 Convention has provided a framework for the protection of millions of refugees, guaranteeing them not only safety but also the social and economic rights necessary to start new lives. However, the human rights agenda out of which UNHCR was born, and on which we depend, is increasingly coming under strain. The global economic crisis brought with it a populist wave of anti-foreigner sentiment, albeit often couched in terms of national sovereignty and national security. At the same time, the changing nature of armed conflict is increasingly limiting the space for humanitarian action.

European immigration policies since the Second World War have reflected a reluctance towards immigration among European countries, which have become migration destination countries "largely unintentionally and reactively, and often against the explicit will of sizable parts of both the political elite and the native population" (Koopmans 2005: 5). Contemporary research on migration, border regimes, and refugee movements in Europe has critically analysed the current policies and practices affecting the rights of migrants and persons with refugee experience in Europe (Hess & Schmidt-Sembdner 2021). Furthermore, historical research on European migration has highlighted how concerns regarding the control over mobility have always been linked to struggles over labour control and public anxieties about "uncontrolled masses", leading to the racialization of immigration as well as the intersection of race, ethnicity, or religion with socioeconomic and legal status (Anderson 2013). This historical development is reflected in current right-wing and populist attempts at othering and dehumanizing migrants and persons with refugee experience, which are having a detrimental impact on immigration policies across Europe (Nowak & Razum 2022).

The following letter to the editor appeared on 27 January 2019 in the German newspaper *Der Tagesspiegel:*

Try to guess who I am! I am more in the media than Donald Trump and his tweets, Erdogan and his democracy, Putin and his politics. I was the main reason for the failure to form a government in Germany and for the rise of the right in Europe. I am the great concern of many citizens in this country, because I am more dangerous than poverty in old age, abuse in families, environmental pollution, drug use, climate change, lack of carers and educators. I am the one who always feels guilty for the mistakes of other people. People they don't even know. I am the one who is always ashamed to greet neighbours when something happens again somewhere. I'm liable for everyone's mistakes and feel threatened by every report in the media.

Did you recognise me? I am the refugees! And it's not a grammatical error due to a lack of knowledge of German. I am the refugees! And I mean all refugees. I'm not a doctor, a lawyer, a farmer, a journalist, an artist, a salesperson, a taxi driver or a teacher – I'm the refugees. Although I come from a small town in Syria and the people in Damascus were already foreign to me, since I have been in Europe, I have become one of hundreds of thousands of refugees from Syria, Pakistan, Afghanistan, Iraq, Iran and Africa. Although we speak different languages, have different religions and pasts, not to mention different world views and opinions. But who cares about such differences, we are all refugees in the end. I lost friends and relatives, my flat, my job, my car, my past and my home because of the war. But one loss that I only felt later was my individuality, which I left behind on the rubber dinghy at the borders of Europe (Gouma 2019: own translation into English).

It was written by Syrian lawyer, Vinda Gouma, who now works as a legal researcher at the German Institute for Human Rights.

It is essential that health professionals relate to persons with refugee experience as fellow human beings, despite the persistence of racist and xenophobic discourses, which have been shown to have a negative impact on clinicians by creating biases that compromise the quality of care (Rousseau et al. 2017). Recent studies point to a correlation between negative attitudes and agreement on restricting access to healthcare for persons with refugee experience (Vanthuyne et al. 2013; Rousseau et al. 2017). On the other hand, positive attitudes correlate with greater agreement with maintaining or expanding access to healthcare for persons with refugee experience, based on arguments such as compassion, recognition of the legality of refugee status, the increased cost of delayed provision of health services, and the recognition of persons with refugee experience as future citizens and access to healthcare as a fundamental human right (Rousseau et al. 2017).

While the right to health for all, including persons with refugee experience, is promoted by international organisations such as the United Nations and the World Health Organization as an effective approach to improving individual and societal well-being globally, national governments are exacerbating existing health disparities by introducing different levels of healthcare coverage that negatively affect migrants with precarious status and persons with refugee experience (Rousseau et al. 2017). This warrants strong criticism, as empirical research has documented the negative impact of these policy changes not only on those excluded from mainstream healthcare services, but also on overall health expenditure (Bozorgmehr & Razum 2015).

The situation of persons with refugee experience is precarious due to the serious reasons for fleeing, and, although ideally temporary, refugee status often becomes permanent. Nevertheless, being labelled a refugee is not desirable as it implies a contrast to the situation of a regular citizen. Beyond their legal status, persons with refugee experience constitute a highly heterogeneous group with diverse resources and needs. Health professionals encounter not only officially recognized refugees, but also individuals who have experienced forced displacement at some point in their lives but do not (or no longer) hold refugee status. Current humanitarian crises evoke memories of forced displacement for many people across different European countries, linking to their personal histories. Furthermore, some individuals who arrived as refugees many years ago now consider their country of arrival their home and may no longer identify with the refugee status.

Ali's story demonstrates the resilience, resourcefulness, and adaptability of persons with refugee experience, as well as the vital role of support in improving their circumstances and forging new identities.

When I was in Pakistan, I had communication with the People with Refugee Experience Project – Interprofessional (PREP IP) team members. They honestly and strongly supported me and my family to resettle in a third country. Thankfully, their hard work, and sacrifice, made big changes in our lives. In December 2023, we landed in our new home in Canada. Now, because of the PREP IP team, we are in the safest country in the world where we can live with respect and dignity, and without fear of bomb blast, torture, deportation, inequality, discrimination, persecution, or massacre. Our family was reunited because my older brother settled in Canada one year earlier than us. Now we are all living together. My mom is going to school to learn English and my sister just finished school and next year is planning to start college to study to become a nurse in the future to help communities. I am also working in the health sector as a home support worker with two organizations. I love to help people which is why I have chosen this career. We are all trying to make new friends here and we have a beloved teacher, she and her husband are always beside us and we are so proud that we have them, and they are more than family to us.

The social integration of persons with refugee experience into their new country is crucial for both them and for society as a whole. Facilitating their access to healthcare and public health services has been shown to enhance their integration into society by improving their ability to work, study, and engage with community life (Bozorgmehr et al. 2020). Ensuring that persons with refugee experience have access to appropriate health services is an important element of the recognition of their full human rights.

While, these arguments underscore the relevance of a human-rights-based approach to healthcare, and the moral and practical imperative to protect the health of persons with refugee experience for the benefit of both the individuals concerned and the societies in which they live, Ali's lived experience remind us that by recognizing and addressing the rights of refugees as fundamental human rights, we can foster environments where asylum seekers and refugees not only survive but thrive, contributing meaningfully to their new communities.

Home is not where you were born; home is where all your attempts to escape cease. (Naguib Mahfouz)

References

Anderson, Bridget. 2013. *Us vs. Them? The Danger Politics of Immigration Control* (Oxford: Oxford Academic).

Atapattu, Sumudu. 2020. 'Climate Change and Displacement: Protecting "Climate Refugees" within a Framework of Justice and Human Rights', *Journal of Human Rights and the Environment,* 11.1: 86–113, https://doi.org/10.4337/jhre.2020.01.04

Arendt, Hannah. 1994. 'We Refugees', in *Altogether Elsewhere: Writers on Exile, ed. by Robinson, Marc* (Boston and London: Faber and Faber), pp. 110–119, https://archive.org/details/hannah_arendt_we_refugees

Bade, Klaus. 2008. *Migration in European History* (John Wiley & Sons).

Bast, Jürgen, Frederik von Harbou, and Janna Wessels. 2020. *Human Rights Challenges to European Migration Policy (REMAP)*, 1st edn (Stiftung Mercator), https://www.stiftung-mercator.de/de/publikationen/human-rights-challenges-to-european-migration-policy/

Benhabib, Seyla. 2004. *The Rights of Others: Aliens, Residents, and Citizens* (Cambridge etc.: Cambridge University Press) (The John Robert Seeley Lectures 5).

Bozorgmehr, Kayvan and Oliver Razum. 2015. 'Effect of Restricting Access to Health Care on Health Expenditures among Asylum-Seekers and Refugees: A Quasi-Experimental Study in Germany, 1994–2013', *PLoS ONE*, 10: e0131483, https://dx.plos.org/10.1371/journal.pone.0131483

Bozorgmehr, Kayvan, et al. 2020. *Health Policy and Systems Responses to Forced Migration*, 1st edn (Cham: Springer International Publishing AG).

Bozorgmehr, Kayvan, Lousie Biddle, and Nora Gottlieb. 2022. 'Gesundheitssystem zwischen Krise und Integration: Lehren aus 30 Jahren Fluchtmigration' [Health Care System between Crisis and Integration: Lessons Learnt from 30 Years of Forced Migration], *GGW (G+G Wissenschaft)*, 22: 15–26, Zugriff auf: https://www.wido.de/fileadmin/Dateien/Dokumente/Publikationen_Produkte/GGW/2022/wido_ggw_0322_bozorgmehr_et_al.pdf

Chetail, Vincent. 2014. 'Are Refugee Rights Human Rights? An Unorthodox Questioning of the Relations between Refugee Law and Human Rights Law', in *Human Rights and Immigration*, ed. by Rubio-Marín, Ruth (Oxford: Oxford University Press) (Collected Courses of the Academy of European Law).

Emcke, Carolin. 2013. *Weil es sagbar ist: Über Zeugenschaft und Gerechtigkeit* [*Because it can be said: On witnessing and justice*] (Frankfurt am Main: Fischer).

Emcke, Carolin. 2023. *Für den Zweifel: Gespräche mit Thomas Strässle* [*For the doubt: Conversations with Thomas Strässle*] (Frankfurt am Main: Fischer Taschenbuch).

European Commission Directorate-General for Migration and Home Affairs. n.d. *Temporary Protection*, https://home-affairs.ec.europa.eu/policies/migration-and-asylum/common-european-asylum-system/temporary-protection_en

European Council. 2001. *Council Directive 2001/55/EC of 20 July 2001 on minimum standards for giving temporary protection in the event of a mass influx of displaced persons and on measures promoting a balance of efforts between*

Member States in receiving such persons and bearing the consequences thereof, https://eur-lex.europa.eu/eli/dir/2001/55/oj/eng

European Union Agency for Fundamental Rights. 2022. *Fleeing Ukraine: Displaced People Experiences in EU,* https://fra.europa.eu/sites/default/files/fra_uploads/fra-2023-ukraine-survey_en.pdf

Farmer, Paul. 2018. *Pathologies of Power: Health, Human Rights, and the New War on the Poor, First World Congress on Migration, Ethnicity, Race and Health, 2018 Edinburgh Declaration* (Berkeley: University of California Press, 2004).

Fiddian-Qasmiyeh, Elena. 2021. 'The Right and Role of Critiquing the Contemporary Patchwork of Protection', *International Migration,* 59: 261–264, https://doi.org/10.1111/imig.12892

First World Congress on Migration. 2018. *Ethnicity, Race and Health, 2018 Edinburgh Declaration,* http://www.merhcongress.com/welcome/edinburgh-declaration/

Gatrell, Peter. 2016. '65 Jahre Genfer Flüchtlingskonvention' [66 Years Geneva Refugee Convention], *Aus Politik und Zeitgeschichte,* 66: 25–32, https://www.bpb.de/shop/zeitschriften/apuz/229825/flucht-historisch/

Gouma, Vinda. 2019. 'Leserbrief', *Der Tagesspiegel,* 28 January https://www.tagesspiegel.de/gesellschaft/lesermeinung-ich-bin-die-fluechtlinge/23917406.html

Guterres, António. 2011. *Remarks at the Opening of the Judicial Year of the European Court of Human Rights,* Strasbourg, 28 January 2011, UNHCR, https://www.unhcr.org/publications/antonio-guterres-united-nations-high-commissioner-refugees-remarks-opening-judicial

Hathaway, James C. 2005. *The Rights of Refugees under International Law* (Cambridge: Cambridge University Press), https://doi.org/10.1017/cbo9780511614859

Hess, Sabine and Matthias Schmidt-Sembdner. 2021. 'Perspektiven der ethnographischen Grenzregimeforschung: Grenze als Konfliktzone' [Perspectives of Ethnographic Border Regime Research: Border as Conflict Zone], *Zeitschrift für Migrationsforschung – Journal of Migration Research,* 1: 197–214, https://doi.org/10.48439/zmf.v1i1.105

Jenni, Karen, and George Loewenstein. 1997. 'Explaining the identifiable victim effect', *Journal of Risk and Uncertainty,* 14: 235–257, https://doi.org/10.1023/A:1007740225484

King, Martin Luther Jr. 1963. *Letter from a Birmingham Jail,* African Studies Center –University of Pennsylvania, 16 April 1963, https://www.africa.upenn.edu/Articles_Gen/Letter_Birmingham.html

Koopmans, Ruud, et al. 2005. *Contested Citizenship: Immigration and Cultural Diversity in Europe, NED—New edition,* Vol. 25 (University of Minnesota

Press: JSTOR) (Social Movements, Protest, and Contention), http://www.jstor.org/stable/10.5749/j.ctttsd0w

McAdam, Jane and Tamara Wood. 2021. 'The Concept of "International Protection" in the Global Compacts on Refugees and Migration', *Interventions*, 23: 191–206, https://doi.org/10.1080/1369801X.2020.1854105

Menjívar, Cecilia. 2023. 'State Categories, Bureaucracies of Displacement, and Possibilities from the Margins', *American Sociological Review*, 88.1: 1–23, https://doi.org/10.1177/00031224221145727

Nowak, Anna Christina, Oliver Razum, and Claudia Hornberg. 2023. 'Exploring the Significance of Legal Status on Refugees' and Asylum Seekers' Access to Health Care in Germany—A Mixed-Method Study', *International Journal of Public Health*, 68, https://doi.org/10.3389/ijph.2023.1605578

Nowak, Anna Christina and Oliver Razum. 2022. 'The Concept of Othering: Definitions and Challenges from the Perspective of Members of the PH-LENS Research Unit', *PH-LENS Working Paper Series No. 3, Version 1.0*, https://doi.org/10.4119/unibi/2967024

Office of the High Commissioner for Human Rights and World Health Organization. 2008. *Fact Sheet No. 31: The Right to Health*, https://www.ohchr.org/en/publications/fact-sheets/fact-sheet-no-31-right-health

O'Flaherty, Michael. 2023. 'Tolerance of Human Rights Violations against Refugees Has Reached Alarming Levels in Europe', *Commissioner for Human Rights*, https://www.coe.int/en/web/commissioner/-/tolerance-of-human-rights-violations-against-refugees-has-reached-alarming-levels-in-europe

Pogge, Thomas. 2005. 'World Poverty and Human Rights', *Ethics & International Affairs*, 191:1–7, https://doi.org/10.1111/j.1747-7093.2005.tb00484.x

Qi, Haodong and Tuba Bircan. 2023. 'Modelling and Predicting Forced Migration', *PLoS ONE*, 18: e0284416, https://doi.org/10.1371/journal.pone.0284416

Rousseau, Cécile, et al. 2017. 'Encouraging understanding or increasing prejudices: A cross-sectional survey of institutional influence on health personnel attitudes about refugee claimants' access to health care', *PLoS ONE*, 12.2: e0170910, https://doi.org/10.1371/journal.pone.0170910

Rudolf, Beate. 2023. 'Die Allgemeine Erklärung der Menschenrechte: Grundlage und Motor des Menschenrechtsschutzes' [The Universal Declaration of Human Rights: The Basis and Driving Force of Human Rights Protection], *Aus Politik und Zeitgeschichte*, 73: 4–10, https://www.bpb.de/shop/zeitschriften/apuz/allgemeine-erklaerung-der-menschenrechte-2023/

Slovic, Paul. 2007. '"If I look at the mass I will never act": Psychic numbing and genocide', *Judgment and Decision Making*, 2.2: 79–95, https://doi:10.1017/S1930297500000061

Small, Deborah A., George Loewenstein, and Paul Slovic. 2013. 'Sympathy and callousness: The impact of deliberative thought on donations to identifiable and statistical victims', in *The Feeling of Risk,* ed. by Slovic, Paul (Routledge), pp. 51–68.

UN High Commissioner for Refugees (UNHCR). 2010. *Convention and Protocol Relating to the Status of Refugees,* https://www.unhcr.org/media/convention-and-protocol-relating-status-refugees

UN High Commissioner for Refugees (UNHCR). 2024. 'Refugee data finder', https://www.unhcr.org/refugee-statistics/

United Nations. 1948. *Universal Declaration of Human Rights* (Paris: United Nations), https://www.un.org/en/about-us/universal-declaration-of-human-rights

United Nations. 1965. *International Convention on the Elimination of All Forms of Racial Discrimination* (New York: United Nations), https://www.ohchr.org/en/instruments-mechanisms/instruments/international-convention-elimination-all-forms-racial

United Nations. 1966a. *International Covenant on Economic, Social and Cultural Rights* (New York: United Nations), https://www.ohchr.org/en/instruments-mechanisms/instruments/international-covenant-economic-social-and-cultural-rights

United Nations. 1966b. *International Covenant on Civil and Political Rights* (New York: United Nations), https://www.ohchr.org/en/instruments-mechanisms/instruments/international-covenant-civil-and-political-rights

United Nations. 1979. *Convention on the Elimination of All Forms of Discrimination against Women* (New York: United Nations), https://www.ohchr.org/en/instruments-mechanisms/instruments/convention-elimination-all-forms-discrimination-against-women

United Nations. 1989. *Convention on the Right of the Child* (New York: United Nations), https://www.ohchr.org/en/instruments-mechanisms/instruments/convention-rights-child

United Nations. 1990. *International Convention on the Protection of the Rights of All Migrant Workers and Members of Their Families* (New York: United Nations) https://www.ohchr.org/en/instruments-mechanisms/instruments/international-convention-protection-rights-all-migrant-workers

United Nations. 2016. *New York Declaration for Refugees and Migrants* (New York: United Nations), https://www.un.org/en/development/desa/population/migration/generalassembly/docs/globalcompact/A_RES_71_1.pdf

World Health Organization. 1948. *Constitution of the World Health Organization* (Geneva: World Health Organization), https://www.who.int/about/governance/constitution

World Health Organization. 2019. *Global Action Plan on Promoting the Health of Refugees and Migrants (2018–2030)* (Geneva: World Health Organization), https://www.who.int/publications/i/item/9789240093928

World Health Organization. 2023. *Fact Sheet Human Rights and Health* (Geneva: World Health Organization), https://www.who.int/news-room/fact-sheets/detail/human-rights-and-health

Background information on the photo:

The mural in Red Hook, New York City, was commissioned in 2010 by the Dutch Human Rights Lawyers group Miles4Justice. It was painted by young adults from the Red Hook Community Justice Center and after-school program run by Groundswell Mural Projects. The photo was taken by Sandra Schiller in 2013.

II. Including Refugee Experience in the Provision of Health and Social Care

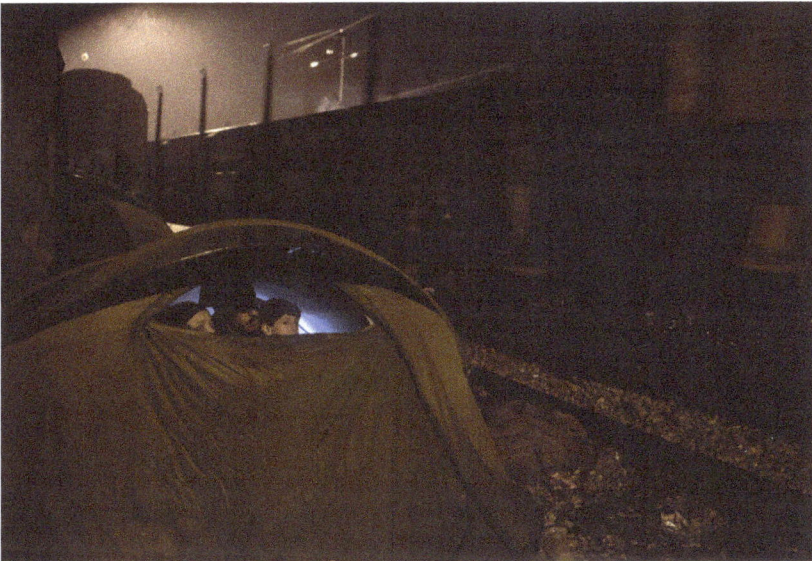

3. Providing Person-Centred Care, Creating Therapeutic Space and Recognizing the Needs of Service Users

Emer McGowan, Sarah Quinn and Rolf Vardal

It is very important to listen to the people with refugee backgrounds. Some of them have come from very difficult situations. Sometimes they are carrying the experiences of what they have gone through. It is making them sick. Sometimes, these refugees, they don`t need medical treatment, they only need somebody that can listen. So out of listening, also knowing this person.

— Male economist from Kenya living with refugee status in Norway

The health needs of refugees, and the barriers and challenges that can prevent them from accessing health and social care, differ from those of the host population over the life-course (WHO 2021). By addressing these physical and mental health needs, health and social care professionals can play a significant role in supporting the resettlement of refugees. Taking a person- or people-centred approach is central to this aim. Adaptable, well-trained and culturally competent health and social care workers are needed to provide services that are responsive to the unique health requirements of refugees (WHO 2021). Provision of person-centred care can help to build trust between health professionals and refugees, both at the time of arrival and more importantly during longer-term refugee settlement (Procter 2016). This chapter explores how health professionals can take a person-centred approach when

   https://doi.org/10.11647/OBP.0479.03

providing care and services for people with refugee experience. It discusses the concept of therapeutic space and how this can help to facilitate communication and build effective working relationships with service users. This chapter is aimed at health professionals who are new to the field of refugee health or those with an interest in the area who have not yet gained practical experience.

The concept of patient-centred care was first discussed by Balint in 1969, where it was described as "understanding the patient as a unique human being" (Balint 1969). Since then, patient-centred care has been an evolving concept and has been described using an array of different terms, including relationship-centred care, personalized care and user-/client-centred care (Santana et al. 2017). In this chapter, we use the term person-centred care as opposed to patient-centred care, in keeping with Ekman et al. who distinguished person-centred care as refraining from reducing the person to just their symptoms or disease (Ekman et al. 2011). A person-centred approach is concerned with human connectedness: the capacity for thought and feeling to be received, and lives to be revealed (Procter 2016). When working with refugees, person-centred care will involve:

- Being open to the way a person explains, understands, or interprets her or his or someone else's health problems or illness.

- Taking into account a person's cultural beliefs, and understanding that these will influence the way in which symptoms are presented.

- Considering the person's understanding of health difficulties and becoming aware of differently perceived causes of illness or disease, optimal care, and culturally appropriate support and treatment.

A conceptual framework for the provision of person-centred care was developed by Santana et al. (2017) based on the Donabedian model for healthcare improvement (Donabedian 1988). This model (Figure 3.1) is based on three categories, "Structure," "Process" and "Outcome". The framework demonstrates the need to target interventions and address challenges at different levels (healthcare system, healthcare provider, and patient) in order to provide person-centred care.

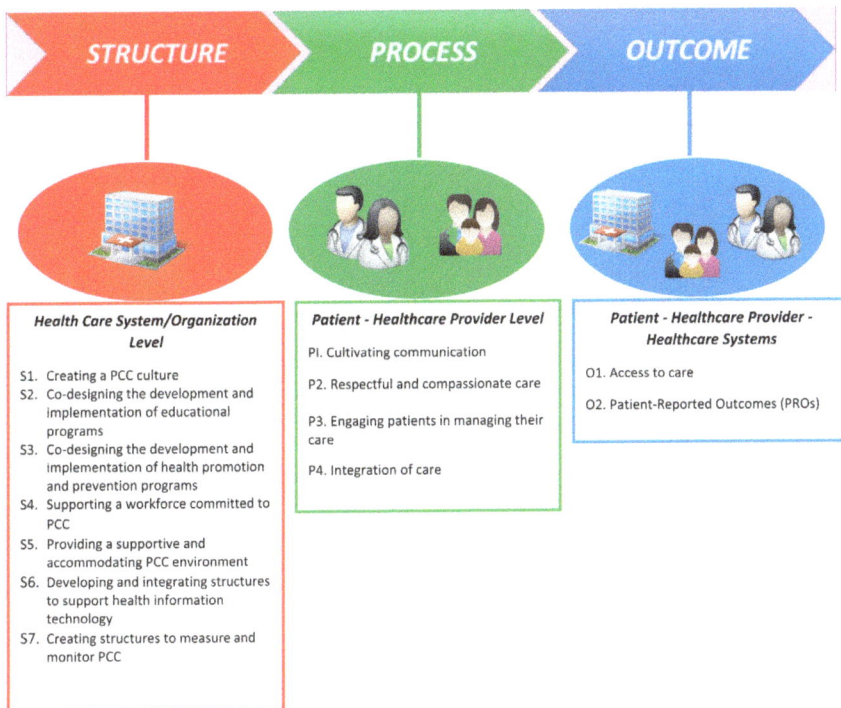

Fig. 3.1 Framework for Person-Centred Care. Reproduced from Santana et al. (2017), CC BY.

The framework lists four Process domains for health professionals to employ to ensure delivery of person-centred care. These are cultivating communication (listening to patients, sharing information, discussing care plans with patients), respectful and compassionate care (being responsive to preferences, needs and values, providing supportive care), engaging patients in managing their care (co-designing care plans with patients), and integration of care (communication and information sharing for coordination and continuity of care across the continuum of care). This framework clearly conveys the importance of not only incorporating the patient perspective but of ensuring that care is also patient-directed, whereby patients have sufficient information and understanding to make decisions about their care (Santana et al. 2017). It also highlights the need to address diversity (including race, ethnicity, gender, sexual identity, religion, age, socio-economic status, and disability), to respect individual patient beliefs and values, and thus to promote dignity and anti-discriminatory care.

Filler et al. (2020) outlined practical strategies that health and social care professionals can implement to aid the delivery of person-centred care in a scoping review, which explored barriers and facilitators of patient-centred care for immigrant and refugee women. A friendly, courteous, and comfortable relationship can be established by assuming a non-judgemental manner, taking time to chat informally, being present, and focusing on the service user (not the computer), becoming familiar with the service-user's culture and migration journey, and potentially learning a few words of the service-user's native language.

The clinical work of any health or social care professional, no matter how willing or keen to help, will be compromised if they do not consider ways to ensure they take a person-centred approach. This approach will also involve family members and caregivers, as well as prevention and health promotion activities (Santana et al. 2017). Service users and communities should play a key role in co-designing health promotion and prevention interventions. These programmes will be better able to meet the needs of all people if they are developed through collaboration with and empowering service-users, patient advisory groups, organisations, and communities (Santana et al. 2017).

One of the four Process domains in the Framework for Person-Centred Care is the provision of respectful and compassionate care (Santana et al. 2017). Compassion is a deep feeling that stems from witnessing another's suffering coupled with a strong desire to help to alleviate that suffering (Goldberg 2020). There are numerous definitions of compassionate care, but there are elements common to many of these: understanding others, choosing to act to help others, actively imaging what others are going through, and reacting to others' needs selflessly (Bivins et al. 2017). Patients who experience compassionate care have been found to have better clinical outcomes, higher patient experience scores, improved hope for recovery, and safer care (Tehranineshat et al. 2019; Goldberg 2020). However, it should be noted that the delivery of compassionate care depends on more than just individual health professionals, and that the wider healthcare team and organisational context in which the care is delivered are key (Tehranineshat et al. 2019). Caring for patients must be a shared responsibility between professional groups within clinical environments that value and respect each discipline's contribution (Bivins et al. 2017). Despite this, health professionals can face challenges with providing compassionate care in practice due to bureaucratic barriers and time constraints, given the business-like ethos of certain areas of healthcare (Patel et al. 2021).

Mechili et al. (2018) advocated the importance of providing respectful and compassionate care for people with refugee experience. Compassionate care has been defined as "the humane quality of understanding suffering in others and wanting to do something about it" (Halsman 2015). As well as sufficient and appropriate care, vulnerable populations, such as refugees, should be shown acceptance, respect, kindness, empathy, and receive attention to their basic needs. Health professionals need to consider the needs, wishes, and expectations of newly arrived refugees in the context of the transcultural setting. Developing the communication skills and competencies necessary to care for vulnerable groups, and enhancing the cultural competencies of interdisciplinary teams of health and social care professionals present some of the most challenging aspects of providing compassionate care for refugees (Mechili et al. 2018).

In a systematic review of refugee experiences of healthcare consultations in primary care settings, Patel et al. (2021) found that compassionate care aspects of communication were important factors in helping improve comfort and trust between healthcare professionals and refugees. Service users preferred to see health professionals who were kind, patient, and welcoming, and those who took interest in them as a person and were willing to take the time to listen to their stories. Health professionals working with refugees should demonstrate compassion and empathy towards their individual patients, and be aware of their emotions, concerns, and suffering (Patel et al. 2021).The European Refugees-Human Movement and Advisory Network (EUR-HUMAN) project ran for 12 months in 2016 in response to the increased numbers of refugees coming to Europe and the requirement for capacity building among health professionals to meet their needs (Mechili et al. 2018; van Loenen et al. 2018). This project proposed a primary healthcare model for refugee care with an emphasis on the provision of compassionate, comprehensive, person-centred, and integrated care. Factors that enabled the provision of compassionate care included communication skills to better convey adequate healthcare information and psychological support, understanding potential linguistic and cultural barriers, and training to provide tools and empower healthcare professionals in order to enable them to build trust. Barriers to providing compassionate care for interdisciplinary teams include a lack of capacity in terms of time and resources, unclear division of roles, staff changes, insufficient funding, poor coordination, and lack of a comprehensive monitoring system (Mechili et al. 2018).

Key recommendations from this project (Mechili et al. 2018; van Loenen et al. 2018) for the provision of compassionate care included:

- Preparing all health and social care professionals to deliver culturally competent, compassionate, and person-centred care. The multidisciplinary team should be trained to use proactive outreach to identify vulnerable refugees.

- An individual's values, societal beliefs, wishes and experiences should be assessed by health and social care professionals and taken into account when planning sessions and interventions.

- The health needs and personal preferences of individuals should be assessed at all stages and considered in conjunction with applying evidence-informed, disease-specific recommendations.

- Informal interpreters and using children as interpreters should be avoided as much as possible. Instead, quality interpretation services should be provided for all healthcare appointments.

- Health information and all services should to be tailored and suitable according to the level of the individual's health literacy.

Self-reflection exercise:

Reflect on your own experiences of providing compassionate and person-centred care. Choose a specific example and explain how you adapted your approach to foster person-centred and compassionate care. Include any barriers or challenges you experienced in taking this approach and outline how you addressed them.

Developing a Therapeutic Relationship

I think people need more information and more time to explain. Because when a person went to a doctor for example in Kenya, they got the time to explain... But here the doctors will want you to say you have problem. "there and there". They are the one who can ask you the question about it. Most of the refugees find that the doctors maybe don`t have time. Because the personal doctors, they don`t have time. They have 20 minutes and most of the time they are writing, and they can think that this doctor just wants to finish with me and go. — Male economist from Kenya living with refugee status in Norway

It is good that those who work with these refugees are updated. That you get a better understanding of what they have gone through and that they are not here voluntarily. That they have come here to save their lives. Their own or to those closest to them. So, we must try to help them in the best possible way, both physically and mentally.

— Female nurse from Bosnia living with refugee status in Norway

The therapeutic relationship, also referred to in the research literature as a therapeutic alliance, a helping alliance or a working alliance, refers to the interpersonal relationship between the health and social care professional and client (Peplau et al. 1997). In the provision of care for refugees, the therapeutic relationship occurs between two human beings, sometimes three, due to the presence of an interpreter. It involves one person defined as (or having) the role of a health and social care professional and another defined as (or having) the role of a patient/client/service user. The interpreter, when present physically or digitally, is regarded as a neutral entity, merely transmitting information between the two other individuals. However, it is essential to emphasize that the interpreter is also a human being whose presence can influence the relationship in various ways. Notwithstanding this, the focus in the following text will primarily be on the space between the health and social care professional and the refugee using their service.

The importance of the therapeutic relationship in healthcare has been widely recognized (Horton et al. 2021) and has been demonstrated to have an impact on clinical outcomes in rehabilitation (Hall et al. 2010; Ferreira et al. 2013; Fuentes et al. 2014). The quality of therapeutic relationships has been understood to be impacted by the extent to which the dyadic partners perceive the relationship to include particular aspects such as agreement on tasks and goals, interpersonal skills, trust, and shared decision making (Elvins & Green 2008). Relationships that rate highly on these factors are judged to be high-quality therapeutic relationships, and those that rate low on them are perceived to be lower-quality relationships (Elvins & Green 2008).

Developing a therapeutic relationship can be aided by shifting the professional/personal boundary towards the personal end of the spectrum (Finaret & Shor 2006). This shift can be assisted by open communication, an informal work setting (e.g., the client's home) and self-disclosure from the professional (Finaret & Shor 2006). Similarly, Miciak et al. (2018) found that physiotherapists and patients being genuine or themselves during interactions was a necessary condition for building therapeutic relationships. Horton et al. (2021) explored the development of therapeutic relationships between physiotherapists and occupational therapists and their patients, and, specifically, the impact of turning points or critical events on these therapeutic relationships. Constructive turning points that help to develop high-quality therapeutic relationships included progress towards goals, positive feedback from patients, and interpersonal affective bonding with patients. In contrast, non-constructive turning points included setbacks in progress towards goals, interpersonal problems with patients, and negative feedback from patients. These studies highlight the importance of health and social care professionals being open, authentic, and willing to be vulnerable themselves when working with clients to help to develop a positive therapeutic relationship.

Effective therapeutic relationships also demand that health and social care professionals can appropriately respond and manage emotional reactions. To do this they must acknowledge service-users concerns, offer comfort and encouragement during sessions and collaborate with the wider multi-disciplinary team as needed (Filler et al. 2020). It is also important that cultural differences are recognised, accommodated and respected, and that care is personalized to the individual rather than generalized to culture or country of origin (Filler et al. 2020).

Humour may be another strategy that health and social care professionals can employ to cultivate a sense of belonging in the rehabilitation setting (Kfrerer et al. 2023). Humour has been found to improve co-operation, compliance and positive motivation in clients (Leber & Vanoli 2001; Walsh & Leahy 2009) and can help with client engagement in rehabilitation (Gard et al. 2000). In a scoping review exploring humour in rehabilitation professions, humour was found to be a used mainly positively in rehabilitation and was considered to be an effective way to improve client/professional relations (Kferer et al. 2023). Humour was used in a number of different ways to build and maintain the therapeutic relationship, including:

- As a management strategy in therapy—to deflect errors, mitigate awkward situations, distract or restructure interactions, and maintain a frame of joking or light-heartedness during sessions.

- To foster relationships with colleagues within the multi-disciplinary team.

- To negotiate power differentials that can exist as part of the relational dynamics between clients and professionals—humour can be used to either establish power and thus influence the tone of the interaction or to equalize power and break down barriers.

- As a therapeutic modality, particularly in group rehabilitation settings.

- To save 'face'—humour was a way for clients to show that they understand and are aware of their condition and difficulties. It can provide a means to ask for help and laugh at oneself.

- To cope with grim situations—using dark/'gallows' humour to relieve tension during vulnerable or intimate struggles in rehabilitation. It can also provide stress relief when used between health professional colleagues.

- To foster group cohesion—by building trust, emphasizing togetherness and indicating belonging to the group.

Creating therapeutic space

The advice below is from Rolf Vårdal, a physiotherapist in Norway who has extensive experience of treating people with refugee experience. Rolf has been a physiotherapist since the early 1990s and working in refugee health since 1997. He has worked as a member of the team for people who have experience forced migration at the Regional Trauma Centre. Rolf has also been a councillor for people with refugee experience who have resettled in the municipality of Bergen, Norway.

When working with refugees, some factors can create connection, while others may create distance. In the host country, the professional likely resides permanently and generally has a sense of stability and safety that the refugee may not have established. Additionally, the professional holds a certain power in this relationship, which they should be conscious of. The power dynamic stems from the professional's authority due to their profession, representing a service, or even a state, where the patient/ client might feel inferior due to the imbalance in roles. The patient/client has a health issue, either physical or psychological, or both, and seeks or expects help from the professional. It is therefore important to assess how the health and social care professional can ensure that the therapeutic space is open and fosters an atmosphere conducive to healing.

Establishing a framework is crucial. Generally, the patient/client will come to the health professional, at least for the first consultation. Expectations for the consultation may vary significantly between individuals, as some may not be familiar with different services or types of therapy. The professional should take time to introduce themselves and explain their role. It is essential that they ask the patient about the concerns to be addressed during the consultation, but they should also inquire more broadly about their general or personal background beyond the presenting health issues. If the professional possesses knowledge of the patient's/client's country of origin, history, culture, or general conditions, displaying genuine interest in the individual can lay the foundation for further contact and contribute to a positive atmosphere. Additionally, 'mapping' the patient's/client's interests, competencies, and experiences helps to establish balance and reduces the top-down approach. However, some patients/clients accustomed to a more submissive relationship with health professionals may require time to understand this rationale and different approach.

For physiotherapy, the physical touch is crucial and can make a significant impact once a safe relationship has been established. However, it may take time to achieve this. Furthermore, gender must be considered, as some patients/clients with refugee experiences may not feel comfortable with a therapist of the opposite gender, especially during the initial phase.

Maté and Maté (2023) contend that compassion is integral to healing. They have outlined five levels of compassion:

Ordinary compassion: "...when somebody is suffering, I feel bad about that, and I don't want them to suffer."

Compassion of understanding: "...I feel bad that you're suffering, I want to understand why you're suffering."

Compassion of recognition: "...I don't see myself as different from you."

Compassion of truth: "...I'm not trying to protect you from pain. I want you to know the truth because I believe the truth will liberate you."

Compassion of possibility: "...I see them for the full, beautiful human beings that they are."

Healing practices vary considerably across the globe, as illustrated in Kirmayer's article (2004) on the cultural diversity of healing. While it is impossible to be fully competent in all practices, building a relationship of trust and cooperation is vital and can be achieved to a much greater extent by all. By understanding and applying these concepts, therapists can work toward creating a therapeutic space that is open, compassionate, and conducive to healing.

> What is important is to know the situation, and a little more about the country they come from. About what they have been through and try to understand and be able to help them better. In other words, health personnel can improve their professional practice by learning from people with a refugee background.
> — Female nurse from Bosnia living with refugee status in Norway

Case Study

In a previous project on refugee health, Physiotherapy and Refugee Education Project (PREP), Patricia Rocca, who works as a physiotherapist for the Swedish Red Cross, created a video telling the story of Khaled.[1] Khaled is a 45-year-old Palestinian man from Syria who has refugee status in Sweden.

The video explores the interplay between pain and post-traumatic stress disorder (PTSD). It demonstrates the benefits of taking a person-centred approach when working with people who have survived trauma and provides specific examples of how this can be done. The importance of interprofessional collaboration is also highlighted through the close working, co-ordination and communication between the physiotherapist and psychologist. The video acknowledges that the approach presented is one of many methods that can be used when providing care for traumatized individuals with a refugee background. As previously noted, it is important to bear in mind that refugees are a broad and heterogeneous group of people. An individualized approach must be taken, and treatment adapted in response to the client's symptoms, resources, and goals.

The video of this presentation is available here: https://www.youtube.com/watch?v=ug_WEkXeOSo

Abridged case study transcript

Khaled came to Sweden in 2016. In his home country he was politically involved since his teenage years and with that imprisoned three times. The first time for eighteen months and the second time when he was in his late twenties for three years. It was during the second imprisoning that he was tortured. The first year in prison he was tortured daily. He was submitted to suspension by hanging from his wrists, beatings, isolation, forced body positions, waterboarding, and witnessing torture. He lived in a small cell together with 30 other individuals. There was not room for everyone to lay or sit down at the same time, so they had to alternate when resting and sleeping.

The following 11 years he lived in a refugee camp in Syria under very scarce circumstances. At the camp he was kept under close surveillance and was frequently harassed by Syrian military, until he escaped for Sweden. Khaled has no formal education; he only attended school until he was 11. His childhood was marked by poverty and discrimination.

---

1   Khaled is not the client's real name and parts of the story have been changed to hide his identity.

In Sweden, he lives with his wife and three children in an apartment provided by the Swedish social services. He attends an introductory programme for migrants but finds it very hard to concentrate due to sleeping problems and flashbacks from torture. He's very concerned about his and his family's future in Sweden. He wishes very much to find a job.

Before Khaled meets with his physiotherapist for the first time, he has already met with a psychologist at the Red Cross Treatment Centre. He has been diagnosed with PTSD and the psychologist has informed him about the interdisciplinary teamwork at the Centre and that he will have consultations with physiotherapists, a social counsellor, and a medical doctor.

To receive a PTSD diagnosis, one has to have been exposed to trauma. In Khaled's case, he has both experienced a traumatic event himself and been forced to witness the torture of friends and fellow prisoners. Khaled's father, who was also politically involved, was imprisoned and tortured when Khaled was a young boy, so Khaled has been exposed to various traumatic events also as a son.

Torture is an act that violently and intrusively attacks an individual's boundaries, physically and mentally. The subjective experience is lack of control, a high degree of helplessness, no possibility to defend oneself, and unpredictability. It induces fear, stress, and pain. Torture results in bodily injuries: wounds, fractures, burns, muscle strains, as well as psychological harm. The absence of treatment affects the healing in a negative way. Torture seeks to break its victim through the intentional use of pain to destroy and/or damage the physical and psychological integrity of the individual and by extension the integrity of the family and community.

Torture and trauma results in alterations of an individual's body ego; loss of body awareness means loss of the ability to recognize one's body and one's physical experiences or sensations which can impair one's ability to understand one's needs and emotions. Impairment in the ability to trust one's body evokes a negative body image and dissatisfaction with one's body. Reconnecting to the body in a positive way and learning how to use movements to self-regulate a conflicting inner state is a central part of recovery. Understanding the method of torture used can aid the physiotherapist in understanding the injuries, and managing the assessment and treatment appropriately and sensitively.

While most physiotherapists may focus on the outcomes of the torture experience itself—that is, scar tissue, fracture, mal-union, persistent pain—it is also of importance that the physiotherapist understands the impact of torture on a psychological level, and the additional stresses that impact the patient's health status and well-being, for example: unsafe journeys, and, upon resettlement, the experience of many losses e.g., loss of status, identity, family, employment, property.

The physiotherapist prepares for the meeting with Khaled by reading his medical journals and consults with the psychologist. When Khaled enters the physiotherapist's room, the physiotherapist starts by asking Khaled to choose a place to sit and asks whether Khaled is okay to be in the room with the door closed. Khaled chooses to position himself so he can see the door. The physiotherapist introduces herself and informs Khaled that, being a healthcare professional, she works under confidentiality laws but that information about patients is shared within the team.

Khaled has had lumbar back pain and shoulder pain for several years. He went to see a physiotherapist once at his healthcare centre, but when he saw all the workout machines, he became scared and never went back again. The physiotherapist asks Khaled how the trauma has affected his body. Khaled describes symptoms of anxiety and stress, never being able to relax, his heart racing and difficulty breathing when being around people, Syrian men in particular. He only feels safe at home and even there he can get jolted by sudden sounds. His coping strategies are walking around in his apartment, or short walks in close proximity to his apartment, and taking showers.

He sleeps two to three hours a night and always with the light on. He is often woken by nightmares, feeling paralyzed, and has difficulty going back to sleep. He has no appetite and very low levels of physical activity. This is all of the information that Khaled is able to share during the first meeting with the physiotherapist.

The role of the physiotherapist during the first meeting is to start building an alliance with Khaled, not to push too deep into Khaled's story. Khaled keeps repeating that he is tired, and he hardly gives any eye contact, his legs are constantly shaking. He is very tense in his shoulders and he keeps his head bowed; he doesn't take off his jacket. The physiotherapist briefly describes how bodily work can help trauma-affected individuals to relax, and that during coming sessions they will explore self-regulating techniques that might help Khaled to stay present and reduce his anxiety. The physiotherapist describes what they will do next time they see each other so that Khaled feels prepared and to ensure predictability. No examination of his shoulders or back is performed at this point.

At the second assessment, the physiotherapist uses the 'Body Awareness Movement Quality and Experience Scale' to examine Khaled's bodily resources. This is a test that consists of two parts; the first one is an observer-based rating scale where the physiotherapist evaluates the functionality of various visually observed movement patterns. The second part consists of a questionnaire on subjective experiences of the body. Results show that Khaled is very tense in his body; he has poor stability and flexibility. He also shows poor coordination and a shallow breathing pattern. His breath is really never integrated with his movements and Khaled finds it very hard to relax when lying down on the floor. He says it reminds him of how his torturers forced him to lie down on cold floors, sometimes for hours, with the threat of beatings if he moved.

During both assessments, the physiotherapist checks in frequently with Khaled by using questions like, "Is it okay if we continue a bit further, or do you need a pause?", "How are you feeling right now?", "Do you have any questions or reflections on what we just said?" The physiotherapist and Khaled agree on treatment with basic body awareness therapy, an evidence-based treatment form, that aims to establish increased awareness of the body and consciousness in movements, progressing toward less effort and a better function in being, doing, and relating. The physiotherapist also proposes that Khaled should participate in group workouts in order to strengthen his physique, but Khaled feels a bit uncertain about this since he has difficulty trusting other men. The physiotherapist and Khaled decide to delay the group workout until Khaled feels safer. Khaled also meets a social counsellor for psychosocial mapping in order to identify difficulties in his daily life that may become a hinderance for therapy.

He also receives a prescription for sleeping medication from the medical doctor.

Throughout all of the consultations at the treatment centre, the same translator is present in the room with Khaled. She is an elderly Palestinian woman. Early in the treatment process, Khaled, the psychologist, and the physiotherapist make a common healthcare plan. This plan is reviewed every six months, as long as his treatment proceeds. In the plan, Khaled's stress factors and protective factors are described; his recurring flashbacks, insomnia, concentration difficulties, body pains, and a psychosocial situation with no job or income are recorded as stress factors. Protective factors are his permanent residence permit, the support he has from his family, and that he is motivated to engage with treatment.

Khaled's treatment goals are:

- To be able to be around people without fear.

- To sleep five hours a night.

- To be able to concentrate at school so he can learn Swedish.

It is decided that Khaled will attend physiotherapy directly after sessions with the psychologist for stabilization following the trauma-exposing treatment. When you encounter an individual that has been exposed to severe trauma, torture, or any other interpersonal violence, it is essential that extra consideration is given to building an alliance with that individual. Trauma-informed care is an approach that recognizes that experience of trauma can affect all aspects of care, from communication to clinical reasoning.

In trauma-informed care, it is important to make the first encounter with the patient an encounter where the patient feels safe. A good start is to explain the purpose of the meeting and describe how the meeting will progress, if you are working with a translator, let the translator introduce him or herself, explain that you as a healthcare professional, and the translator, are bound by confidentiality laws. Make the patient feel that they are in control during the meeting, for example by letting the patient choose where they want to sit in the room or whether the door should be closed or not. Take time to answer their questions. Allow the patient to take breaks and to decline answering questions and be ready to pause the assessment at any point if the patient shows high levels of anxiety or distress. Check in frequently on the patient and ensure you have their consent to continue asking questions or examining their bodies during the physical examination. Explain every step beforehand to ensure safety and a sense of control. Avoid rushing the patient or asking questions too quickly because this may recreate a feeling of an interrogation.

Many patients with PTSD suffer from concentration difficulties and it is therefore crucial to portion the amount of information given. Repetition might be of great help to the patient. Continuity in terms of using the same room and same translator creates a space that is safe and predictable. Strong physiological reactions can be triggered in a traumatized individual by different stimuli, for example smells, sounds, touch, body positions, but also inanimate objects such as an examination bed or medical equipment. Therefore, be aware of the patient's bodily reactions, don't be afraid of asking, "I see that you're tensing. How are you feeling right now?".

Every session starts with the physiotherapist checking in with how Khaled's week has been, how he is feeling, and how his body is feeling. Khaled is given the opportunity to discuss the content of the session. At the end of a session, Khaled is invited to reflect on how it went. The physiotherapist noticed that Khaled often is very shaky when sitting in the waiting room and that he avoids eye contact with other people. He sits in a slumped position; his legs are shaking, and he points his gaze onto the floor.

In the room with the physiotherapist, Khaled shows the same pattern. He reacts to sudden sounds and often looks behind his shoulder. The physiotherapist tries to guide Khaled verbally into a more upright position, where he will experience more space for his breath and a reduction of muscle tension in his neck and back. There are a lot of trauma triggers coupled to different movements and positions. The physiotherapist normalizes and validates Khaled's reactions, and a lot of time is spent on letting Khaled reflect on his experiences in the room and how increasing contact with the body and movements can help Khaled regain and reconquer his body after consulting with Khaled's psychologist.

The physiotherapist learns that during the psychological sessions Khaled loses contact with his body; his legs become numb and he can't feel the floor or the chair he's sitting on. The physiotherapist and

Khaled therefore explore different grounding exercises that Khaled can use during the sessions with the psychologist to break dissociation. Education on bodily reactions to trauma memories, and on persistent pain and its relation to PTSD, is given continuously during Khaled' treatment to better his understanding of his reactions and thereby reduce his anxiety and worries about what is happening in his body.

PTSD and persistent pain are frequently seen in the aftermath of a traumatic experience. Torture survivors have an increased risk of suffering from persistent pain. What factors contribute to the development of persistent pain? Factors that are believed to play a role are: initial pain severity, extent of injury, and the level of emotional stress at pain onset, all of which are present at a high degree in a torture situation. Several factors contribute to persistent pain: continued emotional stress, poor sleep, and avoidance behaviour. Pain can remind the patient of the torture situation and therefore many torture survivors try to avoid pain-provoking activities. This can lead to physical deconditioning, social withdrawal, and minimal involvement in daily activities, and can also contribute to physical deconditioning. Catastrophizing, imagining the worst outcome, can lead to increased stress and arousal and enhance the pain experience. Pain-related fear can cause guarding movements such as tensing of the body.

To treat Khaled's back pain, core exercises are introduced. Firstly, only verbal guidance is used but with a growing feeling of safety; more organic guiding is added in order to help Khaled find a more stable and grounded posture.

A few months later Khaled feels that he is ready to try out the group workout. In the beginning, he stands apart and doesn't interact with other participants but slowly he begins to be more confident. The group activity later inspires Khaled to start working out on his own.

Interprofessional collaboration in person-centred care

Integrated healthcare strategies directed at both psychological and physical health, as well as rigorous control of risk factors, are likely to improve the quality of life of traumatized individuals. As the psychologist approaches Khaled's memories of torture, Khaled experiences bodily reactions in terms of numbing but also back and neck pain. The psychologist encourages Khaled to use body awareness exercises to stay present during their exposure therapy.

The psychologist and physiotherapist always try to have a short talk in between each other's sessions to reinforce each other's treatment strategies. Khaled says that he's found having physiotherapy during and directly after his sessions with a psychologist to be very helpful. He becomes more present and connected to his body. He describes that his head becomes silent when practicing basic body awareness. The safer Khaled feels with the physiotherapist, the more they work with building trust and confidence through couple exercises, for example guiding each other in the room with open and closed eyes.

Khaled is improving; he can now better understand and put words to his physical sensations, and he uses coping strategies when he gets flashbacks or nightmares. Khaled feels more and more that his body can be a resource to stay present even during the toughest trauma-exposing sessions with the psychologist. He also begins putting himself into situations that he avoided before. He can now reach the common laundry room that lies in the basement of his building complex. He walks in the middle of the pavement instead of close to building walls and he dares to close his eyes in public spaces. At school he explores sitting at the front of the classroom and raises his hand to ask questions. It is clear that Khaled is building resilience and expanding his experience of his surroundings.

In reading this transcript/watching the video, please consider the questions below:

1. What are your first impressions about working with a client like Khaled?

2. What practical strategies could you employ in your practice to accommodate the needs of someone who has experienced trauma?

3. Which of your colleagues would you work with to ensure comprehensive care for a client like Khaled? Do you need to broaden your professional network to enable comprehensive care?

This case study provides an example of multiple ways that health and social care professionals can demonstrate person-centred care for a person with refugee experience. The care plan developed for Khaled considers his physical, psychological, and social needs. Instead of focusing solely on his physical pain, the health and social care team addressed his PTSD, trauma history, and struggles with integration. His treatment was tailored to his specific experiences and comfort levels. For example, he initially avoided group workouts due to trust issues, so the team waited until he felt ready. Shared decision making was evident in the way that Khaled was actively involved in his care decisions, such as choosing where to sit, whether the door should be open, and when to begin group therapy. The health and social care professionals demonstrated effective interprofessional collaboration through a treatment plan that was well co-ordinated and aligned with Khaled's evolving needs.

Conclusion

A person-centred approach to care is concerned with human connectedness. When working with people with refugee experience this means acknowledging the unique needs, experiences, and challenges experienced by displaced individuals. Health and social care professionals need to demonstrate openness to the way that someone understands and interprets their health problems. Many refugees have experienced trauma, loss, and disruption, which can impact their physical and mental well-being. A person-centred approach ensures that healthcare services are tailored to their cultural, emotional, and medical needs, fostering trust, establishing a positive therapeutic relationship, and improving health outcomes.

References

Balint, Enid. 1969. 'The possibilities of patient-centred medicine', *The Journal of the Royal College of General Practitioners*, 17: 269–276.

Bivins, Roberta, et al. 2017. 'Compassionate care: not easy, not free, not only nurses', *BMJ Quality & Safety*, 26:1023–1026.

Donabedian, Avedis. 1988. 'The quality of care: how can it be assessed?', *JAMA*, 260.12: 1743–1748.

Ekman, Inger, et al. 2011. 'Person-Centered Care — Ready for Prime Time', *European Journal of Cardiovascular Nursing*, 10.4: 248–51, https://doi.org/10.1016/j.ejcnurse.2011.06.008

Ferreira, Paulo H., et al. 2013. 'The Therapeutic Alliance between Clinicians and Patients Predicts Outcome in Chronic Low Back Pain,' *Physical Therapy*, 93.4: 470–78, https://doi.org/10.2522/ptj.20120137

Filler, Tali, Bismah Jameel, and Anna R. Gagliardi. 2020. 'Barriers and Facilitators of Patient Centered Care for Immigrant and Refugee Women: A Scoping Review,' *BMC Public Health*, 20.1, https://doi.org/10.1186/s12889-020-09159-6

Finaret, Andrea Eini, and Ron Shor. 2006. 'Perceptions of Professionals about the Nature of Rehabilitation Relationships with Persons with Mental Illness and the Dilemmas and Conflicts That Characterize These Relationships,' *Qualitative Social Work*, 5.2: 151–66, https://doi.org/10.1177/1473325006064252

Fuentes, Jorge, et al. 2014. 'Enhanced Therapeutic Alliance Modulates Pain Intensity and Muscle Pain Sensitivity in Patients with Chronic Low Back Pain: An Experimental Controlled Study,' *Physical Therapy*, 94.4: 477–89, https://doi.org/10.2522/ptj.20130118

Gard, Gunvor, et al. 2000. 'Physical therapists' emotional expressions in interviews about factors important for interaction with patients', *Physiotherapy* 86.5: 229–240, https://doi.org/10.1016/S0031-9406(05)60908-X

Goldberg, Michael J. 2020. 'Compassionate Care: Making It a Priority and the Science Behind It', *Journal of Pediatric Orthopaedics*, 40: S4–S7, https://doi.org/10.1097/BPO.0000000000001502

Hall, Amanda M., et al. 2010. 'The Influence of the Therapist-Patient Relationship on Treatment Outcome in Physical Rehabilitation: A Systematic Review,' *Physical Therapy*, 90.8: 1099–1110, https://doi.org/10.2522/ptj.20090245

Haslam, David. 2015. '"More than Kindness"', *Journal of Compassionate Health Care*, 2.1, https://doi.org/10.1186/s40639-015-0015-2

Horton, Ayana, Gail Hebson, and David Holman. 2021. 'A Longitudinal Study of the Turning Points and Trajectories of Therapeutic Relationship Development in Occupational and Physical Therapy,' *BMC Health Services Research*, 21.1, https://doi.org/10.1186/s12913-021-06095-y

Kfrerer, Marisa L., Debbie Laliberte Rudman, Julie Aitken Schermer, Marnie Wedlake, Michelle Murphy, et al. 2022. 'Humor in Rehabilitation Professions: A Scoping Review,' *Disability and Rehabilitation*, 45.5: 911–26, https://doi.org/10.1080/09638288.2022.2048909

Kirmayer, Laurence J. 2004. 'The Cultural Diversity of Healing: Meaning, Metaphor and Mechanism,' *British Medical Bulletin*, 69.1: 33–48, https://doi.org/10.1093/bmb/ldh006

Leber, Donna A., and Elizabeth G. Vanoli. 2001. 'Therapeutic Use of Humor: Occupational Therapy Clinicians' Perceptions and Practices', *American*

Journal of Occupational Therapy, 55.2: 221–26, https://doi.org/10.5014/ajot.55.2.221

Maté, Gabor, and Daniel Maté. 2022. 'In Four A's and Five Compassions: Some Healing Principles', in *The Myth of Normal: Trauma, Illness, and Healing in a Toxic Culture*, ed. by Maté, Gabor, and Daniel Maté (New York: Avery), pp. 374–389.

Mechili, Enkeleint-Aggelos, et al. 2018. 'Compassionate Care Provision: An Immense Need during the Refugee Crisis: Lessons Learned from a European Capacity-Building Project,' *Journal of Compassionate Health Care*, 5.1, https://doi.org/10.1186/s40639-018-0045-7

Miciak, Maxi, et al. 2018. 'The Necessary Conditions of Engagement for the Therapeutic Relationship in Physiotherapy: An Interpretive Description Study,' *Archives of Physiotherapy*, 8.1, https://doi.org/10.1186/s40945-018-0044-1

Patel, Pinika, et al. 2021 'Communication experiences in primary healthcare with refugees and asylum seekers: a literature review and narrative synthesis', *International Journal of Environmental Research and Public Health*, 18.4: 1469.

Peplau, Hildegard E. 1997. 'Peplau's Theory of Interpersonal Relations,' *Nursing Science Quarterly*, 10.4: 162–67, https://doi.org/10.1177/089431849701000407

Procter, Nicholas G. 2016. 'Person-centred Care for People of Refugee Background,' *Journal of Pharmacy Practice and Research*, 46.2: 103–4, https://doi.org/10.1002/jppr.1222

Santana, Maria J., et al. 2017. 'How to Practice Person-centred Care: A Conceptual Framework,' *Health Expectations*, 21.2: 429–40, https://doi.org/10.1111/hex.12640

Tehranineshat, Banafsheh, et al. 2019 'Compassionate care in healthcare systems: a systematic review', *Journal of the National Medical Association*, 111.5: 546–554.

World Health Organisation. 2021. 'WHO releases two publications to promote people-centred health services for refugees and migrants', https://www.who.int/news/item/21-10-2021-who-releases-two-publications-to-promote-people-centred-health-services-for-refugees-and-migrants

van Loenen, Tessa, et al. 2018. 'Primary Care for Refugees and Newly Arrived Migrants in Europe: A Qualitative Study on Health Needs, Barriers and Wishes,' *European Journal of Public Health*, 28.1: 82–87, https://doi.org/10.1093/eurpub/ckx210

Walsh, Irene P, and Margaret M Leahy. 2009. '"Cajoling" as a Means of Engagement in the Dysphagia Clinic,' *Seminars in Speech and Language*, 30.01: 037–047, https://doi.org/10.1055/s-0028-1104533

4. Recognizing the Needs of Refugees: A Healthcare Access Lens

Ganzamungu Zihindula

Introduction

The number of refugees in the world is rising at an alarming rate. At the beginning of 2022, there were 35.3 million refugees, 62.5 million internally displaced people, 5.4 million asylum seekers, and 5.2 million people in need of international protection. In September 2023, it was estimated that more than 114 million individuals were forcibly displaced worldwide (UNHCR 2024: 2). This escalating number means that the challenge of meeting the needs of refugees has also greatly increased. To illustrate this, the UNHCR required a budget of 10,622 billion US dollars to provide life-saving assistance, protection, and solutions for a projected figure of 130.8 million forcibly displaced and stateless people by the end of 2024 (UNHCR 2024). In line with the projected figure, at the end of year 2024 there were 123.2 million FDPs globally. Both the 2024 counting of forcibly displaced and stateless persons (123.2 million) and their projected number (130.8 million) exclude other forms of displaced persons like economic migrants and those who have already naturalized to become citizens of their host countries. This chapter explores the healthcare needs of refugees and discusses best practices for health and social care professionals' recognition and response to these urgent needs. Specific factors that health and social

    https://doi.org/10.11647/OBP.0479.04

care professionals should be aware of to improve the accessibility of the care they provide are highlighted. The chapter also provides details for how health and social care professionals can ensure that they respond effectively to the different needs of people living with refugee experience. The discussion focuses on important issues that health and social care professionals need to recognize and incorporate into their daily practice to improve the quality of care they provide and reduce potential triggers of psychological distress.

Refugee Needs for Consideration by Healthcare Professionals

The needs of refugees can differ from those of citizens in host communities in many ways. The World Health Organisation (WHO) conducted a review of the common health needs and vulnerabilities of refugees and migrants. The impact of migration on physical and mental health, along with low levels of health literacy, experiences of discrimination and restricted access to mainstream health services can mean that refugees' health needs go unmet (WHO 2021). Similarly, children with experiences of forced displacement may have worse health outcomes related to infectious diseases, chronic diseases, and mental health issues compared with local residents or undisplaced children in high-income countries (WHO 2021: 6). In a comparison between refugees and the host population in Uganda, a UNHCR study found that 51% of refugee households were defined as "in need of healthcare services and other basic human right needs", compared to 17% of host households (UNHCR 2022: 3 cited in King et al. 2022). A similar observation was made by the Royal College of Physicians in Ireland, revealing that asylum seekers and refugees had health needs that differed from those of the local Irish population or the citizen thereof, and which should be taken into consideration by healthcare professionals when providing services to the latter. According to the physicians' observations, infectious diseases, including but not limited to Hepatitis B, HIV, and TB, are more common in asylum seekers and refugees following higher background rates of such health conditions in their home countries. This drives the need for screening upon arrival of asylum seekers whose primary needs remain shelter, food, and healthcare services (UNHCR 2022: 2). The health-seeking behaviours of refugees and asylum seekers mirror their differences in health needs (Zihindula 2015) and are influenced by cultural practices and religious beliefs across communities and countries of origin. These factors need to be recognized by a healthcare professional providing services to forcibly displaced persons.

Refugees can require mental health and psychosocial support due to traumatic experiences endured in their country of origin, during transit to their destination, as well as after arriving in the host country due to re-traumatizing events. These factors mean that refugees should receive a thorough needs assessment and identification of health and social care requirements. Such assessments should take into consideration all the effects of psychological trauma including, but not limited to, changes in relationships, reliving traumatic incidents, anger and frustration, euphoria, isolation, sadness, guilt and shame, helplessness, fear, disbelief, and bewilderment, as well as emotional disconnection and distance. In a study of refugee healthcare needs in New Zealand, readily accessible interpreters (language needs), culturally competent and sensitive health practitioners (cultural sensitivity training), and availability of clear and accurate information were found to help refugees access the healthcare services they required (Bafreen Sherif et al. 2022: 5). Studies in South Africa had previously yielded similar results, yet also found that traumatic experiences, especially for refugees and asylum seekers coming from conflicts zones, fear of disclosing their status due to stigma and discrimination, and refugee perceptions of healthcare professionals, are potential barriers to accessing healthcare (Ganzamungu Zihindula et al. 2015; Alfaro-Velcamp 2017; Meyer-Weitz Asante & Lukobeka 2018). To provide appropriate healthcare services for refugees, healthcare professionals should recognize that many refugees arrive from settings where healthcare facilities have been destroyed by war (such as the Democratic Republic of Congo, Palestinian territories, and South Sudan), and have experienced exacerbated vulnerabilities due to economic instability and discrimination based on cultural and traditional practices (Alfaro-Velpimo 2017; WHO 2021). In such environments, interruption of access to health services for chronic health conditions exists in advance of forced migration patterns, thus leaving individuals predisposed to deteriorating physical health and, by extension, mental health. It is worth noting the complexities of the health needs of refugees when they present to a healthcare facility for care. The long-term physical and psychological problems experienced by refugees can date back to their pre-immigration experiences and can be later exacerbated by post-migration factors (RACGP 2023), including discrimination, stigmatisation, racism, gender issues, hostility of the host community, and access barriers to socio-economic and basic human rights opportunities like higher education, healthcare services, and documentation.

The context and geographic location within which a person with refugee status is seeking health services will impact their needs. For example, a refugee located in any country or region in sub-Saharan Africa will have different needs compared to a refugee in a high-income country Europe, North America, or Oceania (Emansons Guntars 2023: 4). In the setting of a high-income country, refugees have access to basic health services (which are sometimes covered by national health insurance policies), healthcare settings regulated by sanitation requirements and adequate equipment, and safety, all of which have positive impacts on mental wellbeing, compared to their counterparts in many sub-Saharan African countries where these remain an issue (WHO 2021). While such services may not be without fees in some high-income countries, such as the USA, the vast majority offer the services free even in low- and middle-income countries (LMICS), e.g., South Africa, Uganda, Kenya, and Zimbabwe. Beyond the actual health service given between clinicians and refugees, safety within facilities is an additional aspect to consider that differs from the general security measures of health institutions. Refugees face a heightened risk of stigma and discrimination by healthcare workers and or other patients. Moreover, their emotional and mental safety during the interaction with healthcare workers is of critical importance. Such safety measures are rooted in cultural awareness, a conscious effort to overcome language barriers, and the intentionality to provide a thorough exam to screen, diagnose, manage, and treat the refugee comprehensively and at the earliest engagement with the facility. At present, the likelihood of discrimination raises questions of whether safety is equally distributed.

Recognizing Dynamic Socioeconomic Needs of Refugees

Refugees can face additional social, educational, and economic challenges in their host communities, including rejection, hostility from the host population, and social class acceptability based on perceptions of race, ethnicity, and identity. Scientific evidence suggests that, in Ireland, refugees from Ukraine who present as white are received more hospitably, with positive emotions, compared to refugees who present as people of colour from Asian and African countries such as the Democratic Republic of Congo, Sierra Leone, Somalia, and Syria (Xuereb 2023). Ukrainians have been referred to as 'brothers' by most European Union states, and particularly in Ireland, where the host communities have been mobilized to receive Ukrainian refugees in solidarity. This 'social solidarity cause' has not been the case for other nationalities, irrespective of the dire situations in which they find themselves, thus exacerbating their risk of mental and emotional harm.

This 'selective solidarity' approach applies to service delivery and access to fundamental human rights. There are radical differences among different refugee groups regarding their access to higher education or the financial support they receive in the form of monthly stipends. For example, Ukrainian refugee undergraduate students at any university in Ireland receive a monthly stipend of 1150 Euros, while all other asylum seekers and refugee groups studying toward a similar undergraduate degree within the same institutions receive a rate that is eight times less than that, at 155.2 Euros a month (Irish Universities Association 2023; Irish Refugee Council 2023). Such unequal consideration and resource distribution have negative effects on the mental health and psychological wellbeing of the recipient refugee, leading to potential sadness, a sense of isolation, helplessness, anger, frustration, and all other effects of psychological trauma. Knowledge of the overarching discriminatory approaches applied to refugees across the many private and public institutions within host countries should be essential for healthcare workers. Adopting a sensitive approach to the lived realities of refugees as central to their health and well-being may reduce the risk of re-traumatisation. This knowledge, along with cultural competency training, are key to providing appropriate healthcare services to asylum seekers and refugees.

Healthcare providers working directly with asylum seekers and refugees must be aware that these populations may have pre-existing perceptions of being structurally and systematically excluded from financial and educational benefits that may have been provided to other forcibly displaced groups. Understanding this dynamic and taking it into consideration when offering healthcare services will prevent the beneficiary from perceiving the healthcare system as a similar institution that applies a 'selective solidarity approach' in the provision of care. Experiences of discrimination can impact the psychological well-being of asylum seekers and refugees, affect their social relationships, increase psychiatric symptoms, lower self-esteem, reduce perceptions of optimism, reduce treatment adherence, and can cause escalating challenges in the work, home, or school environment (Singhal 2024). If not taken into consideration by healthcare providers, pre-existing experiences of discrimination and inequities in social services can lead to reluctance and/or resistance from refugees related to the uptake of health services at healthcare facilities. Not only can this have negative clinical outcomes for patients, but it increases the risks faced by those in their immediate households and communities. In the case of infectious disease, the implications are a cause for concern. Further, poorly managed health conditions will ultimately lead to greater dependence on and cost for the state to manage chronic health conditions and their impact on individuals and families.

Gender, Identity, and Sexual Orientation Care Need Dynamics for Refugees

Women, children, and people who identify as Lesbian, Gay, Bisexual, Transgender, Intersex, or Questioning (LGBTIQ+) are among the most marginalized within refugee communities (Denise Venturi 2023). Age, gender, and sexual identity all have the potential to influence access to healthcare services, and healthcare professionals must recognize that they will experience a vast range of healthcare needs. Sawadogo et al. (2023: 7) conducted a scoping review of barriers and facilitators of access to sexual and reproductive health services among migrants, internally displaced persons, asylum seekers, and refugee women. Limitations that asylum seekers and refugees regularly report include a lack of autonomy in decision-making, discrimination, stigma, delays due to related administrative factors within the health system, availability of healthcare services, the geographic location of health facilities, and the quality of communication or patient-provider relationship, which ultimately determines the quality of services received. Healthcare providers must recognize that all these barriers could potentially result in determinants of sexual and reproductive health services for women, youth, or members of the LGBTIQ+ community. The Women Refugee Commission (2021: 1) cited in Sawadogo et al. (2023), reports that the limited access to reproductive health services for refugee women and girls results in increased risks of unintended pregnancy, complications of pregnancy, diseases, disability, and deaths that could be prevented. A WHO (2022) report highlights issues of abuse, sexual assaults, and violence which are common in the context of forced displacement. Additionally, instances of torture and trauma during the forced migration process and the impact of the resettlement process have been documented (WHO 2021: 11) and may or may not intersect with other issues related to gender, age, and identity. Women, young people, and members of the LGBTIQ+ community may endure specific challenges in accessing services due to social issues and gender-related stigmatisation, related to their cultural background (Diab et al. 2024). Therefore, for women within the refugee community, 'gender-sensitive' health services are routinely reduced to perinatal care and gender-based violence (GBV) support, often overlooking more comprehensive sexual and reproductive health needs (Keygnaert et al. 2014). Importantly, gender-sensitive health services have fallen short in comprehending the inherent heterogeneity of both women and LGBTIQ+ individuals within the refugee community, at times failing to make important distinctions between the specific healthcare concerns of non-heterosexual and non-cisgender refugees who are confronted with policies, norms, and systems in the host community, and some healthcare providers, as well as other social services providers, who interact with them very differently. National legal and policy frameworks within the host country have long determined the accessibility of services for refugees, particularly regarding gender-sensitive services. Importantly, the criminalisation of migration, as well as the precarious legal standing host countries impose on refugees with a specific gender identity such as agender, cisgender, genderfluid, non-binary, genderqueer and transgender within their borders, impacts their realisation of their right to access adequate healthcare (Martinez et al. 2015). When providing healthcare services to refugees, it is essential that healthcare personnel acquire a baseline understanding of these dynamics and remain aware that refugee populations are not a homogenous group with the same vulnerabilities and needs.

Cultural Misunderstandings and Communication Breakdown

There is a pervasive assumption that if a patient, in this case, a refugee patient, is quiet, uncomplaining, and compliant, this means that they are okay. Yet, it is equally possible that this refugee patient has been silenced, rejected, and feels unable or unempowered to communicate their needs. In some cultures, around the world, communities have a wide range of social healing practices, which refugees may be unable to practice or access in host countries. Additionally, they may feel silenced due to unequal treatment or feelings of non-belonging or being unwelcome in the host community. Additionally, there exists the risk of assumptions around the level of awareness and knowledge migrants have about the health systems of the host country, their own health status, and their willingness to adopt prescribed clinical approaches readily. The knowledge, attitudes, and practices of individuals and how they respond to care pathways is rooted in their cultural practices, and in familiarity with health systems in their home countries which are context-specific, inclusive, and responsive to socio-cultural norms. In the absence of practices to create an inclusive and safe environment, there remain ongoing risks of avoidable barriers to access care, non-compliance with prescribed treatment plans, and refugees dropping out of the system.

A Case Study on Refugee Social Integration

As a person with lived experience of forced migration, living in Ireland at the time of writing this chapter, I have worked with refugee populations in both direct provision centres and as a facilitator in English language classes. In these volunteer-led classes, hosted at the Centre of Forced Migration Studies at Trinity College Dublin (TCD), small groups of learners practice every-day English speaking and literacy skills, while also experiencing an informal and welcoming opportunity for intercultural exchange. In my conversations with participants, I gathered personal stories and information about the dynamic needs expressed by the community.

I can further witness that refugees' knowledge and information regarding health systems in their host country is limited. Sometimes the information is made available but in languages unknown to refugees, or other times, it is provided through platforms that are not accessible to a vulnerable group. For example, information provided through electronic devices that many refugees in the global south cannot afford, will not serve them. Some information on Sexual and Reproductive Health (SRH) is provided through social media links, yet many of the refugee groups do not necessarily have access to them, for example older persons, children, and those who were less privileged in terms of basic education. In my case, and for my host country, the language in which information was provided and how this reached the refugee community were the two main issues.

Another aspect of misinformation is linked to refugees not being briefed about the model of the health system in a particular country. Usually, asylum seekers and refugees rely on their fellow migrants who arrived in the host country before them to provide necessary information about the functionality of the health system, and access barriers or facilitators. Being new in the host country, my attention was focused on lived experiences shared by fellow forced migrants. It did not come to my attention at any point that their experiences were individual cases that could differ from one person to another. Furthermore, most of their information was also something that they had heard from a fellow forced migrant. Almost none used trusted sources such as an information document from the government or private sector like a

Non-Governmental Organisation (NGO) working in the healthcare service in the country. The same issue of miscommunication and limited access to credible information applies to a forced migrant living in the Global North: if they remain uninformed, they may miss a treatment opportunity due to misinformation. For example, in Ireland, an asylum seeker or refugee must consult their general practitioner/family doctor before going to the hospital for treatment, whereas in South Africa, for instance, the public healthcare system is structured in a different way.

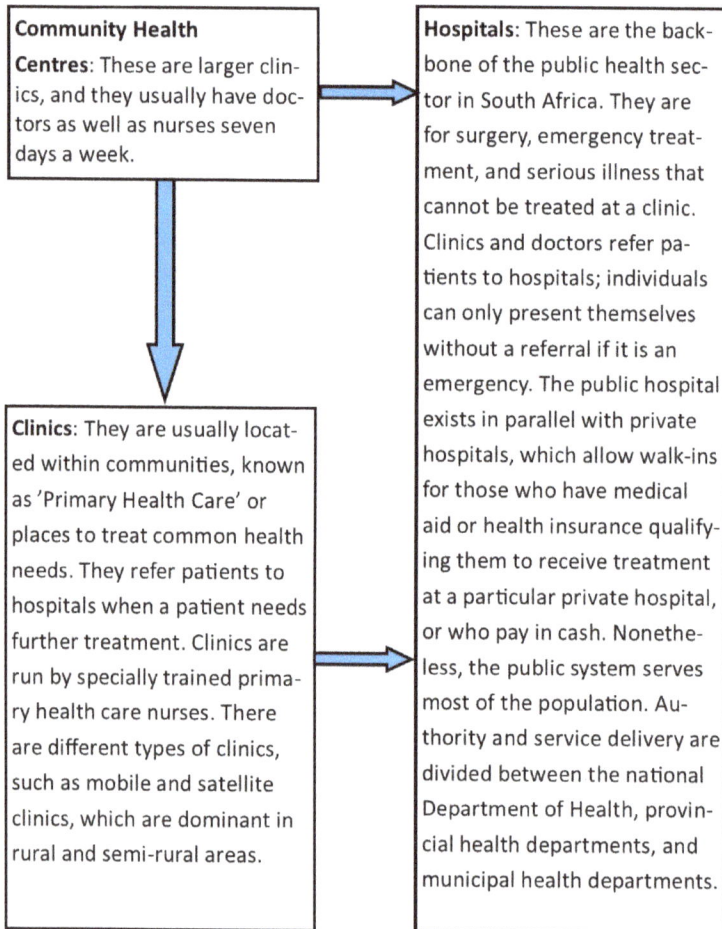

Community Health

Centres: These are larger clinics, and they usually have doctors as well as nurses seven days a week.

Clinics: They are usually located within communities, known as 'Primary Health Care' or places to treat common health needs. They refer patients to hospitals when a patient needs further treatment. Clinics are run by specially trained primary health care nurses. There are different types of clinics, such as mobile and satellite clinics, which are dominant in rural and semi-rural areas.

Hospitals: These are the backbone of the public health sector in South Africa. They are for surgery, emergency treatment, and serious illness that cannot be treated at a clinic. Clinics and doctors refer patients to hospitals; individuals can only present themselves without a referral if it is an emergency. The public hospital exists in parallel with private hospitals, which allow walk-ins for those who have medical aid or health insurance qualifying them to receive treatment at a particular private hospital, or who pay in cash. Nonetheless, the public system serves most of the population. Authority and service delivery are divided between the national Department of Health, provincial health departments, and municipal health departments.

Fig. 4.1 Structure of health service provision in South Africa.

Different countries hosting refugees have different healthcare models and operating systems. It is imperative for refugees to have an orientation session upon their arrival, to inform them about how a particular country's health system operates. This assists in timely access to preventative care and reduces the risks of missing an opportunity for treatment. This system (see Figure 4.1) is different for a country in the Global South such as Malawi, Kenya, DRC, Zimbabwe, or Chad, where refugees live in camps and receive their individualized health services there.

In addition to this summary in Figure 4.1, healthcare professionals ought to recognize that refugees have issues specific to their country of origin and their migration and settlement experiences, making it necessary to understand everyone's unique migration journey and the systemic barriers they have experienced in accessing care (RACGP 2023). A quote from a private correspondent with a lived experience of forced migration and who is currently a medical manager at a hospital providing care to refugees advises that: "Health providers involved in offering healthcare to the refugees must be intentional in addressing the health needs of the refugees and avoid retraumatizing experience" (Dr Lwabanya).

In many contexts, stereotyping is the factor that most hinders both sides in achieving better health outcomes for refugee patients and in building trust between healthcare professionals (HCPs) and patients from refugee groups. Dr Lwabanya reports that HCPs can perceive that patient with refugee experience complain a lot, a perception that does not help them to dig deep and better understand the patient's problems. Thus, they may miss the opportunity to provide better treatment. On the other hand, patients from refugee groups can perceive that they are undervalued in the host country. Consequently, when they visit health facilities, they are in an alert mode, and scrutinize the health provider's attitude to them, e.g., the words used, the tone of the words, how promptly they respond to their requests. Each action taken toward the refugee can positively or negatively affect their relationship with HCPs and ultimately result in a positive or negative impact on the patient's healthcare outcome(s). My experience of training in trauma-informed care (TIC) in the fragile context of the Eastern Democratic Republic of Congo (DRC) has highlighted the need for health providers to complete this training and recommend it to their colleagues to help them improve health outcomes for their patients, especially those with refugee experience, internally displaced people, and victims of sexual violence or rape.

Key Messages that Need to Be Recognised

Differences in culture and expectations: Cultural competence is central to proper healthcare provision in regular settings. However, its significance becomes even more obvious and compelling when healthcare is targeted at refugee populations in which beneficiaries mostly share no cultural background and understanding with service providers. Lack of cultural competence may lead to frustration on the side of the provider and inability to access healthcare on the side of the refugees. Hence, **cultural competence** is certainly a key goal as it takes a lot of time and experience with a particular cultural group. Nevertheless, cultural humility and openness can be keys to the initiation of proper **communication** with culturally diverse groups (WHO 2021). Rapport building and active listening prove to be effective ways to gain trust and ensure the appropriateness of services for refugees. Also, an increase in the ethnic diversity of healthcare providers whenever possible, providing services through healthcare providers who share the same ethnic background as refugee groups, appears to help ensure cultural competence with less time and in a more efficient way.

Patient-provider relationship: In the implementation of trauma-informed care intervention, a series of simulation workshops is conducted using a translational/ transformational simulation approach. Healthcare providers report fewer challenges with socially excluded persons (homeless persons, refugees, asylum seekers, and undocumented persons) when they start building rapport through active listening, connecting before correcting, and offering options, to strengthen such relationships (Vallières et al. 2023). This relates to the importance of communication and interpretation services and the provision of culturally appropriate and respectful care, facilitating the refugee patients to receive appropriately tailored information and health promotion, illness prevention, and preventive care (RACGP 2023: 3). In brief, the patient-provider relationship is nurtured by communication, which permits HCPs to learn more about the refugee patient's history before their migration to the current host country, building a rapport and clearly recognizing the refugee patient's expectations.

Time constraints: Health visits and consultations create an extremely important opportunity for providers to respond to the healthcare of refugees, especially in terms of mental health. Since these vulnerable groups have an additional disease burden compared to regular patients (WHO 2021; UNHCR 2022; Vallières et al. 2023), they require specific attention to "past experience of healthcare, exposure to traumatic experiences, languages, and cultural differences" before and during appointments. Adopting an approach in which some important steps are incorporated into healthcare delivery necessitates more effort and time allotted to appointments with refugee populations. A study conducted with refugees and asylum seekers in Canada to explore the experiences of immigrants who are new mothers with symptoms of depression reported that patients could not share the feelings of depression with their doctors as they were always rushed, and yet, their emotional issues were not covered in the check-up or at the health facility's reception (Ahmed et al. 2008). Healthcare providers need to invest time in building trust with refugee populations to be able to cover all their health-related needs. Also, it is important for them to take time to achieve cultural understanding, and to explain medical concepts and services that are made available to refugees in a way that is culturally sensitive. To improve communication during medical visits, providers must make sure that they employ appropriate strategies to inform refugees clearly about various topics of health, although they are certainly time-consuming.

Lack of knowledge and skills: The importance of informing refugees about the health system and their right to health in the receiving country is extremely important. Support through training and guidance for providers is usually neglected; the need for more training for healthcare providers who are ill-equipped to deal with the difficulties of refugees in service provision is equally crucial. Regarding the health coverage of refugees, providers can totally be unaware of the refugee entitlement for health in the receiving country. With limited time to prepare for medical encounters with culturally diverse groups and inadequate training opportunities, healthcare providers usually lack enough knowledge of refugee culture and good communication skills. Consequently, they worry that in their encounters, they may be misunderstood and offend refugee patients in certain ways that are unknown to them. This can even go as far as fearing accusations of racism due to miscommunication and lack of cultural, religious, and general background understanding.

System-related obstacles: The health systems determine the ways in which internal and external factors can strongly interfere with proper service provision. When the systems fall short of responding to the uniqueness of refugee and asylum seekers needs, this reflects a providers' avoidance of cases and eventually leads to poor health outcomes. Limited financial resources for refugee health support programs, which hinders any attempts to improve care, is an added challenge to the health system. Other obstacles include limited flexibility, despite the heterogeneity of refugee groups. The difficulty of refugees in navigating the health system results in compromised care and increased costs, which affect both health seekers and providers in an unfavourable way.

Policy Implications for Refugee Health

The goal of policies in general is to ensure a structured and orderly approach to managing the complex needs of the population, aligned with key national goals and values. The value of human life, and the need for good life outcomes central to human rights, inform how governments design and implement programmes. The intersection between health outcomes and service delivery are both interdependent and unavoidable. While migration remains a global phenomenon, irrespective of its root cause, the case of refugees and persons exposed to violent and harsh realities in countries experiencing war and extreme poverty warrant that context-specific interventions be adopted. This would ensure inclusive approaches that are respectful of human rights, and considerate to the intersections between physical and mental health, and their impact on the individual, their households, and communities. The United Nations Higher Commission of Refugees (UNHCR), the International Organization for Migration (IOM), and other relevant branches of the UN, in collaboration with governments hosting refugees, can support programmes to improve the quality of care for HCPs and refugees.

Forming this public-private partnership (PPP) and including refugee representatives in the design and implementation of health promotion interventions can positively improve the health and well-being of refugees and their communities. It also makes the health service delivery process safer and more manageable for healthcare workers. Capable public-private partnerships offer an opportunity for the co-creation of approaches that reflect the national mandate, its values and intentions, as well as the voices of refugees to shape systems that are responsive to all stakeholders. Community-led approaches have showed promise in achieving sustainable outcomes across different spheres of governance-related actions. Buy-in from affected persons, and consideration for their needs and expectations, allows for flexible and adaptive systems to be designed that have long-term benefits, reduce risk, and allow for accountability.

Given the diverse social, cultural, and educational needs, and other varied complexities of refugee populations, creating a safe and interactive approach will allow for opportunities for refugee communities to establish and implement behavioural approaches that are conducive to more effective engagement with the healthcare system. This could also improve how healthcare workers and refugees engage during consultations, with positive impact on how data is captured and reported, thus surfacing more information that allows for better understanding of trends and patterns. It could also serve as an opportunity for better collaboration between home and host countries regarding public health approaches and pave the way for improved understanding at regional and global levels about the impact of forced migration on health systems and refugees as independent and interdependent elements. This will ultimately promote integrated actions to accelerate progress for migration health by working across the United Nations system, including the United Nations Network on Migration and other intergovernmental mechanisms (WHO 2021). Lastly, a well-founded health response rooted in the health matters raised in this chapter urges collective efforts to encourage proper policymaking, capacity building, and resource mobilization through a country's own means and that of its partners. This chapter aligns with the WHO (2021) call on policymakers' involvement and support in building the healthcare capacity for service provision, affordable and non-discriminatory access to health with reduced communication barriers, and training of the healthcare workforce in culturally sensitive service delivery for refugees and asylum seekers, particularly those with different forms of disabilities.

Best Practices in Healthcare Delivery for Refugee Populations

Globally, some countries have made progress toward removing healthcare access barriers for asylum seekers and refugees, and, where known, these can be used as benchmarks. To avoid disease complications among refugee patients, a comprehensive post-arrival health assessment is recommended, to be offered to all newly arrived asylum seekers and refugees, preferably within one month of arrival. In places like Australia, such assessment commonly takes place in general practice and involves a comprehensive history and physical examination, pathology screening, catch up immunisation, further management, and referrals as appropriate (Australian Society for Infectious Diseases, and Refugee Health Network of Australia 2016). Comprehensive primary care that is responsive to the diversity of backgrounds and experiences people have had in their refugee journeys offers an essential first step to address many immediate and long-term healthcare needs (RACGP 2023).

Conclusion

For healthcare professionals to respond promptly and effectively to the healthcare needs of refugees, there are a range of individual and systemic improvements that can potentially have a significant impact on people, or, when implemented collectively, have the potential to greatly impact positive health outcomes. Such improvements are: cultural competency training within a trauma-informed care package for healthcare providers serving refugee populations' embedding translators within the care environment; and embracing diversity in the workplace to promote inclusive health to achieve an improved quality of care for both staff and refugees. The healthcare system must diversify its human resource for health staffing to include people from refugee backgrounds who should form part of healthcare service delivery. The latter are likely to be aware of the specific needs of refugees, and are thus able to respond to them, and to consider the cultural sensitivity and religious ethos of their colleagues, all of which matter in health services provision. This chapter calls for refugee host countries and their health systems to develop mechanisms that can adjust their healthcare systems to the needs of refugees and asylum seekers, or any other person from a socially excluded background. This will contribute positively towards improving the health status of refugees in different forms and contexts. These mechanisms and models or approaches should include a variety of public health interventions, including capacity building through ongoing training of healthcare workers and the employment of trained and well-equipped interpreters, as well as the hiring of professionals from different cultural and racial backgrounds, and ultimately to establish a refugee-friendly health service provision.

Dr Lwabanya and I both have lived experiences of forced migration, and we are Global Atlantic Fellows for Health Equity, based at Oxford University, UK. Together with other Atlantic Fellows based in the USA, the Philippines, and the UK, we are conducting Trauma Informed Care TIC training using a translational simulation approach, with HCPs who provide services to refugees and forcibly displaced persons FDPs in the Eastern Democratic Republic of Congo (DRC). The team is aiming to generate a toolkit adaptable to the DRC context and which each of the trainees can use to train fellows in other hospitals located in the war-torn zone in the sub-Saharan Africa region.

References

Ahmed, Amal, et al. 2008. 'Experiences of Immigrant New Mothers with Symptoms of Depression,' *Archives of Women S Mental Health*, 11.4: 295–303, https://doi.org/10.1007/s00737-008-0025-6

Australian Society for Infectious Diseases, and Refugee Health Network of Australia. 2016. 'Recommendations for Comprehensive Post-Arrival Health Assessment for People from Refugee-like Backgrounds', Australasian Society for Infectious Diseases, Survey Hills, https://www.rch.org.au/uploadedFiles/Main/Content/immigranthealth/ASID-RHeaNA%20 screening%20guidelines.pdf

Diab, Jasmin Lilian, et al. 2024. 'Gender Identity as a Barrier to Accessing Adequate and Inclusive Healthcare for Syrian Refugees in Lebanon's Northern Regions,' *Frontiers in Human Dynamics*, 5, https://doi.org/10.3389/fhumd.2023.1205786

Ermansons, Guntars, et al. 2023. 'Refugee Mental Health and the Role of Place in the Global North Countries: A Scoping Review,' *Health & Place*, 79: 102964, https://doi.org/10.1016/j.healthplace.2023.102964

lfaro-Velcamp, Theresa. 2017. '"Don't Send Your Sick Here to Be Treated, Our Own People Need It More": Immigrants' Access to Healthcare in South Africa,' *International Journal of Migration Health and Social Care*, 13.1: 53–68, https://doi.org/10.1108/ijmhsc-04-2015-0012

Irish Refugee Council. 2023. '(A) VTOS (Voluntary Training Opportunities Scheme)—for Protection', *Applicants & People with Stamp 4 (IRC)*, p. 4, https://www.irishrefugeecouncil.ie/what-state-funding-is-available-to-you

Irish Universities Association. 2023. 'Government Arrangements for Displaced Ukrainian Students for September 2023 Entry and Beyond', Irish Universities Association, https://www.iua.ie/press-releases/ukraine/guidance-for-displaced-ukrainian-students-for-sept-2023-entry-and-beyond/

Keygnaert, Ines, et al. 2014. 'Sexual and Reproductive Health of Migrants: Does the EU Care?', *Health Policy*, 114.2–3: 215–25, https://doi.org/10.1016/j.healthpol.2013.10.007

King, Jessica, et al. 2022. 'Assessing Equity of Access and Affordability of Care among South Sudanese Refugees and Host Communities in Two Districts in Uganda: A Cross-Sectional Survey', *BMC Health Services Research*, 22.1, https://doi.org/10.1186/s12913-022-08547-5

Martinez, Omar, et al. 2013. 'Evaluating the Impact of Immigration Policies on Health Status among Undocumented Immigrants: A Systematic Review', *Journal of Immigrant and Minority Health*, 17.3: 947–70, https://doi.org/10.1007/s10903-013-9968-4

Meyer-Weitz, Anna, Kwaku Oppong Asante, and Bukenge J. Lukobeka. 2018. 'Healthcare Service Delivery to Refugee Children from the Democratic Republic of Congo Living in Durban, South Africa: A Caregivers' Perspective', *BMC Medicine*, 16.1, https://doi.org/10.1186/s12916-018-1153-0

RACGP Specific Interests. 2023. 'Healthcare for People from Refugee Backgrounds and People Seeking Asylum', The Royal Australian College of General Practitioners, https://www.racgp.org.au/advocacy/position-statements/view-all-position-statements/health-systems-and-environmental/healthcare-for-refugees-and-asylum-seekers

Sawadogo, Pengdewendé Maurice, et al. 2023. 'Barriers and Facilitators of Access to Sexual and Reproductive Health Services among Migrant, Internally Displaced, Asylum Seeking and Refugee Women: A Scoping Review', *PLoS ONE*, 18.9: e0291486, https://doi.org/10.1371/journal.pone.0291486

Sherif, Bafreen, Ahmed Awaisu, and Nadir Kheir. 2022. 'Refugee Healthcare Needs and Barriers to Accessing Healthcare Services in New Zealand: A Qualitative Phenomenological Approach', *BMC Health Services Research*, 22.1, https://doi.org/10.1186/s12913-022-08560-8

Singhal, Nikhita. 2024. 'Stigma, Prejudice and Discrimination Against People with Mental Illness', American Psychiatric Association, https://www.psychiatry.org/patients-families/stigma-and-discrimination#:~:text=Harmful%20Effects%20of%20Stigma%20and%20Discrimination&text=Effects%20can%20include%3A,increased%20psychiatric%20symptoms

UNHCR. 2019. *Uganda Country Refugee Response Plan: The integrated Response Plan for Refugees from South Sudan, Burundi and the Democratic Republic of the Congo* (Geneva: UNHCR), https://reporting.unhcr.org/sites/default/files/Uganda%20Country%20RRP%202019-20%20%28January%202019%29.pdf

UNHCR. 2024. 'Global Appeal 2024', UNHCR Global Focus Operations Worldwide, https://reporting.unhcr.org/global-appeal-2024#:~:text=In%202024%20it%20is%20predicted,and%20respond%20to%20internal%20displacement

Vallières, Frédérique, et al. 2023. 'Co-Developing, Piloting, and Evaluating a Translational Simulation (TS) Delivery Model for the Promotion of Psychological Trauma-Informed Care (TIC) to Improve Service Delivery within Acute Hospital Settings: A Research Protocol', *HRB Open Research*, 6: 27, https://doi.org/10.12688/hrbopenres.13727.1

Women's Refugee Commission. 2023. *Sexual and Reproductive Health and Rights*, https://www.womensrefugeecommission.org/focus-areas/sexual-reproductive-health-rights/

World Health Organisation. 2021. 'Common Health Needs of Refugees and Migrants: Literature Review', World Health Organisation, https://iris.who.int/bitstream/handle/10665/346743/9789240033108-eng.pdf?sequence=1

Xuereb, Sharon. 2023. 'Emotions, Perceived Threat, Prejudice, and Attitudes towards Helping Ukrainian, Syrian, and Somali Asylum Seekers', *PLoS ONE*, 18.9: e0290335, https://doi.org/10.1371/journal.pone.0290335

Zihindula, Ganzamungu, Anna Meyer-Weitz, and Olagoke Akintola. 2015. 'Access to health care services by refugees in Southern Africa: A review of literature', *Southern African Journal of Demography*, 16.1: 7–35.

5. Pathways to Healing: Expressive Arts Practice with Adolescent Refugees

Rachel Hoare

Introduction

Adolescent refugees,[1] including both accompanied and unaccompanied minors,[2] face a unique set of challenges that make them particularly vulnerable. They bear the 'double burden' of forced displacement from their homeland and the transition from childhood to adulthood. Both experiences are characterized by profound losses, including home, family, friends, country, language, identity, trust, life as it was, and future dreams (Papadopoulos 2002; Tefferi 2007). Furthermore, these young refugees encounter significant barriers in accessing mental health and psychosocial support (MHPSS) services in their destination countries. Beyond the issue of poor appointment availability in overburdened systems, these barriers comprise culturally and socially diverse understandings of mental health, mental health stigma, and differing perceptions of traumatic experiences and loss within broader social and cultural contexts (Bartolomei et al. 2016; Namer et al. 2022).

---

[1] The term 'refugee' is used here to refer to both 'refugee' and 'asylum seeker' and 'adolescent' refers to 10-to-19-year-olds as per the World Health Organization's definition.

[2] Unaccompanied minors are children and adolescents who have been separated from both parents and other relatives and are not being cared for by an adult who by law or custom is responsible for doing so (UNHCR 2020).

    https://doi.org/10.11647/OBP.0479.05

Given these complex challenges, it is crucial for psychological therapy professionals and other health professionals[3] involved in the daily lives of adolescent refugees to adopt a trauma-informed therapeutic approach. This approach should be sensitive to the unique experiences and cultural backgrounds of these young individuals. Moreover, integrating expressive arts and visual tools into practice can significantly enhance therapeutic interventions, offering alternative means of expression and healing. These creative modalities can help bridge language barriers and cultural differences, and provide non-verbal outlets for processing trauma and emotions. By combining trauma-informed care with expressive arts, professionals can create a more inclusive and effective healing environment that addresses the multifaceted needs of adolescent refugees.

This chapter presents a structured yet flexible approach to therapeutic expressive arts work with adolescent refugees, drawing from Herman's (1992) trauma healing framework and Jalonen and Cilia La Corte's (2017) practical guide to therapeutic work with refugees as well as the author's expressive arts practice. The approach incorporates elements of safety, stabilisation, the processing and integration of traumatic experiences and identity development, into distinct yet permeable stages that align with the roles of different professionals. The stages reflect key principles from these frameworks, emphasizing cultural sensitivity, adaptability, and the non-linear nature of healing. Importantly, each intervention is carefully aligned with the cognitive, emotional, and social developmental stages of adolescence, ensuring effective age-appropriate support.

The following sections outline these stages, distinguishing between those that can be implemented by health professionals and those requiring the expertise of psychological therapy professionals. This distinction ensures that each professional group operates within its specific scope of practice. Throughout these stages, the integration of expressive arts plays a crucial role in facilitating healing and communication. To illustrate this approach in practice, the latter part of the chapter presents a case study of Axmed, an unaccompanied

---

3   The term 'psychology therapy professionals' will be used to refer to psychologists and psychotherapists with a clinical role and all other clinicians will be referred to as 'health professionals'.

minor refugee from Somalia who claimed asylum in Ireland. This case study serves as a practical example, demonstrating how expressive arts techniques are applied within this therapeutic framework.

Health professionals should engage primarily in:

- stabilisation and relationship-building;
- psychoeducation;
- bearing witness.

Psychological therapy professionals can address all stages of the healing process encompassing the above and:

- trauma memory processing;
- integration of trauma memories;
- identity development.

As these stages are interconnected, health professionals may occasionally engage with elements typically addressed by psychological therapists. In such instances, health professionals can still provide valuable support by fostering a safe and supportive environment, recommending available resources such as self-help materials, and referring the adolescent refugee to community support groups or counselling services where possible.

Using the Expressive Arts with Adolescent Refugees

'But I'm no good at art': embracing the use of the expressive arts

Whether you are a social care worker supporting separated adolescent refugees in a residential setting as they navigate everyday life and strive for independence, a frontline humanitarian worker assisting families, a teacher supporting refugee adolescents, an occupational therapist helping them develop skills for daily living and work, or a therapist looking to introduce expressive arts and play into working with refugee adolescents, you may have reservations about incorporating expressive arts into your practice. Common concerns include: "I'm not good at art, how can I use this approach", "I'm worried that they just won't engage with the materials", or "how do I know which approach to adopt?".

You are not alone in these concerns. Many professionals in this field have faced similar uncertainties when beginning their journey with the expressive arts. Research conducted by George Land, for NASA (National Aeronautics and Space Administration), found that rather than being indicative of a lack of innate talent, difficulties with artistic expression in professional settings are the result of educational systems that prioritize rationality and conformity over creative exploration: non-creative behaviour is learned. This systematic suppression of the natural creative instincts prevalent in early childhood is documented in his 1992 work with Beth Jarman (Land & Jarman 1992).

A good way to start on your creative journey is by introducing simple tools like fidget toys and playdough in the spaces where you engage with adolescent refugees. You may be surprised at how effectively these materials can help young people to alleviate their own anxiety, serving as an excellent introduction to the power of the expressive arts and play (Schaefer & Drewes 2014). The expressive arts techniques showcased in the case study presented here are intended to enhance, rather than replace, your current skill set. By incorporating these creative and innovative strategies, healthcare professionals can enrich their existing approaches and provide more comprehensive support to adolescent refugees.

The Expressive Arts as a Path to Healing

Art and creativity define our humanity, allowing us to connect with and assist others, regardless of age, gender, or cultural background. The healing powers of the visual arts, storytelling, drama, comedy, dance, music, play, poetry, and communal rituals—collectively known as the expressive arts—have been integral to ancient civilizations and the cultures of indigenous peoples (Malchiodi 2020). These practices, which are instinctive responses to grief, loss, and trauma, continue to be used to celebrate and honour new life and life's transitions (Linklater 2014). For example, Navajo healers still include sandpainting and music in their healing rituals (Degges-White 2011). Rites of passage such as coming-of-age initiations, marriages, and burial and mourning traditions all use forms of the expressive arts (Archibald & Dewar 2010).

In his powerful foreword to Cathy Malchiodi's (2021) book on creative interventions with traumatized children, Bruce Perry, child psychiatrist, researcher, and educator emphasizes the enduring nature of these ancient traditions. He views them as fundamental to healing from trauma and loss:

> Amid the current pressure for 'evidence-based practice' parameters, we should remind ourselves that the most powerful evidence is that which comes from hundreds of separate cultures across the thousands of generations independently converging on rhythm, touch, storytelling and reconnection to community.

The increasing recognition of the therapeutic benefits of the arts is reflected in the World Health Organization (WHO) Arts and Health Program, which organizes events, supports research, and raises awareness of the potential value of the arts in promoting good health (World Health Organization 2019).

The Expressive Arts for Healthcare Professionals Working with Adolescent Refugees

Expressive arts modalities are particularly valuable for healthcare professionals working with adolescent refugees. The universal and non-verbal nature of various forms of artistic expression make them ideal for transcending language barriers and cultural differences. Activities such as drawing, painting, music, and dance enable adolescent refugees to safely express emotions and experiences that may be difficult to articulate verbally, thereby fostering emotional healing, resilience, and a sense of agency. Moreover, expressive arts can be easily integrated into various healthcare settings, making them accessible and adaptable tools for professionals working with this population.

Integration of the Expressive Arts into Psychotherapy Modalities

The expressive arts serve not only as a distinct psychotherapy modality but also significantly enhance the skill sets of psychological therapy professionals across various therapeutic approaches. By incorporating these techniques into existing psychotherapy practices, therapists and their clients can move beyond the constraints of verbal communication. This advancement facilitates deeper therapeutic engagement and progression (Degges-White 2011). This is made possible through the integration of visual, tactile, synchronous, rhythmic, and other intuitive expressive processes which promote the integration of sensory-oriented and brain-focused aspects of arts-based expression into the therapeutic process (Rappaport 2014; Malchiodi 2023).

Activating these creative processes not only unlocks new pathways for individual self-expression, but also expands and enriches the therapeutic opportunities afforded by the therapy process. According to Degges-White (2011), the expressive arts are suitable for psychotherapists working with clients of all ages and have been effectively applied in various clinical settings including private practice, educational establishments, and residential treatment centres. This adaptability makes expressive arts a versatile tool across all psychotherapy modalities, capable of enhancing the therapeutic experience in diverse clinical environments.

Interconnected Phases of Healing for Health Professionals

Stabilisation and Relationship-Building

Many adolescent refugees have experienced or witnessed conflict and extreme violence in their home countries (pre-flight) and during their escape to safety (flight). Some may never have known the feeling of safety. Therefore, the focus during the stabilisation stage is on helping the adolescent refugee feel safe in the world, within their body, and in their relationships, while exploring ways to calm their nervous system. Establishing a sense of security during this crucial initial stage lays the groundwork for the development of a trusting relationship within a supportive environment. This foundation enables deeper emotional healing to occur in subsequent phases of healing.

Psychoeducation

Following the initial stabilisation phase, psychoeducation serves as a crucial step in empowering adolescent refugees. At this stage we may only have a "thin" version of their story and an understanding of some of their main concerns (Kohli 2006). Based on this limited information and our knowledge of common challenges faced by refugee adolescents, we can begin to provide valuable psychoeducation support.

Psychoeducation involves delivering information through therapeutic collaboration and wellbeing activities, helping to build choices and understanding. This information can be divided into practical and psychological support. Practical supports help in the navigation of areas such as education, primary care, and leisure pursuits in their new environment. Psychological support focuses on normalizing their experiences and providing general information about stress responses and coping strategies.

Age-appropriate psychoeducation about trauma responses can help refugee adolescents to understand that experiences such as flashbacks and the inability to sleep are normal reactions to abnormal events. By explaining that difficulties with sleep, concentration, and feelings of overwhelm are common for those who have experienced traumatic events, we reassure them that their responses are valid and that they are not alone. This understanding forms the basis for introducing coping strategies such as specific techniques to improve sleep quality, enhance concentration, and manage emotional responses, thereby empowering adolescents with both knowledge and tools to support their wellbeing.

It is important to deliver this information in an age-appropriate manner, using visual formats where possible to support different learning preferences, enhance comprehension and improve memory retention. This approach can be particularly beneficial for those who have experienced trauma or are communicating in a non-native language. By providing this initial psychoeducation, we lay the groundwork for the next phase of bearing witness, where adolescents may feel more comfortable sharing their "thicker" stories and experiences (Kohli 2006).

Bearing Witness

Building upon the foundation of safety and psychoeducation, the next critical step is bearing witness to the stories of adolescent refugees (Kohli 2006). This process deepens the developing trusting relationship, allowing these young people to feel secure enough to share fuller versions of their experiences. The expressive arts, introduced in the stabilisation and relationship-building phase, provide a safe medium for expression, especially when trauma has impacted their linguistic abilities or when communication occurs in a non-native language. Health professionals play a vital role in this process by authentically bearing witness to these narratives and validating diverse means of expression.

The act of bearing witness is crucial, as it acknowledges refugee adolescent experiences, promotes healing, and reinforces their sense of identity and belonging. Jalonen and Cilia La Corte (2017) emphasize the importance of understanding the psychosocial context that shapes these interactions. This aligns with Bronfenbrenner's socio-ecological framework, highlighting the dynamic interplay between individuals and their multiple environmental systems, and underscoring the importance of a supportive, coordinated approach (Bronfenbrenner & Morris 2006). Health professionals, therefore, need to be well-informed about refugee adolescent entitlements, and able to signpost them to organisations providing essential services.

Bearing witness extends beyond recognizing the traumatic impacts of loss, separation, acculturation, and identity development. It also nurtures the resilience that enables these adolescents to overcome their challenges (Shakya et al. 2014). This approach builds on coping strategies introduced during psychoeducation, reinforcing and expanding upon them in the context of each individual's unique experiences.

Blackwell (2005) advises practitioners to maintain a balanced approach, avoiding both detachment and over-involvement, to prevent alienating or disempowering refugees. He stresses the importance of allowing them to express overwhelming experiences rather than focusing solely on consoling them. Recent neuroscience research (e.g., Schore 2012; Van der Kolk 2015) validates and builds upon Winnicott's (1965) concept of "holding" through emotional understanding, and Bion's (1984) principle of "containing" often unbearable projected feelings. Applying these concepts, Jalonen and Cilia La Corte (2017) use the metaphor of a practitioner as a sea-going ship with a stabilizing keel and strong hull providing safety even in the worst emotional weather. This image reinforces the idea of the practitioner as a stable, containing presence throughout the healing process.

Phases of Healing for Psychological Therapy Professionals

Trauma Memory Processing

Trauma memory processing is a fundamental aspect of healing that addresses the psychological, emotional, and physiological impact of trauma, thereby fostering recovery and well-being (Levine 2010; Van der Kolk 2015). It enables adolescent refugees to express their emotions and to start the process of grieving their losses and integrating their memories. Expressive arts activities such as drawing (Annous, Al-Hroub, and Zein 2022) or creating and listening to music (Bensimon, Amir, and Wolf 2008) can facilitate the externalisation and processing of traumatic memories and provide a non-verbal outlet for difficult emotions and experiences.

For example, an adolescent refugee might start to process trauma by drawing or painting scenes of fear or sadness, or by sculpting them from clay. In a safe and supportive environment, they can be guided to add symbols of safety and hope, helping them to reframe their traumatic memories into a coherent personal narrative (Malchiodi 2021).

This process also reinforces the development of self-soothing techniques (stabilisation) and the normalisation of their experiences (psychoeducation), allowing them to understand that their reactions are a natural response to their circumstances, rather than feeling that there is something inherently wrong with them (Perry & Szalavitz 2006; Jalonen & Cilia La Corte 2017).

Integration of Trauma Memories

Integrating traumatic memories into a coherent narrative is a crucial step in the healing process for adolescent refugees. Once they have mastered body-based grounding and stabilisation techniques to manage intense feelings and sensations (Levine 2010; Van der Kolk 2015) and have processed trauma memories through expressive arts within a therapeutic relationship, they can begin to integrate these memories into their current self-awareness. By transforming fragmented and distressing memories into a coherent narrative, the emotional impact is reduced, promoting stability and self-acceptance. However, it is also important to recognize that some individuals may not feel ready to engage at this level during the time that you have with them, and this must always be respected.

Peter Levine's therapeutic "titration" technique is critical for pacing and modulating this process to prevent re-traumatisation. It involves gradually introducing potentially triggering topics, allowing the adolescent to engage and withdraw as needed, thus prioritizing their safety and well-being during the integration process (Levine 2010). Cathy Malchiodi's work in expressive arts therapy aligns with this approach by providing creative methods for externalising, processing, and integrating trauma at a controlled and manageable pace (Malchiodi 2021). She demonstrates how activities such as drawing, painting, sculpting, making music, and engaging in drama help individuals to view their experiences from different perspectives and integrate them into their broader life stories.

The combined use of body-based therapies and expressive arts ensures a holistic approach to trauma integration. Engaging in creative activities helps adolescent refugees transform fragmented memories into a coherent and manageable narrative. These culturally sensitive methods are particularly relevant for adolescent refugees, aiding in the processing and integration of traumatic experiences while fostering resilience and developing a stronger sense of identity.

Identity Development

Identity development is a key task of adolescence, as young people navigate the complex process of understanding who they are and how they fit into the world (Ferrer-Wreder & Kroger 2020). For refugee adolescents who bear the double burden of being forcibly displaced and transitioning from childhood to adulthood, this period involves forming both an ethnic identity tied to their heritage and a national identity connected to their new country (Hayes & Endale 2018). The development of such a dynamic, multifaceted identity, which integrates both ethnic and national aspects encompassing feelings of belonging and emotional connections to various groups, is vital to ensure effective cultural transition and has been shown to positively impact the adjustment and well-being of refugee adolescents (Nguyen 2013).

Expressive arts enable adolescents to explore different aspects of their identity, share their unique experiences and build a cohesive self-concept. The creative processes involved not only supporting emotional healing but also empowering adolescents to embrace their individuality and cultural heritage. By doing so, they develop a more confident and integrated sense of identity as they transition into adulthood. The creative expression of identity issues related to migration and cultural minority status through expressive arts can help adolescent refugees adapt to their new environment.

Expressive arts techniques offer powerful tools for adolescent refugees to explore and articulate their evolving identities. Rousseau et al. (2005) describe drama workshops which offer a safe space for identity exploration through storytelling and dramatic play. Meyer-Demott et al. (2017) present movement exercises where participants share and mirror movements, affirming individual identities while fostering group acceptance. Rubesin (2016) describes a collective "I Am" poem activity as an identity-focused approach. Drama, movement and poetry each empower adolescent refugees by highlighting their multifaceted identities, encouraging creative self-expression, and cultivating supportive peer networks. In addition to processing experiences and promoting healing in group settings, these tools offer varied approaches to navigating complex identity issues.

The Case Study

Construction of the Case Study

This case study features a composite character constructed from the author's clinical notes compiled over six years of therapy sessions with 42 adolescent unaccompanied minor refugees. Sessions with individuals took place over a period of between several months and a year depending on individual needs. By creating this composite, the author preserves UM anonymity while capturing both common and unique experiences, ensuring the character's multidimensionality. The case study begins by detailing the refugee adolescent's context, background and trauma responses, viewed through Urie Bronfenbrenner's socio-ecological framework, which recognizes the complex range of social interactions impacting individuals at various levels (Bronfenbrenner 1979; Bronfenbrenner & Morris 2006).

The case study is informed by research in neuroscience (how our brain and nervous system work), interpersonal neurobiology (how our brains grow and change through interactions with others) and traumatology (the study of the impact of trauma on individuals) and draws on Van der Kolk's (2015) comprehensive integration of these fields to explain trauma's complex effects on the brain and the body. These concepts are made accessible through simple visual explanations which provide psychoeducation for practitioners to help adolescent refugees to normalise, understand, and connect with their feelings.

After presenting the background of the composite character, Axmed, the case study is divided into two sections. The first section, relevant for all health professionals, focuses on stabilisation, relationship-building, psychoeducation, and bearing witness. The second section, designed for psychological therapy professionals, concentrates on trauma memory processing, the integration of trauma memories, and identity development. Throughout both sections, examples from a wide range of expressive arts are provided, although these represent only a small selection of possible approaches given the rich variety of expressive modalities available in therapeutic practice. It is important to reiterate that while the case study presents these stages sequentially, in practice they are often interconnected and overlapping. Furthermore, given the length and complexity of the therapeutic process, this case study can only describe small segments of what is typically a much longer and more nuanced journey.

Axmed's Experiences: Pre-flight, Flight and Post-flight

Axmed (15) travelled to Europe alone from his war-torn home country, Somalia, where he had been part of a persecuted minority group. As the eldest of six siblings, he was the only one his family could afford to send to Europe with people smugglers. His journey to Europe was fraught with danger, spanning seven countries and including six months in prison where Axmed was routinely beaten. After his family paid for his release, Axmed continued his perilous journey, surviving a capsized dinghy in the Mediterranean Sea where he witnessed many drownings, including those of young children. He spent six months in mainland Europe before being smuggled to Ireland in a lorry. Axmed had never heard of Ireland and thought that he was going to the UK.

Upon claiming asylum in Ireland, Axmed was immediately assessed by the Social Work Team for Separated Children Seeking Asylum and assigned a social worker. His initial meeting, conducted in a busy open-plan office, left him feeling unsafe and reluctant to share his story fully. After two weeks in emergency accommodation, Axmed was placed in a residential unit for UM where he was assigned Laura as his social care worker and keyworker.

Health Professionals: Relationship-building and Stabilisation Using a Mental Health Toolkit

Relationship-building

Careful preparations were made to ensure that Axmed's arrival at the residential unit and his first meeting with Laura would be characterized by clear communication and an environment that was conducive to building trust. Laura coordinated with Axmed's social worker beforehand to select an appropriate interpreter based on Axmed's ethnicity and gender preferences. Initially, Axmed had expressed concerns about interpreter confidentiality and Laura addressed these worries by explaining the strict confidentiality measures in place, clarifying exactly what this meant for their interactions. Reassured, Axmed agreed to proceed with the interpreter. To ensure that the meeting ran smoothly, Laura briefed the interpreter on confidentiality protocols and arranged post-meeting debriefings for both Axmed and the interpreter.

Creating a safe and welcoming environment was of utmost importance from the start. Axmed's initial meeting with Laura took place in a secure confidential space—a crucial consideration given the abuse and betrayed trust he had experienced during displacement. This safe setting, often overlooked in other services for refugee adolescents, proved vital for Axmed, helping him feel physically safe and welcomed in the residential unit. During their first encounter, Laura cultivated a collaborative atmosphere using inclusive language and maintaining direct engagement with Axmed, despite the presence of the interpreter and his social worker. Her use of the pronoun "we" to show that issues would be tackled together was particularly effective.

Cultural sensitivity is crucial when building a therapeutic relationship with a refugee adolescent. Recognizing this, Laura approached her interactions with Axmed with open-mindedness and cultural curiosity. She engaged with communities from Axmed's cultural background to gain a deeper understanding of their traditions and practices, attending events and engaging with members of his community who had been living in Ireland for a number of years. This engagement highlighted the profound cultural significance of names, prompting Laura to pay particular attention to pronouncing Axmed's name correctly. This consideration was especially meaningful to Axmed, who had previously felt as though his identity had been dismissed when other service providers mispronounced or anglicized his name. Laura also acknowledged Axmed's use of multiple names, a practice rooted in his culture as protection against authorities, rebel groups, and perceived threats from evil spirits.

By respecting these cultural nuances and embodying a hospitality attitude (Jalonen & Cilia La Corte 2017), Laura established a foundation of trust and understanding essential for their developing relationship. Her empathic, collaborative approach created an environment in which Axmed felt respected, understood and safe—key elements in building a positive therapeutic relationship with refugee adolescents. This culturally sensitive foundation not only facilitated their initial interactions but also paved the way for effective therapeutic work in the future whilst demonstrating the importance of cultural competence in working with diverse populations.

Stabilisation: Developing a Mental Health Toolkit for Axmed

During Axmed's initial weeks in the residential unit, Laura observed his withdrawn behaviour and how he struggled with emotional regulation. She also noticed that he had difficulties remembering things and often found it hard to concentrate. Axmed confided in Laura that he was haunted by the events that had happened during the journey from his home country. Recognizing these challenges, Laura prioritized developing a mental health toolkit for Axmed, based on Lahad's (1992) BASIC Ph model of coping and resiliency, later refined by Lahad et al. (2013).

Lahad's model, designed for assessing and developing coping skills and building resilience in the wake of natural and man-made disasters, identifies coping resources across six dimensions: Belief, Affect, Social, Imagination, Cognition, and Physical pathways. Laura and Axmed collaboratively constructed the toolkit, focusing on strategies most likely to provide Axmed with additional support when needed. As a result,

Axmed could metaphorically open up the toolkit and see what might help him at any particular moment.

Axmed chose to build his toolkit in his phone's notes app, finding it the most accessible resource when feeling anxious or hopeless. While younger children often prefer creating a physical toolkit, adolescents typically opt for digital versions on their phones. Axmed found it beneficial to photograph items that he identified for his toolkit and add these images to his phone's notes. Visual cues resonate more strongly with trauma survivors than written or spoken words as our brains process images more efficiently. Moreover, images can help anchor individuals in the present moment, a particularly valuable benefit for those who have experienced trauma. Axmed's toolkit included the following components that helped him to stabilize and stay grounded.

Regulating the Body Using Breathing Techniques

Deep breathing is a powerful tool for managing anxiety and stress. To maximize its effectiveness, individuals need to understand how and why it works—this is where psychoeducation comes in. The combination of practical techniques and educational approaches exemplifies how stabilisation methods and understanding work together to support psychological well-being. Laura, Axmed's keyworker, applied this integrated approach when teaching him deep breathing techniques. She not only showed Axmed how to perform deep breathing but also explained its physiological effects, demonstrating the close connection between coping strategies and comprehending their impact.

In her explanation, Laura introduced Axmed to the concept of the autonomic nervous system. She described how stress activates the Sympathetic Nervous System, triggering the 'fight or flight' response. In contrast, deep breathing stimulates the Parasympathetic Nervous System—often called the 'rest and digest' system.

Laura explained that when Axmed practises deep breathing, especially during exhalation, his body responds in the following ways:

- His blood pressure lowers.

- His heart rate decreases.

- His pupils constrict.

By providing both the technique and science behind it, Laura empowered Axmed with a comprehensive tool for managing his anxiety and stress. Building on this foundation, Laura introduced Axmed to a specific deep breathing exercise known as the 7/11 technique (Figure 5.1). This method provides a structured approach to deep breathing, making it easier for Axmed to implement in his daily life:

The Seven-Eleven Breathing Technique Practised by Axmed:

- Breathe in for a count of 7.
- Breathe out for a count of 11.

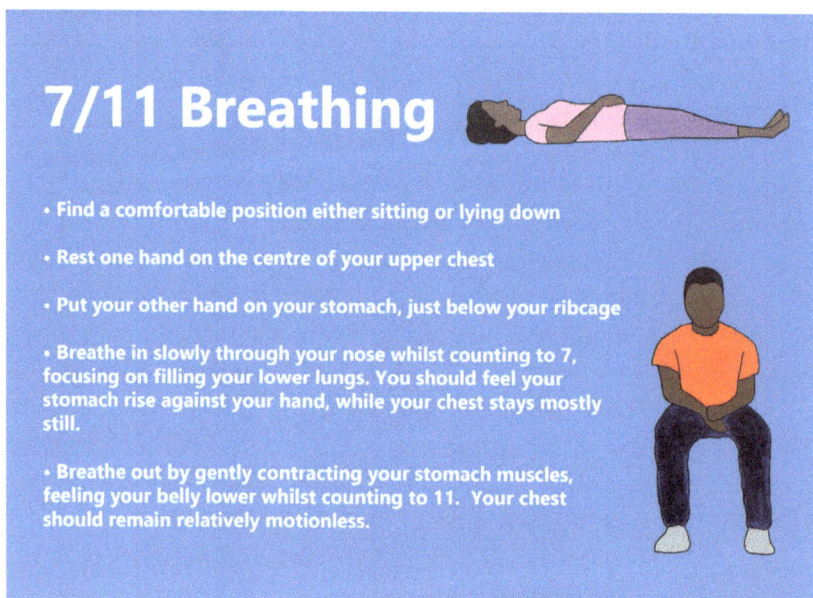

Fig. 5.1 The seven-eleven breathing technique.

It is important to note that Laura demonstrated deep 'diaphragmatic breathing' to Axmed, emphasizing the expansion of his stomach rather than his chest during inhalation. As Axmed consistently practised these techniques under Laura's guidance, he discovered their effectiveness in managing his daily stress and anxiety. He particularly valued how this method provided him with a sense of control during intense moments of stress. To reinforce this practice, Laura supplied Axmed with the following instructions which he stored in his phone's notes for easy reference:

Cultural Comforters

Axmed uploaded pictures of an inspirational verse from the Qur'an, his prayer mat, his home town and a cat he had befriended there. He considered uploading pictures of the family he had left behind but felt that he was not ready to do that yet as he found it too upsetting. Axmed also decorated a stone using acrylic paint pens with his favourite quotation from the Qur'an which he then kept in his pocket. He found that holding it and taking it out when he was feeling anxious provided comfort.

Nourishing Items

Axmed kept a hot water bottle in his room which he would fill and cuddle when he was feeling low. He uploaded pictures of all these items to the toolkit on his phone to remind himself to use them when needed. Axmed also ensured that he always had access to an electronic version of the Qur'an on his phone. Additionally, he found that a walk in nature helped him feel better, so he included an image of the park near his home.

Calming and Grounding

When Laura first met Axmed, he was struggling to manage and express his anger in a healthy and constructive way. According to Sunderland (2016), the root causes of anger in adolescents often mask deeper feelings of hurt, sadness, or fear, and it is therefore important to address these underlying emotions to prevent destructive behaviours. Axmed needed a safe outlet for his anger, so Laura and himself explored various healthy ways in which he could express anger and frustration.

Axmed discovered that writing down his feelings was particularly effective. He kept a private journal in his native language, finding that handwriting gave him a greater sense of empowerment than typing. In their book, *Opening it Up by Writing it Down*, James Pennebaker and Joshua Smyth highlight the psychological and health benefits of expressing emotions through writing (Pennebaker & Smyth 2016).

Exercise also proved beneficial for Axmed. When feeling particularly angry, he would engage in speed walking around his local park, allowing his body to release anger in a healthy manner rather than suppressing it. These strategies helped Axmed manage his levels of cortisol, often referred to as the 'stress hormone'. Without such outlets, elevated cortisol levels in his body could lead to quicker, more intense and uncontrollable anger responses. Maintaining balanced cortisol levels is crucial in preventing various negative health effects (Sunderland 2016).

Axmed downloaded an app that played various rain sounds, which he found very calming as they reminded him of the different types of rain in his home country. He created a playlist of music for calming and another for letting off steam. Additionally, he included a link to a motivational speaker whom he found uplifting.

Friends and Other Human Supports

Axmed also added the phone numbers of several of his friends to his toolkit—people he could call when he was feeling low—as well as emergency helpline numbers. Axmed and Laura also worked on the wording for text messages that he copied and pasted into the toolkit so that he always had them ready if he was unable to think of what to say to his friends when he was feeling low. With Axmed's permission, Laura informed the other staff in the residential unit that Axmed had the toolkit in the notes section of his phone so that they could direct him to it when they felt he might benefit from it.

Psychoeducation

Psychoeducation formed the cornerstone of Laura's approach in supporting Axmed during the stabilisation phase of his healing process. Her role was vital in providing Axmed with a comprehensive understanding of how psychological trauma affects his thoughts, emotions, and physical responses. By breaking down complex concepts into accessible explanations, Laura enabled Axmed to draw connections between his past experiences and current challenges. Laura firstly emphasized that a trauma or stress response is a normal reaction to an abnormal event. She explained that the responses illustrated in Figure 5.2 are typical, while the traumatic experience itself is not normal. Axmed kept this visual in his phone as a reminder that his responses were normal and that he was not 'going crazy'. It also served to reinforce the importance of engaging with his stabilisation techniques.

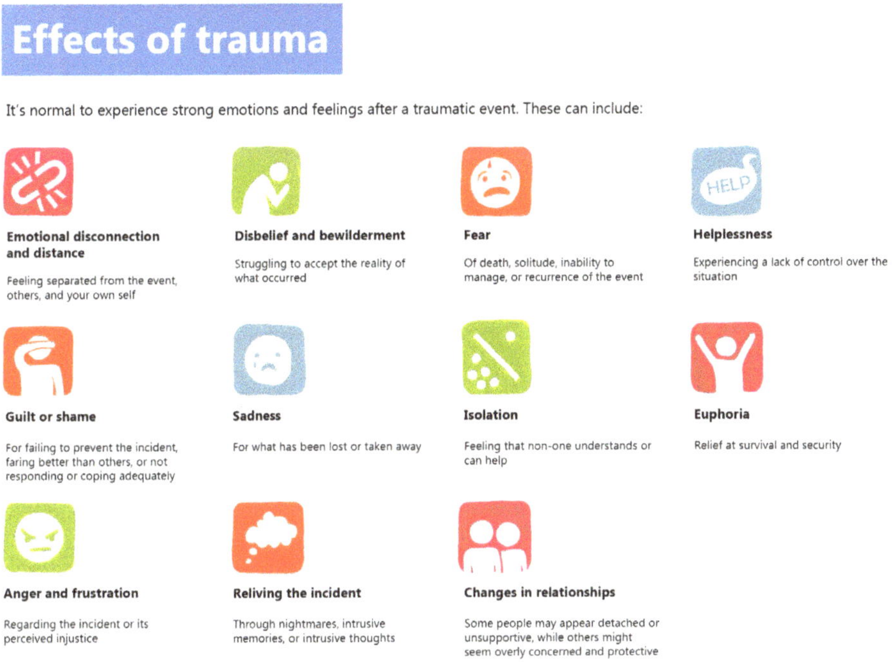

Effects of trauma

It's normal to experience strong emotions and feelings after a traumatic event. These can include:

Emotional disconnection and distance

Feeling separated from the event, others, and your own self

Disbelief and bewilderment

Struggling to accept the reality of what occurred

Fear

Of death, solitude, inability to manage, or recurrence of the event

Helplessness

Experiencing a lack of control over the situation

Guilt or shame

For failing to prevent the incident, faring better than others, or not responding or coping adequately

Sadness

For what has been lost or taken away

Isolation

Feeling that non-one understands or can help

Euphoria

Relief at survival and security

Anger and frustration

Regarding the incident or its perceived injustice

Reliving the incident

Through nightmares, intrusive memories, or intrusive thoughts

Changes in relationships

Some people may appear detached or unsupportive, while others might seem overly concerned and protective

Fig. 5.2 Effects of trauma.

Recognizing Axmed's specific difficulties with memory and concentration, as well as his interest in understanding his own emotional experiences, Laura focused on these aspects of his cognitive and emotional functioning. This approach aligned with typical adolescent development which often involves increased self-reflection and the desire to understand one's internal experiences (Meeus 2019). Laura explained where important cognitive and emotional processes were situated in the brain and was then able to connect Axmed's personal experiences to the underlying neurobiology (see Figure 5.3).

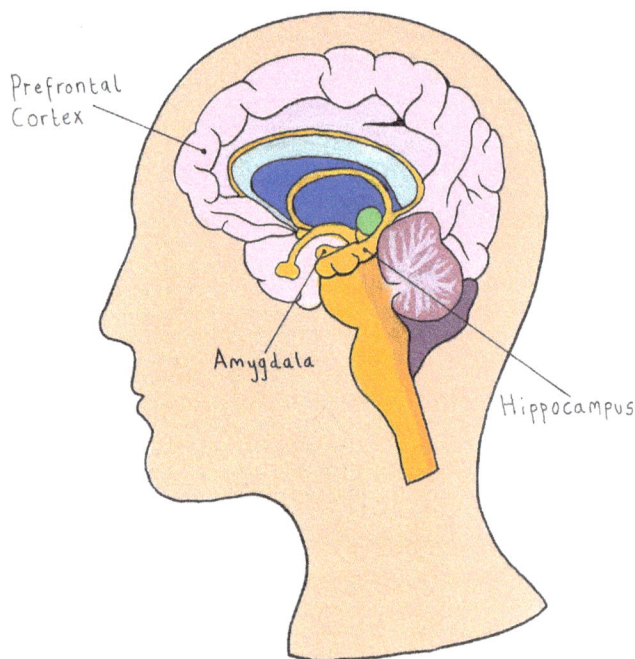

Fig. 5.3 The brain and traumatic stress.

Laura described how trauma affects key brain areas using clear analogies and simple, accessible explanations:

- The amygdala, the brain's alarm system, activates quickly when danger is perceived. After a traumatic event, this alarm can get stuck in the 'on' position, causing feelings of nervousness even in safe situations.

- The hippocampus, which acts as a memory storage cabinet, can be disrupted by scary events, resulting in memories that are too overwhelming to file neatly away. This can cause them to feel jumbled or to resurface unexpectedly.

- The prefrontal cortex, the brain's control centre, helps with thinking and emotional regulation. Traumatic events can overwhelm this centre, making it harder to focus or manage feelings. However, Laura explained that the prefrontal cortex can be strengthened through practices like calm breathing, engaging in good sleep hygiene, taking regular exercise and learning new skills.

- Drawing on this brain-based psychoeducation, Laura introduced practical stabilisation tools in the form of the 7/11 breathing exercise and mandala colouring. A mandala is a sacred, circular, geometric design that is symbolic in Buddhist and Hindu cultures. See Figure 5.4 below for examples of uncoloured and coloured mandalas. Printable uncoloured mandalas are available at https://mondaymandala.com/m/

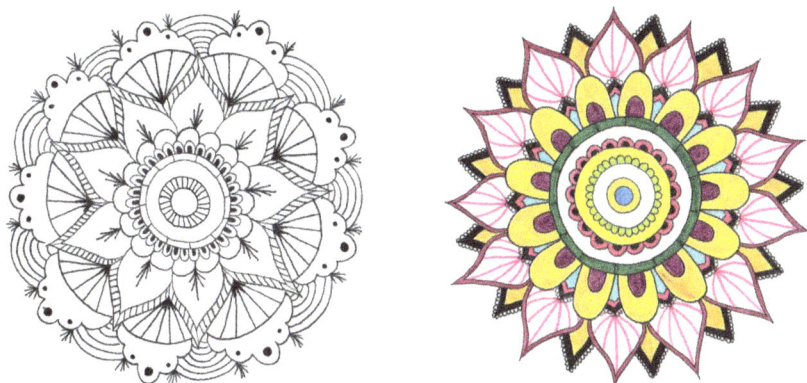

Fig. 5.4 Examples of mandalas.

Laura explained how these methods directly apply the neurobiological principles they had discussed, helping to calm the nervous system and provide a non-verbal outlet for processing emotions. Laura showed Axmed examples of mandalas and explained their centuries-old use across various cultures for meditation and healing. She emphasized how the act of colouring these patterns induces a state of mindfulness, which can help regulate the brain areas they had discussed.

Laura then demonstrated how to synchronize rhythmic breathing with the colouring process, creating a powerful, multi-sensory experience of self-regulation. She explained that this combination of activities could help calm intrusive thoughts, reduce anxiety, and ground Axmed when he felt overwhelmed by traumatic memories or stress. By engaging in these practices regularly, Axmed could not only manage immediate stress responses but also build long-term resilience, reinforcing the healthy coping mechanisms they had discussed.

Bearing Witness

Given Axmed's early openness to creative expression, Laura introduced the strengths-based 'Tree of Life' intervention as an effective way for him to share his story and be witnessed in the process. Originally developed to support vulnerable young people in Zimbabwe, this intervention is now used globally with children, adolescents, and adults, individually and in groups. This approach uses the tree and its constituent parts as metaphors to represent different aspects of an individual's life. Aligning with storytelling traditions, this approach helps adolescents to externalize their narratives and create psychological distance from their experiences. This is particularly beneficial for refugee adolescents like Axmed because it:

- Reduces feelings of overwhelm by offering a more objective perspective on their life story.
- Provides a culturally sensitive framework for expressing complex emotions and experiences.

The intervention enhances feelings of belonging in the host country while respecting diverse cultural viewpoints, family structures, and traditions. Initially designed for clinicians, it has been adapted for broader professional use through appropriate training. Axmed created his personal Tree of Life, with each element symbolizing a part of his journey:

- Roots: origins, ancestry and culture.
- Ground: current place of residence.
- Trunk: skills and abilities.
- Branches: hopes and dreams.
- Leaves: important people.
- Fruits: gifts received (material and non-material).

This process enriched Axmed's narrative, emphasizing supportive relationships, talents, and aspirations rather than focusing on loss and trauma. It provided a safe space for him to address challenges and celebrate his unique story, with Laura witnessing and validating his experiences (see Figure 5.5 below).

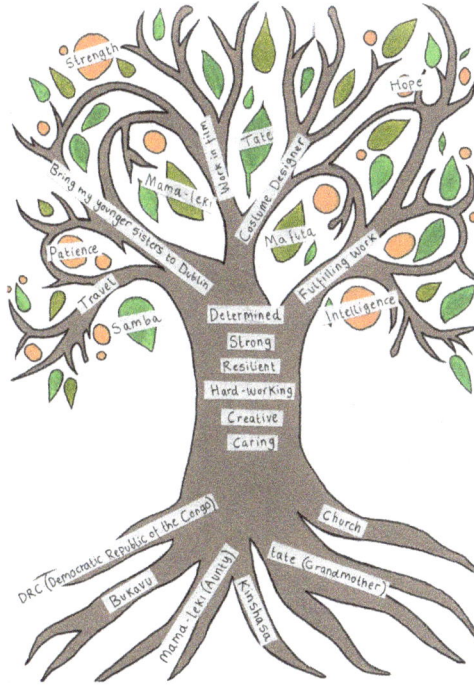

Fig. 5.5 Axmed's Tree of Life.

Creating the tree allowed Axmed to rediscover himself, recognize his agency, and take ownership of his life story. Often, individuals are defined by their experiences, a concept known as "thin description" (Jacobs 2018). By drawing the tree, Axmed could "thicken" or enrich his narrative, highlighting positive aspects that might otherwise be overlooked due to a focus on problems (Azarova et al. 2018). Through this process, Axmed reconnected with his whole identity, including its positive aspects, and considered his challenges without risking re-traumatisation. He felt seen, acknowledged, and validated by Laura's attentive witnessing of his experiences. For those interested in using this approach, REPSSI (2016) provides a comprehensive rationale and clear instructions.

Psychological Therapy Professionals

Trauma Memory Processing

Recognizing Axmed's struggle with emotional regulation after his traumatic experiences, his therapist, Rosie, ensured that she had a range of materials available in the therapy room, including coloured pencils, paints, markers, and clay. Axmed was drawn to the tactile nature of the clay and Rosie guided him through a brief grounding exercise, encouraging him to feel its coolness and malleability. She then invited him to create a physical representation of a trauma memory that had been troubling him, explaining that there was no right or wrong way to do this.

As Axmed worked with the clay, Rosie observed his process, noting how he initially created small, tightly formed balls before gradually moulding them into more abstract shapes. She encouraged him to notice any physical sensations or emotions that arose as he manipulated the clay, particularly those associated with the traumatic memory so that they could address them with grounding techniques. After a while, Rosie expressed interest in understanding Axmed's creation, inviting him to share his reflections if he felt comfortable doing so.

Responding to her genuine curiosity, Axmed explained that the smaller more compact shapes represented the intense feelings of fear and helplessness he experienced during the traumatic event. He described how one shape symbolized the paralyzing fear he felt when hearing gunshots near his home, while another represented the helplessness of being unable to contact his family during their forced separation. Axmed explained that the larger, more fluid forms symbolized moments of resilience and survival. One of the shapes represented the strength he found in comforting younger children during their dangerous journey, while another symbolized the hope he felt upon safely reaching the refugee camp.

Rosie then introduced a technique called "transformative sculpting" (Bat Or 2010). She asked Axmed to choose one of the shapes representing a difficult aspect of the traumatic memory and slowly transform it into something that felt more manageable or empowering. As Axmed reshaped the clay, Rosie guided him to focus on his breathing and the sensations in his body, helping him to connect the physical act of transforming the clay with the internal process of reframing and integrating the traumatic memory.

Throughout the session, Rosie maintained a calm accepting presence, validating Axmed's experiences and emotions related to the traumatic event. She encouraged him to take breaks when needed and to express any discomfort or resistance he felt during the process. At the end of the session, Rosie and Axmed discussed how the clay work could relate to his healing journey. They explored how Axmed might apply the idea of 'reshaping' to his traumatic memories when they felt overwhelming, identifying specific coping strategies he could use to help manage flashbacks or intrusive thoughts in his daily life. This hands-on metaphorical approach allowed Axmed to externalize and process his traumatic memories in a safe, contained manner, while also practising emotional regulation skills that he could apply outside of therapy.

While Axmed chose to verbalize his experience, it is important to recognize that not all individuals feel comfortable or ready to discuss their creative expressions in detail. Rosie routinely explains to the refugee adolescents she works with that there is no obligation to explain or interpret their work. She affirms that the creative process itself is a powerful tool for healing and self-discovery, with therapeutic value extending beyond verbal expression. The physical manipulation of the clay, the focus required, and the externalisation of internal experiences all contribute to bringing unconscious material into conscious awareness, an embodied process that can be healing without the need for verbal interpretation.

Integration of Trauma Memories

As Axmed's healing journey progressed to the integration of the trauma memories, Rosie introduced several expressive arts techniques, each chosen to address different aspects of this integration process and grounded in the safety of the secure base of the therapeutic relationship. One particularly effective method was the creation of a collage for which Rosie provided Axmed with a variety of materials—magazines, coloured paper, postcards, fabric scraps, and paint. She invited him to create representations of 'inside me', focusing on feelings and sensations rather than actual events. This non-linear approach allowed Axmed to express the complex, often fragmented nature of his traumatic memories in a safe and contained environment (Stallings 2015). Through this medium, Axmed was able to integrate the chaos of fleeing his home country, the fear he experienced during his migration journey, and the confusion related to navigating life in a new culture.

Recognizing that trauma is often stored in the body, Rosie also guided Axmed through exercises that allowed him to express his experiences through physical movement. This helped him to release tension held in his body and to connect with emotions that were difficult to verbalise. As he moved, Axmed sometimes found words or images emerging, which himself and Rosie would then explore further through art or discussion. Music became another tool for memory integration. Rosie introduced Axmed to the concept of creating soundscapes that represented his emotional journey. Using various instruments and digital tools, Axmed created compositions that captured the intensity, rhythm, and tonal qualities of his experiences. This auditory expression provided a new dimension through which he was able to process his memories, allowing him to engage with them in a non-verbal, sensory way.

Throughout this process, Rosie maintained a stance of compassionate witness, validating Axmed's experiences and emotions without judgement. She helped Axmed to recognize the strength and resilience he demonstrated in surviving his traumatic experiences, thereby cultivating a sense of empowerment and agency. As Axmed engaged with these various expressive arts techniques, he began to notice a shift in how he related to his traumatic memories. While they remained a part of his history, they began to feel less fragmented and overwhelming. He developed a greater capacity to hold the complexity of his experiences—acknowledging the pain and loss while also recognizing his resilience and growth.

Through this multi-modal, expressive arts approach, embedded within a strong therapeutic relationship, Axmed was able to gradually integrate his traumatic memories into a more coherent sense of self. Furthermore, Rosie emphasized that the integration of trauma memories is an ongoing process and she encouraged Axmed to continue using expressive arts as a tool for self-regulation and processing outside of their sessions. Drawn particularly to collaging and working with clay, Axmed continued to engage in these two activities at home, empowering himself with strategies to manage future challenges and to continue his healing journey beyond the confines of formal therapy.

Identity Development

As Axmed progressed in his therapy, Rosie recognized the importance of supporting him in developing an identity that would embrace both his Somali heritage and his new life in Ireland. As an unaccompanied minor without a family supporting him, it was crucial for Axmed to find a sense of belonging and continuity amidst the profound changes he had experienced. Rosie therefore introduced a series of expressive arts activities designed to explore and integrate different aspects of Axmed's identity.

One especially powerful exercise was the creation of a 'personal flag'. Rosie provided Axmed with a large piece of paper, paints, markers, and different craft materials and invited him to design a flag that represented different aspects of his identity—his Somali roots, his Muslim faith, his refugee journey, and his new experiences in Ireland. Axmed divided his flags into sections. He incorporated the star from the Somali flag, symbolizing his homeland, and used Islamic calligraphy to represent his faith, which had been a source of strength and coping throughout his journey. The section representing his life in Ireland included the green, white and orange of the Irish tricolour interwoven with African patterns, symbolizing his emerging bicultural identity. Large swathes of blue paint tinged with red, representing his very difficult journey across the Mediterranean were woven into both sections. He took a picture of the flag and stored it in the notes section of his phone.

Music also played a significant role in Axmed's identity development. Rosie encouraged him to create a personal soundtrack, incorporating both traditional Somali music and contemporary music that he heard in Ireland. This musical fusion became a powerful metaphor for Axmed's evolving identity, demonstrating the harmonisation of his different cultures. He added it to his invisible toolkit as he found that listening to it helped to ground him when he was missing his family and struggling with feelings of non-belonging.

Rosie maintained a supportive and curious stance throughout this process, always validating Axmed's experiences and emotions. She helped him to recognize the strength inherent in his bicultural identity, framing it as a unique asset rather than a source of confusion or conflict. As Axmed engaged with these expressive arts techniques, he began the slow process of developing a more integrated sense of self, starting to see his identity as incorporating elements of both cultures rather than having to make a choice between them. This was a slow process with frequent challenges and setbacks, but overall, this shift allowed him to feel more grounded in his present life while maintaining a strong connection to his roots.

Through this expressive arts-based approach to identity development, embedded within a strong therapeutic relationship, Axmed was able to move towards a more coherent and flexible sense of self. Throughout the process, Rosie encouraged Axmed to reflect on how these different aspects of his identity coexisted and influenced each other. She helped him to see that rather than abandoning his roots, his new life meant that he was adding new dimensions to his identity. Rosie emphasized to Axmed that identity development is an ongoing, lifelong process and she encouraged him to continue exploring and expressing his evolving sense of self beyond their sessions.

Conclusion

Axmed's journey through therapy illustrates the power of expressive arts in supporting UM through the complex processes of stabilisation, trauma memory processing, and integration and identity development. His case study demonstrates how a culturally sensitive, multi-modal approach can effectively address the unique challenges faced by unaccompanied minors arriving in Ireland. Through the skilled guidance of professionals like Laura and Rosie and the use of the expressive arts, Axmed was gradually able to build resilience, process traumatic memories, and develop a more integrated sense of self. This holistic approach, grounded in a strong therapeutic relationship, not only helped Axmed to navigate his immediate challenges but also equipped him with valuable tools for ongoing healing and growth. Axmed's story underscores the importance of flexible creative interventions in supporting the mental health and well-being of UM as they adapt to life in their host countries.

References

Annous, Nadia, Anies Al-Hroub, and Farah El Zein. 2022. 'A Systematic Review of Empirical Evidence on Art Therapy with Traumatize Refugee Children and Youth', *Frontiers in Psychology, 13: 1–10,* https://doi.org/10.3389/fpsyg.2022.811515

Archibald, Linda, and Jonathan Dewar. 2010. 'Creative Arts, Culture and Healing: Building an Evidence Base', *A Journal of Aboriginal and Indigenous Community Health,* 8.3: 1–25.

Azarova, Vera, et al. 2018. 'Celebrating heritage: A mixed-method approach to explore the experiences of refugee children and young people', *Psychotherapy Section Review,* 61: 50–67, https://doi.org/10.53841/bpspsr.2018.1.61.50

Bartolomei, Javier, et al. 2016. 'What are the barriers to access to mental healthcare and the primary needs of asylum seekers? A survey of mental health caregivers and primary care workers', *BMC Psychiatry,* 16: 1–8, https://doi.org/10.1186/s12888-016-1048-6

Bat Or, Michal. 2010. 'Clay sculpting of mother and child figures encourages mentalization', *The Arts in Psychotherapy,* 37.4: 319–327, https://doi.org/10.1016/j.aip.2010.05.007

Bensimon, Moshe, Dorit Amir, and Yuval Wolf. 2008. 'Drummin through trauma: Music therapy with post-traumatic soldiers', *The Arts in Psychotherapy,* 35.1: 34–48, https://doi.org/10.1016/j.aip.2007.09.002

Bion, Wilfred R. 1984. *Learning from Experience* (London: Routledge).

Blackwell, Dick. 2005. *Counselling and Psychotherapy with Refugees* (London: Jessica Kingsley Publishers).

Bronfenbrenner, Urie. 1979. *The Ecology of Human Development* (Cambridge, Massachusetts: The President and Fellows of Harvard College).

Bronfenbrenner, Urie, and Pamela A. Morris. 2006. 'The Bioecological Model of Human Development', in *Handbook of Child Psychology: Theoretical Models of Human Development,* ed. by Lerner, Richard M. and William Damon (New Jersey: John Wiley & Sons), pp. 793–828.

Degges-White, Suzanne. 2011. 'Overview of the Expressive Arts', in *Integrating the Expressive Arts into Counseling Practice: Theory-Based Interventions,* ed.

by Degges-White, Suzanne and Nancy L. Davis (New York: Springer Publishing Company), pp. 30–35.

Ferrer-Wreder, Laura, and Jane Kroger. 2020. *Identity in Adolescence,* 4th edn (Oxford and New York: Routledge).

Hayes, Sherrill W., and Etsegenet Endale. 2018. '"Sometimes my mind, it has to analyze two things": Identity Development and Adaptation for Refugee and Newcomer Adolescents', *Peace and Conflict: Journal of Peace Psychology,* 24.3: 283–290, http://dx.doi.org/10.1037/pac0000315

Herman, Judith. 1992. *Trauma and Recovery: The Aftermath of Violence—From Domestic Abuse to Political Terror,* 3rd edn (New York: Basic Books).

Jacobs, Suzan F. 2018. 'Collective narrative practice with unaccompanied refugee minors: "The tree of life" as a response to hardship', *Clinical Child Psychology and Psychiatry,* 23.2: 279–293, https://doi. org/10.1177/1359104517744246

Jalonen, Angeline, and Paul Cilia La Corte. 2017. *A Practical Guide to Therapeutic Work with Asylum Seekers and Refugees* (London: Jessica Kingsley Publishers).

Kohli, Ravi. 2006. *Social Work with Unaccompanied Asylum-seeking Children* (New York: Palgrave MacMillan).

Lahad, Mooli. 1992. 'Story-making in assessment method for coping with stress: Six part story-making and BASIC PH', in *Dramatherapy: Theory and Practice 2,* ed. by Jennings, Sue (New York and London: Routledge), pp. 150–154.

Lahad, Mooli, Miri Shacham, and Ofra Ayalon. 2013. *The 'Basic PH' Model of Coping and Resiliency* (London: Jessica Kingsley).

Land, George, and Beth Jarman. 1992. *Breakpoint and Beyond: Mastering the Future Today* (New York: Harper Business).

Levine, Peter. 2010. *In an Unspoken Voice: How the Body Releases Trauma and Restores Goodness* (California: North Atlantic Books).

Linklater, Renee. 2014. *Decolonising Trauma Work: Indigenous Stories and Strategies* (Nova Scotia: Fernwood Publishing).

Malchiodi, Cathy. 2020. 'Expressive Arts Therapy as Self-Regulatory and Relational Interventions with Children and Caregivers', in *The Handbook of Therapeutic Care for Children: Evidence-informed approaches to working with traumatised children and adolescents in foster, kinship and adoptive care,* ed. by Mitchell, Janise, Joe Tucci and Ed Tronick (Philadelphia: Jessica Kingsley Publishers), pp. 289–313.

Malchiodi, Cathy. 2021. *Creative Interventions with Traumatized Children,* 2nd edn (New York, London: The Guilford Press).

Malchiodi, Cathy. 2023. 'What is Expressive Arts Therapy?', in *Handbook of Expressive Arts Therapy*, ed. by Malchiodi, Cathy (New York and London: The Guilford Press), pp. 153–569.

Meeus, Wim. 2019. *Adolescent Development: Longitudinal Research into the Self, Personal Relationships and Psychopathology* (London and New York: Routledge).

Meyer-Demott, Melinda A., et al. 2017. 'A controlled early group intervention study for unaccompanied minors: can expressive arts alleviate symptoms of trauma and enhance life satisfaction?', *Scandinavian Journal of Psychology*, 58.6: 510–518, https://doi.org/10.1111/sjop.12395

Namer, Yudit, et al. 2022. 'Asylum seeking and refugee adolescents's mental health service use and help-seeking patterns: a mixed-methods study', *Mental Health Research*, 18: 1–10, https://doi.org/10.1038/s44184-022-00019-2

Nguyen, Angela-Minhtu D., and Verónica Benet-Martinez. 2013. 'Biculturalism and Adjustment: A Meta-Analysis', *Journal of Cross-Cultural Psychology*, 44.1: 122–159, https://doi.org/10.1177/0022022111435097

Papadopoulos, Renos K. 2002. *Therapeutic Care for Refugees: No Place Like Home* (London: Tavistock Clinic Series).

Pennebaker, James W., and Joshua M. Smyth. 2016. *Opening Up by Writing it Down: How expressive writing improves health and eases emotional pain*, 3rd edn (New York: The Guilford Press).

Rappaport, Laury. 2014. 'Mindfulness, Psychotherapy and the Arts Therapies: Overview and Roots', in *Mindfulness and the Arts Therapies*, ed. by Rappaport, Laury (London and Philadelphia: Jessica Kingsley Publishers) pp. 526–886.

REPSSI. 2016. *Tree of Life: A Workshop Methodology for Children, Young People and Adults* (REPSSI).

Rousseau, Cécile, et al. 2005. 'Playing with identities and transforming shared realities: Drama therapy workshops for adolescent immigrants and refugees', *The Arts in Psychotherapy*, 32.1: 13–27, https://doi.org/10.1016/j.aip.2004.12.002

Rubesin, Hillary. 2016. 'The stories we share: Reflecttions on a community-based art exhibit displaying work by refugees and immigrants', *Journal of Applied Arts and Health*, 7.2: 159–174, https://doi.org/10.1386/jaah.7.2.159_1

Schaefer, Charles, and Athena A. Drewes. 2014. *The Therapeutic Powers of Play* (New Jersey: Wiley).

Schore, Allan. 2012. *The Science of the Art of Psychotherapy* (New York and London: W.W. Norton and Company).

Shakya, Yogendra, et al. 2014. 'Newcomer Refugee Youth as 'Resettlement Champions' for their Families: Vulnerability, Resilience and Empowerment', in *Refuge and Resilience*, ed. by Simich, Laura and Lisa Andermann (New York: Springer), pp. 131–154.

Stallings, Jessica W. 2015. 'Collage as an expressive medium in art therapy', in *The Wiley Handbook of Art Therapy*, ed. by Gussak, David E., and Marcia L. Rosal (New Jersey: Wiley), pp. 163–170.

Sunderland, Margot. 2016. *What Every Parent Needs to Know: Love, Nurture and Play with Your Child* (London: Penguin, Random House).

Tefferi, Hirut. 2007. 'Reconstructing Adolescence after Displacement: Experience from Eastern Africa', *Children and Society*, 21.4: 297–308, https://doi.org/10.1111/j.1099-0860.2007.00101.x

Van der Kolk, Bessel. 2015. *The Body Keeps the Score: Mind, Brain and Body in the Transformation of Trauma* (London: Penguin).

Winnicott, Donald W. 1965. *The Maturational Processes and the Facilitating Environment: Studies in the Theory of Emotional Development* (London: Hogarth Press).

World Health Organization. 2019. *What is the Evidence on the Role of the Arts in Improving Health and Well-being? A Scoping Review. Health Evidence Network synthesis report 67* (Geneva: World Health Organization), https://www.who.int/europe/publications/i/item/9789289054553

6. Promoting Interaction and Mutual Learning Between Local and Refugee Communities

Méabh Bonham Corcoran, Sarah Quinn and Frédérique Vallières

Introduction

This chapter explores the critical role of communities in facilitating the integration of refugees and asylum seekers into their host countries. The first section examines the benefits of community engagement for integration and social inclusion, with particular attention to the role of occupation. Readers are encouraged to reflect on these factors in relation to the populations they serve.

The second section presents a case study of a community garden in Ireland, which serves as a successful model for refugee and asylum seeker integration. The case study highlights the perspectives of committee members involved in the initiative, illustrating the processes and challenges of fostering inclusion. Additionally, it underscores the importance of mutual learning between refugee and local community members.

Although this chapter is framed within an occupational therapy perspective, the concepts discussed have broader relevance. Health and social care professionals across disciplines may find the insights valuable for enhancing their understanding and application of community-based integration strategies in their respective practice settings.

    https://doi.org/10.11647/OBP.0479.06

Communities in the Integration Process

Arriving in the New Community

On arrival to the new host country, the focus of refugee health and integration centres is on meeting immediate needs such as health, housing, employment, and education. While these elements are important facets of the process of integration, the role of community and belonging to said community can often be over looked. Community support and community engagement are of critical importance in the process of integration, and it is through the interactions of refugees and local community members that a sense of belonging and place-making can be found, particularly when participating in community activities or groups (Ager & Strang 2008). This community engagement can increase overall wellbeing and quality of life by increasing feelings of social connectedness within an area (Ager & Strang 2008).

Despite the inclusion of community resources and development in policies surrounding migrant health and integration, the focus has remained on access to health, education, and employment. This has left the final pillar, community, reliant on public initiative and interest (Ager & Strang 2008; Daley 2009; National Social Inclusion Office 2017: 11). The resources available within a community for the newly arrived will vary between countries, cities, and towns, whether the resources are based in urban or rural areas, or if they are facilitated by local governments or local community initiatives. Community supports are often provided through a variety of organisations, ranging from non-governmental organisations, local community organisations, or initiatives such as: schools; libraries; community centres; churches; health centres; or primary care facilities linking in with community supports through programmes such as social prescribing or mother and baby groups, or government funded programmes aimed specifically at integrating refugees into the local community.

The use of community groups at any stage of the integration process can be seen as beneficial in promoting community ties and relationship building between locals and refugees. Communities have been cited as being a contributing factor in reducing the impact of ill health and disease within society, thus improving population health (Public

Health England 2015). MacQueen and colleagues (2001: 1929) defined community as "a group of people with diverse characteristics who are linked by social ties, share common perspectives, and engage in joint action in geographical locations or settings". Further, Scaffa and Reitz (2020: 29) describe community health as referring to "the physical, emotional, social, and spiritual well-being of a group of people who are linked together in some way, possibly through geographical proximity or shared interest". Strang and Ager (2010) emphasized the reciprocal nature of refugee integration, stressing the importance of both refugees' adaptation and host societies willingness to adapt institutions for successful integration.

The Role of Occupation

The role of community in developing a sense of connection, both to oneself and one's place in society, has been highlighted (Wilcock 2006). Further, active community engagement can lead to feelings of acceptance and contentment (Wilcock & Hocking 2015). In occupational therapy and occupational science literature, the importance of activity and occupation for the promotion of overall health and wellbeing has long been understood and linked to community health and wellbeing (Wilcock & Hocking 2015; Hocking & Wilcock 2020).

As human beings, we are seen to engage with our meaningful and purposeful occupations both on an individual and a collective level. Collective occupations are those that take place in and contribute to the meso-level of our social connections and relationships (Kantartzis 2017). Engaging with collective occupations can promote the making of shared meanings among communities, in addition to creating a safe space that fosters diversity and group cohesion (Hocking & Wilcock 2020). Despite evidence supporting community involvement as a means to increase social cohesion and inclusion among asylum seekers and refugees, many migrant programmes group these populations together as a community and do not promote integration into existing host communities or provide any support to bring these communities together (Darawsheh et al. 2022). To foster mutual support and integration there is a need for programmes that are attuned to the specific needs and strengths found in the local context, that consider the cultural backgrounds and experiences of the refugee population, and that utilize the strengths and resources of both local and refugee communities to foster mutual support and interaction (Costigan et al. 2022).

The World Federation of Occupational Therapists (WFOT) (2019: 13) focus on the role of social participation during integration and state that "social participation is about citizenship and human rights". Within occupational therapy and occupational science there is the theory of occupational justice, which addresses the right of all individuals to occupation as a means to promote and support overall health and wellbeing, specifically through the opportunity for choice and freedom in our meaningful and purposeful occupations that are either individual or collective in nature (Wilcock & Hocking 2015). Underlying these beliefs is the concept of equity, that as occupational beings we have the right to equitable access when participating and engaging in our daily occupations (Wilcock & Hocking 2015). WFOT (2014: 1) acknowledges that "human displacement has direct and indirect consequences on occupational opportunities necessary to address human needs, access human rights, and create and maintain health", thus creating situations of occupational injustice (WFOT 2019).

Occupational injustice is present when an individual or group is denied or deprived of the opportunity to engage or participate in their meaningful and purposeful occupations (Wilcock & Townsend 2000). There are five occupational injustices presented in the literature: occupational deprivation; occupational marginalisation; occupational alienation; occupational imbalance; and occupational apartheid (Durocher Gibson & Rappolt 2014). While each can be applicable to refugees, asylum seekers, and other forcibly displaced populations, occupational deprivation is often the most cited of these injustices. Occupational deprivation occurs when the right to choose our occupations has been restricted due to isolated locations, individual ability, or other circumstances outside of our control (Townsend & Wilcock 2004). Due to the nature of seeking asylum or refugee status, there are often many restrictions placed on these individuals that can result in a lack of occupational participation and engagement (Trimboli & Halliwell 2018).

Supporting the Integration Process

Occupation shapes an individual's everyday life through the processes of doing, being, belonging, and becoming. Through their chosen occupations, individuals contribute to the community and engage with others by participating in shared occupations (Wilcock & Townsend 2000). Occupational participation has been found to be essential to the processes of integration and resettlement (Whiteford 2005). Thornton and Spalding (2018) add that this engagement and participation in activities for those seeking asylum or refugee status often contributes to social cohesion by breaking down the language barriers that may be present within these communities. As individuals, we develop through participating in occupations that contribute to our health and social inclusion (Townsend & Wilcock 2004). Often occupational roles and routines are lost due to the processes of migration and restrictions present in the new host country, such as policies relating to employment or access to education (WFOT 2019). This loss can lead to asylum seekers and refugees feeling disconnected, unable to contribute to society as an occupational being, and experiencing a loss of a sense of self and identity (Morville & Erlandsson 2017). Abramovic and colleagues (2019: 707) discuss the importance of the "more-than-human" experiences that enable integration through connections to places or environments. An example of places fostering connection are community gardens. They can provide opportunities for inclusion and integration through creating a sense of belonging, purpose, and identity (Abramovic Turner & Hope 2019).

Strang and Quinn (2021) highlight the need for timely support during the initial stages of the integration process to lessen the risks of social isolation within community settings. Often, within these settings, relationships are built based on dependency and on one-sided sharing of the information and resources available, which can impact negatively on mental health and wellbeing (Strang & Quinn 2021). Examples such as the New Scots Refugee Integration Strategy: 2024 demonstrate an evidence-based model to support policies that can work towards building trust, social connections, and integration between the refugee and the local community by promoting reciprocity and resource exchange in migrant policies, thus enabling work that enhances social networks, lessens stress, and facilitates integration (Strang & Quinn 2021). Within the Irish context, community development initiatives and support for asylum seekers and refugees has been identified as an area that is lacking in resources (Foreman & Ní Raghallaigh 2020). Further, Foreman and Ní Raghallaigh (2020) acknowledge the fact that there are some supports in place, but often these are allocated to those availing of set protection schemes, which is a small percentage of those entering the country.

What is the Role of Community Groups?

Integration can also be a dynamic process, where communities can come together to identify and develop the resources needed and initiate local projects (Daley 2009). Communities that are well supported and have accessible resources for new entrants have the potential to provide timely support to isolated refugees and asylum seekers on arrival to prevent their further withdrawal from said communities and services and lessen their risk of developing or exacerbating mental health issues (Strang & Quinn 2021). However, there may be multiple groups present and active in an area with limited supports or resources. As a result, competition for these groups/resources can lead to the group focus shifting from that of the whole community to the interests of the individual group (Daley 2009). As such, support from government and availability of funding, resources, and supports are necessary for the success and sustainability of these groups.

Within healthcare, the client is often an individual availing of the profession's services; we do not often see groups of individuals or communities as a client. While this book seeks to support health and social care professionals in working with refugees and asylum seekers, this chapter aims also to highlight the importance of the community within the integration process and how the health and social care professional may support such communities. While health and social care professionals practise in community-based settings, the focus of intervention remains on the individual while still considering the contexts in which they reside and the people they engage with, such as fellow refugees, community members, or care providers (Scaffa &

Reitz 2020). The next section of this chapter will present a case study of an urban community garden that has included those with refugee experience as members over the past year. The case study discusses a community-centred initiative that was developed within, for, and by the community, with limited resources at conception to now receiving support and funding from various national and local authorities to continue their work and increase the reach of the garden. The concept of community-centred initiatives is one that health and social care professionals may consider in their area of practice, and they may also consider its application to their caseload. These initiatives classify the whole community as the client and look to address the needs of a community as per its members (Scaffa & Reitz 2020).

Community Garden Project: A Case Study

This case discusses a community garden based in Dublin, Ireland. The garden has been in situ for over 10 years and has been well established as a key resource and place of refuge for the local community from the beginning. The garden has continued to grow since its inception and now holds many annual community events and celebrations on site, alongside its regular opening hours throughout the week. The addition of an indoor space, owned by the local authorities, but available to book free of charge for garden events, has seen the range of activities offered here grow in the past two years. While gardening is the main activity, there are now also knitting groups, repair cafes, English, Irish, French, and Arabic language classes, and many other events taking place. This case explores the role of the garden in welcoming refugees from a newly opened reception centre, the inclusion of multicultural events within the gardens calendar, and the ongoing impacts of the mutual learning opportunities for both local and refugee community members.

Materials for this case study were obtained through observations, correspondence with a garden member who facilitated the English language groups, and a focus group with local residents. The focus group comprised both native Irish residents and migrants from non-forcibly displaced backgrounds who were members of the community garden committee. However, it is important to acknowledge that no participants identified as asylum seekers or refugees.

The purpose of this case study was to explore the impact of including asylum seekers and refugees from the perspective of local residents and to examine how the group approached this process. To deepen this research, insights from individuals with lived experience of seeking asylum or refugee status would be invaluable in understanding integration and inclusion more comprehensively. While this study contributes to our understanding of the topic, it also aims to inspire further exploration among readers.

Background to the Irish Context

Over the past decade, Ireland has seen a significant increase of those seeking asylum within its borders. This increase has resulted in many debates and discussions regarding the country's ability to accommodate these increasing numbers, while simultaneously demonstrating the minimal resources in place to do so, particularly in relation to the inclusion of asylum seekers and refugees within the host community. The recent civil unrest and increased number of anti-migrant protests in Ireland have further highlighted the need for inclusive and safe spaces within communities that enable an informal process of integration. Ireland has seen a surge of community gardens opening across the country, with these often being described as inclusive and welcoming spaces for refugees and asylum seekers. However, to date there has been limited research to investigate the impact of community gardens and their role in supporting refugees and asylum seekers entering Ireland.

On arrival to Ireland, asylum seekers and refugees are required to apply for international protection at the point of entry (i.e., airport or seaport) or go to the International Protection Office (Sweeney 2023). The individual then has the right to remain in Ireland until the outcome of their application is decided. During this time, applicants may avail themselves of temporary services where their needs for accommodation, clothing, food, and healthcare services are met, in accordance with the EU reception conditions directive (Sweeney 2023). Those under the International Protection Accommodation Services receive an expense allowance of €38.80 per week per adult and €29.80 per week per child (Sweeney 2023). However, within the accommodation services there are restrictions placed on asylum seekers and refugees relating to their ability to cook for themselves and their family, to have recreational spaces for socializing or play, and curfews are often implemented within the centres (Moran et al. 2019). This current system increases the risk for occupational injustice to be present within this population due to the lack of choice, freedom, and autonomy in their daily lives. As such, community spaces could be seen as having the potential to reduce these occupational injustices by providing recreational spaces and opportunities for developing social connections and a sense of belonging to the local area.

Context within the Garden

The garden is in an area of Dublin steeped in Irish history and owes its name to the surroundings and stories of the past. The area is now known for its thriving community garden and all the events that take place there. The garden is a volunteer-led initiative within this urban area; however, members view it as more than just an urban community space, but as a growing ecosystem that has flourished since opening in 2011. Prior to 2011, the area where the garden is now situated was a wasteland, surrounded by residential housing. A number of locals petitioned their local authorities to allow the space to be developed into a community garden and were eventually granted just over 300 square metres of land (about the area of a tennis court). Since then, the garden has now doubled in size and includes a hacienda and a walkway around the perimeter. Next to the garden, a dilapidated cottage was renovated and is available for use by the garden members and the local community for different events and groups, such as knitting classes, youth groups, and workshops.

The locals view the garden as more than just a place to grow vegetables, fruits, trees, and flowers; but as a space to foster a sense of community and belonging to the area. It serves as a haven and meeting place for many local groups and like-minded people who enjoy meeting, sharing, and growing with others in its nurturing environment. Members are asked to contribute a small annual fee of five euro per household if unemployed or ten euro if employed. For refugees and asylum seekers this fee does not apply, and a committee member assists those who are interested in joining to create a membership. The garden is run by its committee members, who are elected annually, and it adheres to a constitution, rules, and code of conduct.

To keep the garden running and aid further development, the committee applies for various grants and holds fundraising events throughout the year, such as quiz nights and a cafe on their annual open day. The garden has been recognized locally and nationally through various community awards, environmental initiatives, and placemaking awards. It has been featured on both local and national news and television programmes, highlighting it as a model for successful community gardens that work for the community. The funding received by the garden from local and national government authorities spans the areas of integration and inclusion, sustainability and climate action, and enhancing inner city community spaces. This is testament to the diversity of the garden in how it is serving its community and demonstrating a standard of practice for other settings to start or develop their own community gardens.

Inclusion of Local Refugees and Asylum Seekers from a Local's Perspective

Late 2022 saw the opening of a direct provision centre within the locality of the community garden. The proposed opening of this centre incited unrest and anti-migrant protests among some of the residents living in the area. In response to this, a non-political community group was formed to support the refugees and asylum seekers moving into the area. This group organized donation drop-off points to gather much-needed supplies for the residents, held fundraising events, and organized language classes through an offshoot of their group.

At the beginning of 2023, members of the group, who are also members of the community garden, felt they would like to get involved and support the asylum seekers and refugees. This took the form of a gardening programme for English learners that took place once a week. The initial stages of the programme saw a strong interest and attendance rate from those living in the centre. The structure of the group was as follows: from 10.30am to 12pm gardening for English learners took place (this provided an informal class where participants engaged in conversational English rather than in a classroom-style setting); from

2pm to 3pm a woman-only workshop took place, which included activities such as singing, jewellery making, mindfulness, and painting; from 3pm to 5pm a crochet and knitting group was held in the cottage; and to finish the day from 5pm to 6pm a group of men attended an English class held in the cottage. The programme was very successful and many of its participants are still members of the garden to this day.

However, once the participants gained the right to work, they were less able to attend the programme on a weekly basis and the structure changed to a more simplified 'drop-in' style open space. This change in attendance again saw the garden adapt to the needs of its community, and there was an increase in events celebrating the different cultures and backgrounds of its members. Some of these were led by those with refugee experience, while others showcased Irish culture and history. As previously discussed in this chapter, many of the direct provision centres have limited cooking facilities, with the asylum seekers and refugees included in this case study only having access to limited cooking appliances (e.g., a kettle or a microwave). As such, the garden has hosted multiple 'potluck' events, where residents of the centre were invited into the homes and kitchens of local community members to cook a traditional dish from their country of origin. These dishes were then brought to the garden and shared with all who attended. A year on from the initial programme, many of those initial participants have continued to engage in various aspects of the garden, whether hosting a cultural event, using their skills (i.e., sewing or carpentry) at the repair cafes, or working in the garden during its dedicated gardening days.

Impact of Inclusion of Asylum Seekers and Refugees from a Local's Perspective

The garden has seen an increase in the events and activities on offer since the inclusion of asylum seekers and refugees. A focus group was held in May 2024 to discuss the impact and future of the community garden with committee members who identified as Irish residents and have been actively involved in engaging with refugees and asylum seekers coming to the garden. The focus group discussed how they felt the garden has grown since early 2023 with it now being split between gardening activities and the more social activities and groups taking place. This caused disagreements as to the garden's future, but these have since been resolved. One committee member discussed this growth through shared knowledge and understanding and how this has shaped their view and perception of those joining the garden.

> So just around the exchange of knowledge, so I think that maybe you know there's a certain—this kind of thing that you know you're helping them, and you're sharing knowledge about Ireland and try and make them feel at home and all that kind of stuff. But at the same time there's information coming back, there's an exchange of knowledge. So, like even just small bits, like people will say to you oh, you know when we grow that in wherever it is, whether it's Eastern Europe or North Africa, this is what we do and why they do it.

The sharing of experiences and knowledge was discussed throughout the group and how it has shaped everyone's understanding of different cultures. Committee members felt that this shared learning contributed to a sense of belonging and connection within the community garden, with one member commenting on seeing asylum seekers and refugee members out in the local area asking after the garden and its members.

> They say "ah how are you and how's the garden", so it's a lovely neighbourhood feeling. And then I met another guy in—he's working now...give me a big hug... so they really were thankful for them for being part of the garden.

While other members have returned to the garden after a period of absence and were able to see the work that they had completed in use by garden members, contributing to feelings of pride and joy.

> Actually, one of them came back last week and he saw the glass house and his eyes were like full of spark you know, he was so proud.

Committee members also felt the impact was relevant to other garden members and helped with changing the beliefs and perspectives that local members had of those with a refugee or asylum-seeking background. This was felt both in their own personal experiences and through conversations with other members on their views and understanding of refugees' experiences.

And then we were having a chat in the hacienda, and there was certainly a couple of people who definitely had views that you know some refugees who are more worthy than others. And I know that her attitude has completely changed, yes completely turned around now. So, it's good yeah that's what I'm saying. So, like and sometimes you don't have to have a big debate or discussion or an argument, all you have to do is to engage with people and learn about them, and then within six months or so she was saying "oh my God you won't believe what those people have to go through" so yeah.

Another member reflected on this further and discussed how it impacted on the general narrative of fear and resistance towards refugee and asylum seekers amongst the wider community.

It's really important, I think you're right, because you get inundated with negative things about refugees or asylum seekers, but through the garden and through interacting normally it's just like your...if you walk in the street you're not scared, you're not like oh this person is dangerous, it's like oh I know this person. It's very different.

Overall, committee members reflected very positively on how the garden has grown and developed since the inclusion of refugees and asylum seekers. On visiting the garden or attending any of the events throughout the year, one can see the diversity and pride present within its structures and members. Refugees and asylum seekers have only added to this by sharing their knowledge and culture, showing ingenuity and skill in identifying problems and providing solutions, such as building the greenhouse from recycled windows or the ability to move a sizable plant to a new location. Committee members further confirmed this sentiment during the focus group, stating;

it's like we have a problem they ha- are the solutions for the garden... yeah they've been a huge asset overall, somebody who's come through the asylum system.

What is the Future for the Garden?

The committee expressed the wish for the garden to continue to develop and adapt to the community's needs in the future. The committee continues to apply for grants and funding to support this development, however this is a point of frustration and uncertainty as local authorities continue to send mixed messages as to how long the garden will remain in its current format.

> There's a real disconnect between what the policies are saying at the top and what's actually happening on the ground.

While more support from local authorities and government may ensure the viability of the garden, this may also pose issues with regulations being imposed and the space becoming more like a recreational park rather than a community garden. The current structure of the garden allows for an informal type of involvement, members can come and go as they please within the opening hours and either contribute to the garden or just enjoy the space as it is, an oasis within the city. The addition of the renovated cottage on-site, and recent developments within zoning for the area, have given hope for the future of the garden itself and its place within the community.

> Currently zoned as green, which means the local area office want to keep this space recreational. They've put a lot of money into the cottage, which isn't ours, it's a community facility for everybody and that bodes well for the garden surviving. I think they like the garden.

The importance of ownership of the garden and member contributions was considered a key factor for the garden's future. This is reflected in the recent addition of working groups focusing on different areas of the garden, which is felt to give members a sense of ownership without requiring them to be on the committee, and encourages more members to join. Membership is one of the main concerns for the sustainability of the community garden, with committee members discussing the different groups contributing to this, particularly asylum seekers and refugees volunteering their time while awaiting their work permits. Many of those that began with the weekly programme are still valued members of the community garden and continue to encourage other refugees and asylum seekers in the centre to come to the various events or just to garden and enjoy the space. In summary, this community garden can be seen to illustrate the benefits of community groups and their role in promoting mutual learning and integration between the local and refugee communities on arrival to the new host country.

Putting Learning into Practice

For health and social care professionals working with those with refugee experience, it is important to understand the supports and resources available within the community. It is recommended that health and social care professionals develop and foster relationships with community organisations and services in their locality to maintain up-to-date information and knowledge of their availability and to better serve those accessing their services. It is important to be able to signpost these supports so that people with refugee experience learn who they can contact for assistance with issues or problems they may be having. The support available to people with refugee experience will vary greatly between countries, but also even across different localities within the same country. Consequently, health and social care professionals need to ensure that they have a good understanding and awareness of the different organisations in their localities and keep up to date with changes in these and the services they provide.

To implement the learning gained from this chapter, the reader is first asked to reflect on the following in relation to their practice area:

1. Can you identify relevant organisations or sources of support that are available in your local community for new entrants?

2. Can you give a brief summary as to why each may be useful to someone with refugee experience?

If it is felt that this task is difficult to complete, or that perhaps the reader may be aware of the organisations available but are not clear about what services they provide or how to access them, then this has identified a gap in our knowledge. While as health and social care professionals we cannot be expected to know of all the potential services available, understanding the key ones relevant to your client group/service users would be beneficial to your practice. As such, the reader is now asked to complete the following exercise in relation to their current practice and caseload:

1. Identify two or three organisations/community groups/ programmes that may be useful for those with refugee experience.

2. Investigate what process you would need to follow to refer someone in your care to them or to access the group/service.

3. Reflect on what support is needed from the health and social care professional perspective: is this something that the individual can attend alone, or will they require support/ check ins throughout? How does this fit within your caseload?

Lastly, the reader is asked to consider their own place in promoting interaction and mutual learning between the local and refugee community: what is the health and social care professional's role, what do we need to do/understand/be aware of to best serve these communities and what learning can we gain? Consider how you can better connect with community organisations in your locality:

1. How might you make use of these links to enhance the everyday life of those with refugee experience?

2. Reflect on your practice context. Is there a way that you might connect with another professional and, together with the person from a refugee community, use these supports to promote their sense of inclusion and participatory citizenship?

3. What can you all learn from one another?

References

Abramovic, Jessica et al. 2019. 'Entangled recovery: refugee encounters in community gardens', *Local Environment*, 24.8: 696–711, https://doi.org/10.1080/13549839.2019.1637832

Ager, Alastair, and Alison Strang. 2008. 'Understanding Integration: A Conceptual Framework', *Journal of Refugee Studies*, 21.2: 166–191, https://doi.org/10.1093/jrs/fen016

Costigan, Catherine L. 2022. 'Building community: Connecting refugee and Canadian families', *Cultural Diversity and Ethnic Minority Psychology*, 28.3: 338, https://doi.org/10.1037/cdp0000428

Daley, Clare. 2009. 'Exploring community connections: community cohesion and refugee integration at a local level', *Community Development Journal*, 44.2: 158–171, https://doi.org/10.1093/cdj/bsm026

Darawsheh, Wesam et al. 2022. 'Factors Shaping Occupational Injustice among Resettled Syrian Refugees in the United States', *Occupational Therapy International,* 2022: 2846896, https://doi.org/10.1155/2022/2846896

Durocher, Evelyne, Barbara E Gibson and Susan Rappolt. 2014. 'Occupational justice: A conceptual review', *Journal of Occupational Science,* 21.4: 418–430, https://doi.org/10.1080/14427591.2013.775692

Foreman, Maeve, and Muireann Ní Raghallaigh. 2020. 'Transitioning out of the asylum system in Ireland: Challenges and opportunities', *Social Work & Social Sciences Review,* 18.1: 15–30, https://doi.org/10.1921/swssr.v21i1.1365

Hocking, Clare, and Elizabeth Townsend. 2015. 'Driving social change: Occupational therapists' contributions to occupational justice', *World Federation of Occupational Therapists Bulletin,* 71.2: 68–71, https://doi.org/10.1179/2056607715Y.0000000002

Hocking, Clare, and Ann A. Wilcock. 2020. 'Population Health: An Occupational Perspective' in *Occupational Therapy in Community and Population Health Practice*, ed. by Scaffa, Marjorie E. & Reitz, Maggie S (FA Davis), pp. 59–71.

Kantartzis, Sarah. 2017. 'Exploring occupation beyond the individual: Family and collective occupation' in *Occupational Therapies Without Borders: Integrating Justice with Practice*, ed. by Sakellariou, Dikaios, and Nick Pollard (Elsevier), pp. 19–28.

MacQueen, Kathleen M, et al. 2001. 'What Is Community? An Evidence-Based Definition for Participatory Public Health', *American Journal of Public Health,* 91.12: 1929–1938, https://doi.org/10.2105/ajph.91.12.1929

Moran, Lisa et al. 2019. 'Hoping for a better tomorrow: a qualitative study of stressors, informal social support and parental coping in a Direct Provision centre in the West of Ireland', *Journal of Family Studies,* 25.4: 427–442, https://doi.org/10.1080/13229400.2017.1279562

Morville, Anne-Le, and Lena-Karin Erlandsson. 2017. 'Occupational deprivation for asylum seekers' in *Occupational Therapies Without Borders: Integrating Justice with Practice* ed. by Sakellariou, Dikaios, & Pollard, Nick (Elsevier), pp. 381–389.

National Social Inclusion Office. 2017. *The Migrant Integration Strategy: A Blueprint for the Future* (Dublin: Ireland), https://www.gov.ie/en/publication/5a86da-the-migrant-integration-strategy-2017-2020/

Public Health England. 2015. *A Guide to Community-Centred Approaches for Health and Wellbeing. Full Report* (London: England), https://www.gov.uk/government/publications/health-and-wellbeing-a-guide-to-community-centred-approaches

Scaffa, Marjorie E. and Maggie S Reitz (eds). 2020. *Occupational Therapy in Community and Population Health Practice* (FA Davis).

Strang, Alison, and Alastair Ager. 2010. 'Refugee integration: Emerging trends and remaining agendas', *Journal of Refugee Studies*, 23.4: 589–607, https://doi.org/10.1093/jrs/feq046

Strang, Alison, and Neil Quinn. 2021. 'Integration or isolation? Refugees' social connections and wellbeing', *Journal of Refugee Studies*, 34.1: 328–353, https://doi.org/10.1093/jrs/fez040

Sweeney, Caroline. 2023. *Note 2: Refugees in Ireland. Refugees in Ireland, the EU and Worldwide* (Dublin: Ireland), https://data.oireachtas.ie/ie/oireachtas/libraryResearch/2023/2023-12-11_l-rs-note-refugees-in-ireland-the-eu-and-worldwide-refugees-in-ireland_en.pdf

Thornton, Molly, and Nicola Spalding. 2018. 'An exploration of asylum seeker and refugee experiences of activity: A literature review', *World Federation of Occupational Therapists Bulletin*, 74.2: 114–122,

Townsend, Elizabeth, and Ann A. Wilcock. 2004. 'Occupational justice and Client-Centred Practice: A Dialogue in Progress', *Canadian Journal of Occupational Therapy*, 71.2: 75–87, https://doi.org/10.1177/000841740407100203

Trimboli, Concettina, and Vicky Halliwell. 2018. 'A survey to explore the interventions used by occupational therapists and occupational therapy students with refugees and asylum seekers', *World Federation of Occupational Therapists Bulletin*, 74.2: 106–113, https://doi.org/10.1080/14473828.2018.1535562

Whiteford, Gail. 2000. 'Occupational Deprivation: Global Challenge in the New Millennium', *British Journal of Occupational Therapy*, 63.5: 200–204, https://doi.org/10.1177/030802260006300503

—— 2005. 'Understanding the Occupational Deprivation of Refugees: A Case Study from Kosovo', *Canadian Journal of Occupational Therapy*, 72.2: 78–88, https://doi.org/10.1177/000841740507200202

Wilcock, Ann, A. & Townsend, Elizabeth. 2000. 'Occupational terminology interactive dialogue', *Journal of Occupational Science*, 7.2: 84–86, https://doi.org/10.1080/14427591.2000.9686470

Wilcock, Ann, A. 2006. *An Occupational Perspective of Health* (Slack Incorporated).

Wilcock, Ann, A., and Clare Hocking. 2015. *An Occupational Perspective of Health* (SLACK Incorporated).

World Federation of Occupational Therapists. 2014. 'Position statement on human displacement revised', https://doi.org/10.1179/otb.2012.66.1.005

—— 2019. 'Position Statement: Occupational Therapy and Human Rights', https://www.wfot.org/resources/occupational-therapy-and-human-rights

III. Professional Practice and Interprofessional Collaboration in Refugee Health

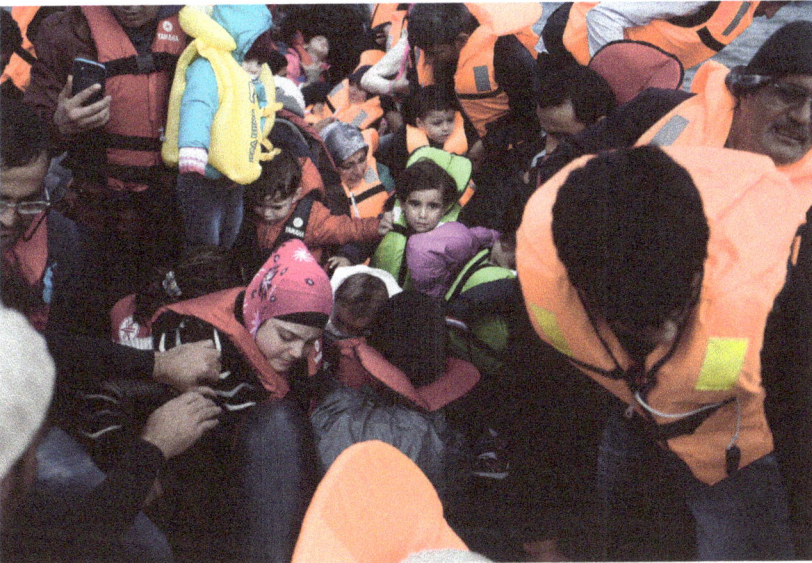

7. Evidence-Informed Practice and Learning Through Critical Reflection

Emer McGowan and Sarah Quinn

I think that health personnel who work with refugees must be aware of which group they are working with. It is a very good feeling when someone comes, and you see that they have received the right treatment. That you have helped them with the problems they had. It creates a very good feeling.
—Female nurse from Bosnia living with refugee status in Norway

Taking an evidence-informed approach and reflecting critically on service provision are two practices that can be employed to ensure quality in the care provided to people with refugee experience. When working with potentially vulnerable populations, like people with refugee experience, evidence-informed practice highlights the importance of attending to the needs of individuals and integrating their narratives into the use of practices that are evidence-based (Nevo & Slonim-Nevo 2011; Kumah et al. 2022). This chapter argues for the adoption of evidence-informed practices in work with people with refugee experience as more appropriate than the traditional and well accepted evidence-based practice model. The complementary practice of critical reflection is an internal process that helps refine understandings of an experience, potentially leading to changes in perspective and future actions (Mann et al. 2009) and supporting the development of services responsive to the needs of people with refugee experience.

 https://doi.org/10.11647/OBP.0479.07

Evidence-Informed Practice

Across the recent past, efforts to improve quality, reliability, and service-user outcome and experiences, have promoted the move away from practices based on tradition and rituals, towards the implementation of best available evidence in guiding interventions (Kumah et al. 2019). Health and social care professionals are expected to apply the best available evidence to inform their clinical decision-making, roles, and responsibilities (Kelly et al. 2015; Andre et al. 2016; Kumah et al. 2022). The many advantages to the service user, professional, organisation, and health and social care systems of the use of best available evidence have been espoused. These include improved outcomes for service users and increased transparency, enhanced cooperation between professionals, greater job practitioner satisfaction, and improved system efficiency (Tickle-Degnen & Bedell 2003; Nevo & Slonim-Nevo 2011; Kelly et al. 2015).

Two main concepts have been associated with the application of evidence into healthcare practice: evidence-based practice and evidence-informed practice. Evidence-based practice (EBP) is well-established in health and social care and regarded as the norm or gold standard for the delivery of effective healthcare (Kumah et al. 2022). The universally accepted definition of evidence-based practice (EBP), adapted from the definition of evidence-based medicine, is "the conscientious, explicit and judicious use of the best evidence in making decisions about the care of the individual patient" (Sackett et al. 1996). In recent times, the concept of evidence-informed practice is increasingly being adopted instead of evidence-based practice (Kumah et al. 2022). Evidence-informed practice (EIP) has been described as the "assimilation of personal judgement and research evidence regarding the efficiency of interventions" (McSherry et al. 2002). It is an approach to care that involves combining research evidence regarding the efficacy of interventions with the professional's experience and judgement and the client's preferences and values, while demonstrating cognisance of the context of the situation (Nevo & Slonim-Nevo 2011).

Best evidence, from an EBP perspective, is categorized in a hierarchy of quality (Evans 2003). Systematic reviews or meta-analyses are considered to be the gold standard in EBP. Randomized controlled trials are thought to provide strong evidence and are rated as second-level evidence. Evidence, believed to hold less value in EBP, include surveys and all forms of qualitative research. In this regard, EBP has been criticized for privileging statistical and meta-analytical techniques over qualitative research and interpretive, discursive, or narrative approaches to knowledge, which can simplify and distort complex situations (Morrell & Learmonth 2015). The term evidence-informed practice (EIP) grew out of a need for a more inclusive understanding of evidence (Davis et al. 2000). This has been contested as the debate about what constitutes best evidence for EBP has become more sophisticated over time and additional forms of evidence in informing the delivery of healthcare have gained recognition (Rycroft-Malone 2008). Acknowledging that EBP traditionally based clinical decision making on empirically supported treatments, protocol adherence, and standardisation, the American Psychological Association (2006) consider the application of EIP to be more comprehensive, describing the process as a synthesis of empirically supported treatments with client characteristics, culture, and preferences. Both EBP and EIP aspire to incorporate evidence to improve quality of care and the terms are often used interchangeably in the literature (Gambrill 2007).

The EBP model described a five-step procedure beginning with the development of an evidence-based clinical question used to guide the search for evidence (Taylor, 2007). The application of such a procedure is dismissed under the EIP model. Instead, EIP is guided by a client-centred question, and advocates a more encompassing, interpretative view of evidence with greater flexibility in its selection for use in guiding practice (Nevo & Sloim-Nevo 2011). The contrast between sources of evidence acceptable in EBP and EIP is presented in Table 7.1. In EIP, evidence is seen to enrich, but not limit, practice (Epstein 2009). Using this lens, findings obtained through case studies, qualitative or mixed methods research, clinical narratives, and experiences are seen as important sources of evidence as well as those arrived at by randomized controlled trials. A wide range of information sources is acceptable in EIP and advised to be used creatively and sensitively in service delivery. The appropriateness of research evidence and clinical protocols or guidelines to the service user's experience and changing needs must be judged by the professional rather than applied objectively and allowed to dominate practice (Nevo & Sloim-Nevo 2011). EIP acknowledges the importance of additional factors in the implementation of evidence such as the therapeutic relationship, service-user motivation, and assessment procedures. While quality is important, EIP evidence is not in a hierarchy. EIP requires a broad knowledge of empirical evidence and clinical experience to be applied to a therapeutic process in a manner that is sensitive and creative, and in this respect it is a more appropriate practice to use with persons who have refugee experience.

What counts for evidence.........		
In evidence-based practice?		In evidence-informed practice?
	Levels of evidence	Many forms of evidence:
I	Systematic reviews or meta-analysis of randomized controlled trials.	• Research articles, both quantitative and qualitative.
II		
III	Randomized controlled trials.	• Clinical guidelines and protocols.
IV	Non-randomized experimental studies.	• Books.
V		• Conferences and webinars.
	Non-experimental studies (e.g., surveys, qualitative research).	• In-service training.
		• Self-generated data e.g., surveys, audits.
	Respected opinion (world leaders).	

Table 7.1 Summary of evidence in EBP and EIP.

Lack of knowledge of their rights and entitlements, combined with unfamiliar professional practices and behaviours, may compound the vulnerability of groups within a system, such as those with refugee experience whose status is compromised and whose options for alternative care are minimal (Rycroft-Malone 2008). Difficulties navigating health and social care systems, language and culture-related differences, and fear of stigmatisation, contribute to barriers this population face in accessing and using services (Asgary & Segar 2011). Although the use of evidence to inform intervention is essential, the process of employing evidence in practice should be flexible and responsive in order to meet the ongoing and changing goals, conditions, experiences, and preferences of service users (Isakson et al. 2015). EIP is driven by a client-centred approach, offering an integrated, inclusive process to the application of evidence into practice, appropriate to the provision of health and social care for people with refugee experience (Nevo & Slonim-Nevo 2011). Working with refugees requires adoption of a socioecological perspective that demonstrates an appreciation for the individual's narrative—their history, culture, community, and current work or school context—and an understanding that, in addition to resettlement stressors, such as language and poverty, the individual may be experiencing secondary stressors like the loss of loved ones and reminders of trauma (Isakson et al. 2015). In EIP, the professional integrates the service user's perspectives, in this case the person with refugee experience, and uses their issues to drive the search for evidence. It does this by emphasizing the development of client-driven questions rather than the search for randomized control trials to answer evidence-driven questions, as in EBP, that may or may not speak to the service user's actual issues (Nevo & Slonim-Nevo 2011).

The cultural competence of health and social care professionals is essential when working with people with refugee experience (Szajna & Ward 2014). Missed cues can occur when the practitioner does not understand the background and cultural practices of a service user or is not cognisant of their own cultural biases. Disconnect between service user and practitioner can result from differing views on health and illness across cultures (Englund & Rydstrom 2012). Addressing cultural preferences is integral to EIP. Recognizing that the priorities of service users and their families are not necessarily those of the professional and having open, culturally sensitive discussions of therapeutic goals in intervention planning facilitates quality care (Isakson et al. 2015). Similarly, measurement of progress may vary across cultures. For example, progress, and a positive outcome from engaging with a service for the service user might mean finding a job, not just feeling well. Such considerations reinforce the importance of culturally sensitive consultation with service users to ensure that the professionals' understanding of evidence for the effectiveness of practice is in line with the experiences of the service user.

Professional expertise is necessary to make decisions that integrate the best available research evidence with client characteristics and preferences. To this end, the professional needs skills to enable them to access, understand, and apply evidence. Developing a level of skill and confidence in accessing and interpreting the best available evidence is required (Brangan et al. 2015). Translating the evidence in a way that is meaningful to the practice context is of particular importance in EIP. The generation of evidence from within a given practice context through the evaluation of practice outcomes offers an alternative means of applying evidence for best practice that does not rely on access to the literature. Adopting best-practice standards can also involve auditing services, conducting satisfaction surveys, using guidelines and outcome measures as deemed appropriate. In the application of clinical guidelines and protocols, cognizance of the dynamic and changing nature of health and social care, the needs of the service user, and the cultural context are required. To ensure that the integration of evidence into practices is flexible, especially with traumatized and vulnerable groups, the expertise and sound clinical reasoning of the professional is crucial.

Evidence is believed to be socially and historically constructed, meaning that it is contextually bound and interpreted to be made relevant to individual contexts. In this respect, evidence is not static or value-free (Rycroft-Malone 2008) but a catalyst to the process of healthcare decision-making and delivery (Gabbay et al. 2003). Several factors including the culture, leadership, and teamwork within the health or social care context plays an important role in the successful implementation of evidence in practice. The barriers to implementation include time and accountability pressures (Metzler & Metz 2010). Given that organisations' values vary in emphasis, factors to consider include the culture of the organisation and professionals' freedom to adapt services to suit the particular needs of service users. Adaptation of services may include the adjustment of an organisation's protocols to better support people new to a health and social care system to attend appointments. Permission from organisational leaders to increase a professional's autonomous use of time to reflect and think creatively around problems, to collaborate, and to search for evidence may need to be negotiated. The professionals' cultural competence and self-awareness can also act to facilitate or inhibit EIP and an individual's use of services (Szajna & Ward 2014). An awareness that our systems and services do not operate in a cultureless environment, a consciousness of the form of health and social care we deliver, and an appreciation of the possibilities for change within services is important when trying to adopt best practices to meet the needs of people with refugee experience. Whole organisational change can be required, in the implementation of EIP, for the construction of a sensitive and culturally aware context with strong consensus-informed governance (Rycroft-Malone 2008). To enhance the success of implementing evidence in practice "the interaction of various ingredients" is required (Rycroft-Malone 2005: 1) and, in EIP, service user, practitioner, and contextual factors drive the identification of relevant evidence and are crucial to its creative and flexible implementation.

Critical Reflection

In healthcare, critical reflection is seen as integral to professional learning as it supports the analysis and evaluation of practice experience (Eaton 2016). Improving critical reflection skills has the potential to improve professional practice and enable better management of complex service users and healthcare systems (Désilets et al. 2022). Reflective writing is a key feature in most healthcare professional portfolios and commonly used as evidence of competence and continuing professional development (Eaton 2016). Reflective practice can lead to better quality care as it can enable better learning (Börjesson et al. 2015), develop emotional competency and communication skills (Harrison & Fopma-Loy 2010), and encourage critical thinking (Kinsella 2006).

Reflection is described as "a metacognitive process including connecting with feelings that occur before, during and after situations with a purpose of developing greater awareness and understanding of self, other, and situation, so that future encounters with the situation including ways of being, relating, and doing are informed from previous encounters" (Wald 2015). Critical reflection contributes to conceptual understanding of health-and-social-care-related issues and has the power to transform experiences into meaningful learning. To reflect critically involves more than pausing, thinking back over events, problem solving, and planning future practice based on what is already known and how issues are typically managed. Additionally, it demands critically appraising the content, process, and premise underlying the experience to make better sense of what has happened and reach a better understanding of the experience. Reflection has scope to give meaning to experience, turn experience into practice, link past and present experiences, and prepare us for future practice.

Why practise the skill of critical reflection?

It encourages independent learning—reflection can help us to identify areas or skills where we require further development. By intentionally evaluating our knowledge, behaviours, and competencies we will be better able to see what we can work on to improve our practice in future.

It helps order our thoughts and problem-solve—as we reflect, we re-order our minds which can make it easier to reframe problems and consider alternative solutions.

It helps achieve deep as opposed to surface learning—thinking over complex issues as we reflect, facilitates abstract conceptualisation which enables deeper learning.

It helps identify our personal strengths as well as areas for development—reflection involves critical self-assessment and should highlight what we're doing well in addition to what we need to improve.

It helps challenge our assumptions and recognize multiple perspectives—critical reflection can help us to become aware of our innate or unconscious biases and how these influence our behaviours. It can also make us more cognisant of the viewpoints of others and the impact that cultural context can have on different situations.

It helps in exploring new ways of doing or thinking about things—reflection can allow you to be more creative in considering possible action plans to address complex problems.

How Critical Reflection Works

Reflection, in helping to improve self-awareness and encourage critical thinking (Ghanizadeh 2017) may improve our ability to learn (Mann et al. 2009). By linking concrete real-world experiences to professional knowledge, it can help make sense of practice situations.

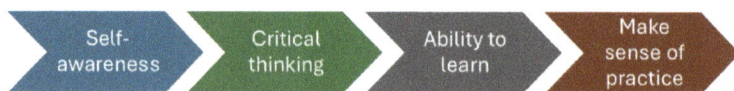

Fig. 7.1 How critical reflection aids learning and sense-making.

Theorists (e.g., Brookfield; Schön; Kolb; Gibb; Mezirow) have each emphasized aspects of the reflection process they consider important and developed methods of reflecting that encourage analysis of experiences to enhance learning. For instance, Schön (1991) emphasizes Reflection-in-Action and Reflection-on Action. Reflection-*in*-action encourages practitioners to think about what is happening during the interaction or event—thoughts, feelings, decisions, actions, consequences, and meaning. Reflection-*on*-action encourages practitioners to consider the events at a later time, allowing time to process experiences, feelings, and actions while taking into account new information and an opportunity to link the experience of theory and knowledge.

Brookfield's reflective theory (Brookfield 1995) requires the identification of significant events within an interaction or experience: it encourages practitioners to think about what happened in the event; feelings, thoughts, and actions during the event; what happened after the event; and the learning from that event. Brookfield also recommends accessing different perspectives and questioning assumptions. Gibbs (1988) highlights the importance of identifying other possible behaviour or action choices. Kolb (1984) proposed the experiential learning cycle, which emphasizes the role of reflection in learning. In this model, learning begins with an event (concrete experience) which the individual reflects upon (reflective observation). The reflection leads to the formation of new ideas (abstract conceptualisation) which can then be applied in the future resulting in new experiences (active experimentation). Knowledge gained from reflection does not arrive in a logical and structured fashion but instead requires an active participatory element (Eaton 2016).

Reflection and Professional Identity

Reflective practice helps people to achieve a deeper understanding of their profession (Ng et al. 2015) and has been found to facilitate healthcare professionals in the development of their professional identity (Binyamin 2017). An individual's professional identity encompasses the beliefs, values, attitudes, motives, and experiences through which they define themselves in a professional role (Ibarra 1999). It reflects the professional's concept of who they are and their perception of what it means to be and act in their professional role (Mackey 2006). As such, it impacts what they do and how they practice their profession (Binyamin 2017). Understanding who one is as a health and social care professional has an impact on the provision of care and influences the effectiveness of service delivery (Best & Williams 2019).

Professional identity formation has been described as a transformative journey from being a lay person to "becoming" a professional (Poole & Patterson 2021). Health professionals' development of their professional identity is moulded by a range of different factors including critical experiences in clinical education, exposure to role models, professional socialisation (transmission of professional values), interactions and relationships with service users and professionals from other disciplines, and ongoing self-enquiry (Binyamin 2017; Poole & Patterson 2021). Identity formation is an ongoing process of reflecting on who one is and who one wants to be (Binyamin 2017). The literature suggests that the most powerful influences on professional identity formation are role models or mentors, and experiential learning in both clinical and non-clinical scenarios (Monrouxe 2016) but that it is reinforced by reflection on these learning experiences (Mann et al. 2009; Cruess et al. 2019). Critical reflection on learning experiences, whether from observing role models or through direct experience, means that information that would otherwise remain tacit becomes explicit (Cruess et al. 2019).

In a study investigating the role of reflection in the development of professional identity, Désilets et al. (2022) conceptualized and implemented a reflection process comprised of four elements: relationship with self (identification with a role), situations (clinical, learning), profession (appropriation of values and norms), and society. To foster the development of reflection skills, they advocated for the importance of providing a safe environment, mentorship, peer support, time to reflect, and helping students to see the potential benefits of reflective practice (Désilets et al. 2022). Being secure and confident in one's professional identity better enables health professionals to collaborate with other professionals in the multidisciplinary healthcare team (Porter & Wilton 2019).

Reflection and Interprofessional Collaboration

Reflective practice has been recognized as central in the development of good collaboration practices for health and social care professionals and is a key aspect of interprofessional education (Richard et al. 2019). It has been recognized by the World Health Organisation as one of the main interprofessional learning domains (WHO 2010). In a review of reflective practice in interprofessional education and practice, Richard et al. (2019) made three recommendations for implementing reflective practice in interprofessional education and collaborative practice (IPECP):

- Use meaningful clinical situations and rely on IPECP theory and evidence (theory to practice).

- Engage a well-trained facilitator during group discussions or two facilitators with complementary expertise (IPECP and critical thinking), where possible.

- Support the reflective approach using a rigorous and explicit process based on precise criteria. To achieve critical reflection, planning and explicit training in critical thinking are key.

The usefulness of reflective practice in complex or challenging situations where there are multiple perspectives and factors to consider has been recognized (Kinsella 2010; Kuipers et al. 2014; Richard et al. 2019). Similarly, the greater the complexity of a clinical situation, the more important it is for healthcare professionals to engage in effective interprofessional collaboration (Kuipers et al. 2014; World Health Organization [WHO] 2010).

Reflective Writing

Thinking reflectively usually involves looking back at something, analysing an idea, experience, or event, and thinking carefully about its meaning. Committing this reflection to paper involves an exploration and an explanation of events, not just a description of them. Reflective writing is not a straightforward description of an event to convey information or support simple decision-making, but a critical practice with a consequent utility to improve health and social care. Reflective writing requires the professional to see and understand what is happening above and below the surface. Situations must be analysed critically to uncover assumptions, biases, motives, and understand others' perspectives, taking time to consider how thoughts and feelings interact to influence behaviour.

Adopting this approach facilitates the professional to learn more about themselves, the situation, their practice, and others.

Application of Reflective Writing in Practice

The event	A student met an asylum seeker in a Direct Provision Centre to prepare a meal together.
Reflective report	So, we met at the centre and I was a little apprehensive. We'd decided to cook together, a meal from her country. I worried that this might be too spicy for me and that I would have to tell her I didn't like it and I would find that difficult to do. I had organized with the centre manager for us to use the kitchen. Usually, residents have all their meals prepared for them.
	I had shopped on my way to the centre for the ingredients of the meal we were to prepare. Once we were in the kitchen my partner examined all the food I had bought. She was disappointed that I couldn't get certain vegetables that she thought were essential, but I explained that I would have needed to go to the Asian shops for those, which I didn't have time to do. Plus, I didn't know what they were so I couldn't get something similar.
	I helped prepare the raw ingredients and then she cooked. I tried to help turn things on the pan but she said she'd better do it so I sat down. The manager came in when we were cooking and complained about the spicy smells. I said there was nothing we could do about it but that we'd be finished soon. My partner told me when the manager had left that the dish needed time to simmer. This was a bit annoying. I wish she had told me that before I had told him we were nearly finished as this didn't make me look very good in his eyes. My partner also got worried that the manager would be angry and take this out on her later somehow. I told her this was unlikely.
	In the end we had a cup of coffee while we waited for the food to be ready, staying in the kitchen out of sight of the manager. It felt as if we were hiding which was a bit strange. After our meal was finished, which I surprisingly liked very much, I brought a plate of food out to the manager by way of apology. It would be nice to cook together again though, because of the manager's attitude, it might be some time before we can.

To summarize the student's reflections	Feelings and thoughts: "I was a bit worried. I didn't think I'd like it because I don't like spicy food."
	Actions: "We cooked together."
	Learning: "I liked this."
	Plan: "I hope we do it again sometime"
Now ask yourself:	Has the report produced new understanding of situations or reinforced knowledge already understood?
	Has the student objectively considered her own thoughts, feelings, and behaviour in the situation and reached new understandings?
	Has the student tried to understand the event from the asylum seeker's perspective?
	Is there learning that can inform the student's practice?
	Will this learning make a meaningful difference to the asylum seeker's life?
	Is this a deep reflection?
What level of depth has this student reached in her reflections?	
	This was a basic reflection.
	Descriptive or/and emotive.
	No useful learning was concluded.
	She did not:
	Ask herself questions about the event.
	Make connections between behaviours, emotions, ideas.
	Assess impact of behaviours, emotions, ideas, & contexts.
	Identify useful learning.
	Consider implications of this learning on practice.
How could the student reflect at a deeper level?	
	She might have asked…
	Might her partner have been worried too?
	Her partner usually has little choice in food—what does that mean for her?
	Might gathering the correct produce have been important & why?

	Her partner usually has little opportunity to cook—what does this feel like?
	How did the manager's interruption impact the activity? Was this interruption justified?
	What she might have learnt...
	Be open minded towards things (even food) that are different to what she's used to.
	Preparation is important—effort is required in setting expectations, in gathering supplies etc.
	The impact & experience of events varies depending on our personal histories/circumstances etc.
	Ideas about things to do differently next time...
	Might they shop together? Much more empowering and inclusive and could lead to higher success.
	Consult with her partner before answering for her. Support her to answer the manager herself.
	Apologize to the manager for not being clear about their expectations and to the partner.
	Ask her partner how she would like to manage the confrontation with the manager.

Table 7.2 Reflective writing in practice.

To ensure reflections are critical and not merely descriptive, the professional might consider applying the guidance in this list:

- Use description only to serve the process of reflection.
- Show awareness of one's thoughts, values, attitudes, assumptions—ask oneself questions about the event.
- Identify the impact of emotion but don't be emotive.
- Make connections between behaviours, emotions, ideas.
- Recognize possible change.
- Show evidence of valuable learning.
- Identify the implications of this learning on practice.

Further prompts that can be used to structure reflective writing, to help ensure reflection goes beyond description and demonstrates critical thinking, are outlined in Table 7.3.

EVENT	OTHER INFLUENCES
What happened? Be specific, relevant, concise in detail.	How did the physical space impact what people did or said?
FEELINGS AND THOUGHTS	How have your cultural norms influenced how you thought & behaved?
How did you feel & what did you think before, during, & after the event?	How might others have experienced the event given their cultural background?
Had you any assumptions about how this event would transpire?	
What are your values & beliefs?	What are the everyday practices of the organisation/community and how did these shape the event?
ACTIONS/BEHAVIOURS	LEARNING
How did you react during the experience? How much of your behaviour is habitual and influenced by your values?	What did you learn about: • yourself as a person (e.g., your privilege, your cultural norms, your values given your age, gender etc);
How did you interact with others? How did your behaviour influence others' experiences of the event?	• others (both service-users and other professionals);
What was the result of your or others' actions/behaviour?	• your professional skills/ knowledge/attitudes from this experience?
What went well or badly? Why?	
What else could you have done? What could have been done differently to improve outcomes?	
PLAN: What would you do if a similar situation arose again?	

Table 7.3 Prompts to aid critical reflection.

Critical Reflection in Refugee Health

Reflective practice is a useful approach to assist in improving treatment outcomes and to enhance clinical practice when working with population groups, like refugees, where there may be increased complexity (Brooks 2018). In the provision of health and social care, professionals need to be aware of a range of personal and contextual factors that can impact the delivery of that care. To be culturally competent and aware, healthcare professionals need to be mindful of and reflect upon the unique context and personal experience of each person to whom they provide a service. When working with people with refugee experience, it is important to consider:

- The impact of power and privilege of a majority/dominant culture (likely the health/social care professional's) on the professional's behaviours—are they collaborative or autocratic—and on the behaviours of the refugee/asylum seeker—are they confused, quiet, subservient, angry?

- How the spaces, regulations and routines of where the refugee/asylum seeker lives might impact behaviours and mood during interactions.

- How the refugee is experiencing difference; think about their norms and how their current situation differs from these.

- How they are experiencing: autonomy, adjustment, assimilation, identification, inclusion, community.

Working in a multi-disciplinary team, professionals need to think critically about how they work with their colleagues and how well they function as a team. When being critical across disciplines, the wellbeing of the refugee remains the central focus. Colleagues' behaviour should be considered in the context of their disciplinary background, experience, professional bias, and expertise. It is important to appreciate the different perspective they bring to any situation so that mutual understanding of the problem can be found. Future interactions should be planned on the basis of what is learned from critical reflection on collaboration.

The environment beyond that of the immediate setting in which an event took place can impact the behaviours and activities within the micro level setting. Cognizance of and reflection on wider contexts in which services operate can assist more meaningful problem solving and future planning. Potential factors to consider at these levels are displayed in Figure 7.2.

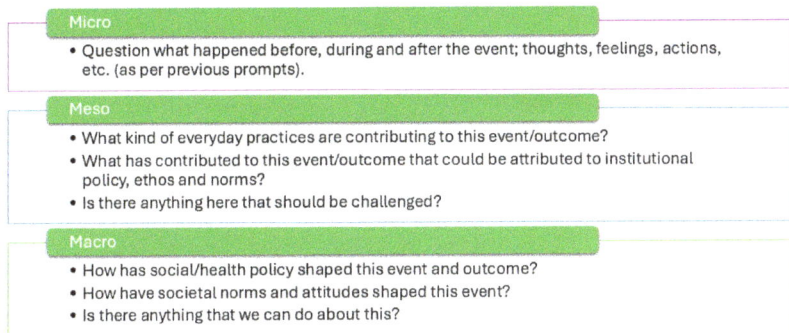

Fig. 7.2 Critical reflection at micro to macro levels.

Below there is a suggested activity to practice critical reflective writing related to interactions with a service user who has refugee experience.

Critical reflection activity:

Use your reflective writing skills to describe and critically appraise how a person from a refugee community might experience your health/ social care work setting. Select three events (points of contact by the person with your work setting), ideally ones in which you were present.

Appraise each event in turn by:

1. Explaining the context of the events, providing an objective account of each,

2. Identifying your thoughts, feelings & behaviours,

3. Recognizing multiple perspectives & influence of cultural factors,

4. Evaluating the learning you have gained,

5. Considering what might be done differently or repeated in the future.

Remember:

Ask yourself questions as you reflect that challenge your values, beliefs, and habitual ways of thinking and behaving.

Be succinct. Use writing to help you decipher your learning but synopsize this before including it in your reflective report.

Conclusion

This chapter has outlined two important practices that health and social care professionals can implement to ensure quality in their practice and to improve the services that they deliver. Through critical reflection on their experiences of working with people with refugee experience, professionals can become aware of areas that work well, in addition to those where further development is needed. Taking an evidence-informed approach enables the individual service user's unique experiences, conditions, goals, and preferences to be taken into account when delivering and planning care. Integrating these approaches into their practice can help to ensure that health and social care professionals are able to strive to deliver optimal care for people with refugee experience.

References

American Psychological Association, Presidential Task Force on Evidence-Based Practice. 2006. 'Evidence-based practice in psychology', *American Psychologist*, 61.4: 271–285, https://doi.org/10.1037/0003-066X.61.4.271

André, Beate, Anne G. Aune, and Jorunn A. Brænd. 2016. 'Embedding evidence-based practice among nursing undergraduates: results from a pilot study', *Nurse Education in Practice*, 18: 30–35, https://doi.org/10.1016/j.nepr.2016.03.004

Asgary, Ramin, and Nora Segar. 2011. 'Barriers to health care access among refugee asylum seekers', *Journal of Health Care for the Poor and Underserved*, 22.2: 506–522, https://doi.org/10.1353/hpu.2011.0047

Best, Stephanie, and Sharon Williams. 2019. 'Professional identity in interprofessional teams: findings from a scoping review', *Journal of Interprofessional Care*, 33.2: 170–181, https://doi.org/10.1080/13561820.2018.1536040

Binyamin, Galy. 2017. 'Growing from Dilemmas: Developing a Professional Identity through Collaborative Reflections on Relational Dilemmas with Role Partners', *Israeli J Occup Ther*, 26.1.

Börjesson, Ulrika, Elisabet Cedersund, and Staffan Bengtsson. 2015. 'Reflection in action: Implications for care work', *Reflective Practice*, 16.2: 285–295, https://doi.org/10.1080/14623943.2015.1023275

Brangan, Joan, Sarah Quinn, and Michelle Spirtos. 2015. 'Impact of an evidence-based practice course on occupational therapist's confidence levels and goals', *Occupational Therapy in Health Care*, 29.1: 27–38, https://doi.org/10.3109/07380577.2014.968943

Brookfield, Stephen. 1995. *Becoming a Critically Reflective Teacher* (San Francisco: Jossey-Bass).

Brooks, Michelle. 2019. 'The importance of using reflective practice when working with refugees, asylum seekers and survivors of torture within IAPT', *The Cognitive Behaviour Therapist*, 12: e16, https://doi.org/10.1017/S1754470X19000023

Cruess, Sylvia R., Richard L. Cruess, and Yvonne Steinert. 2019. 'Supporting the development of a professional identity: general principles', *Medical Teacher*, 41.6: 641–649, https://doi.org/10.1080/0142159X.2018.1536260

Davis, Huw T. O., Sandra Nutley, and Peter C. Smith. 2000. *What Works? Evidence-based Policy and Practice in Public Services* (London: Policy Press).

Désilets, Valérie, et al. 2021. 'Reflecting on professional identity in undergraduate medical education: implementation of a novel longitudinal course', *Perspectives on Medical Education*, 11: 1–5, https://doi.org/10.1007/s40037-021-00649-w

Eaton, Colette. 2016. '"I don't get it"—The challenge of teaching reflective practice to health and care practitioners', *Reflective Practice*, 17.2: 159–166, https://doi.org/10.1080/14623943.2016.1145582

Englund, Ann-Charlotte Dalheim, and Ingela Rydström. 2012. '"I Have to Turn Myself Inside Out": Caring for Immigrant Families of Children With Asthma', *Clinical Nursing Research*, 21.2: 224–242, https://doi.org/10.1177/1054773812438915

Epstein, Irwin. 2009. 'Promoting harmony where there is commonly conflict: Evidence-informed practice as an integrative strategy', *Social Work in Health Care*, 48.3: 216–231, https://doi.org/10.1080/00981380802589845

Evans, David. 2003. 'Hierarchy of evidence: a framework for ranking evidence evaluating healthcare interventions', *Journal of Clinical Nursing*, 12.1: 77–84, https://doi.org/10.1046/j.1365-2702.2003.00662.x

Gabbay, John, et al. 2003. 'A Case Study of Knowledge Management in Multiagency Consumer-Informed "Communities of Practice": Implications for Evidence-Based Policy Development in Health and Social Services', *Health*, 7.3: 283–310, https://doi.org/10.1177/1363459303007003003

Gambrill, Eileen. 2007. 'Transparency as the route to evidence-informed professional education', *Research on Social Work Practice*, 17.5: 553–560, https://doi.org/10.1177/1049731507300149

Ghanizadeh, Afsaneh. 2017. 'The interplay between reflective thinking, critical thinking, self-monitoring, and academic achievement in higher education', *Higher Education*, 74: 101–114, https://doi.org/10.1007/s10734-016-0031-y

Gibbs, Graham. 1988. *Learning by Doing: A guide to Teaching and Learning Methods* (Oxford: Oxford Further Education Unit).

Harrison, Paula A., and Joan L. Fopma-Loy. 2010. 'Reflective Journal Prompts: A Vehicle for Stimulating Emotional Competence in Nursing,' *Journal of Nursing Education*, 49.11: 644–52, https://doi.org/10.3928/01484834-20100730-07

Ibarra, Herminia. 1999. 'Provisional selves: Experimenting with image and identity in professional adaptation', *Administrative Science Quarterly*, 44.4: 764–791, https://doi.org/10.2307/2667055

Isakson, Brian L., John-Paul Legerski, and Christopher M. Layne. 2015. 'Adapting and Implementing Evidence-Based Interventions for Trauma-Exposed Refugee Youth and Families', *Journal of Contemporary Psychotherapy*, 45.4: 245–53, https://doi.org/10.1007/s10879-015-9304-5

Kelly, Michael P., et al. 2015. 'The Importance of Values in Evidence-Based Medicine,' *BMC Medical Ethics*, 16.1, https://doi.org/10.1186/s12910-015-0063-3

Kinsella, Anne E. 2006. 'Poetic resistance: Juxtaposing personal and professional discursive constructions in a practice context', *Journal of the Canadian Association for Curriculum Studies*, 4.1: 35–49.

Kinsella, Anne E. 2010. 'The Art of Reflective Practice in Health and Social Care: Reflections on the Legacy of Donald Schön', *Reflective Practice*, 11.4: 565–75, https://doi.org/10.1080/14623943.2010.506260

Kolb, David (1984). *Experiential Learning: Experience as the Source of Learning and Development* (Prentice Hall).

Kuipers, Pim, Carolyn Ehrlich, and Sharon Brownie. 2013. 'Responding to Health Care Complexity: Suggestions for Integrated and Interprofessional Workplace Learning', *Journal of Interprofessional Care*, 28.3: 246–48, https://doi.org/10.3109/13561820.2013.821601

Kumah, Elizabeth A., et al. 2019. 'PROTOCOL: Evidence-informed practice versus evidence-based practice educational interventions for improving knowledge, attitudes, understanding, and behavior toward the application of evidence into practice: A comprehensive systematic review of undergraduate students', *Campbell Systematic Reviews*, 15.1–2, https://doi.org/10.1002/cl2.1015

Kumah, Elizabeth A., et al. 2022. 'Evidence-informed vs Evidence-based Practice Educational Interventions for Improving Knowledge, Attitudes, Understanding and Behaviour towards the Application of Evidence into Practice: A Comprehensive Systematic Review of Undergraduate Students', *Campbell Systematic Reviews*, 18.2, https://doi.org/10.1002/cl2.1233

Mackey, Hazel. 2006. '"Do Not Ask Me to Remain the Same": Foucault and the Professional Identities of Occupational Therapists', *Australian Occupational Therapy Journal*, 54.2: 95–102, https://doi.org/10.1111/j.1440-1630.2006.00609.x

Mann, Karen, Jill Gordon, and Anna MacLeod. 2007. 'Reflection and Reflective Practice in Health Professions Education: A Systematic Review', *Advances in Health Sciences Education*, 14.4: 595–621, https://doi.org/10.1007/s10459-007-9090-2

McSherry, Robert, Maine Simmons, and Paddy Pearce. 2002. 'An introduction to evidence-informed nursing', in *Evidence-informed Nursing: A Guide for Clinical Nurses*, ed. by McSherry, Robert, Maine Simmons, and Pamela Abbott (London: Routledge), pp. 1–13.

Metzler, Megan J., and Gerlinde A. Metz. 2010. 'Analyzing the Barriers and Supports of Knowledge Translation Using the PEO Model', *Canadian Journal of Occupational Therapy*, 77.3: 151–58, https://doi.org/10.2182/cjot.2010.77.3.4

Monrouxe, Lynn V. 2016. 'Theoretical insights into the nature and nurture of professional identities' in *Teaching Medical Professionalism: Supporting the Development of a Professional Identity*, ed. by Cruess, Richard L., Sylvia R. Cruess, and Yvonne SteinerT, 2nd edn (Cambridge University Press), p. 37–54.

Morrell, Kevin, and Mark Learmonth. 2015. 'Against Evidence-Based Management, for Management Learning', *Academy of Management Learning and Education*, 14.4: 520–33, https://doi.org/10.5465/amle.2014.0346

Nevo, Isaac, and Vered Slonim-Nevo. 2011. 'The Myth of Evidence-Based Practice: Towards Evidence-Informed Practice', *The British Journal of Social Work*, 41.6: 1176–97, https://doi.org/10.1093/bjsw/bcq149

Ng, Stella L, Elizabeth A Kinsella, Farah Friesen, and Brian Hodges. 2015. 'Reclaiming a Theoretical Orientation to Reflection in Medical Education Research: A Critical Narrative Review', *Medical Education*, 49.5: 461–75, https://doi.org/10.1111/medu.12680

Poole, Claire, and Aileen Patterson. 2021. 'Fostering the Development of Professional Identity within Healthcare Education-Interdisciplinary Innovation', *Journal of Medical Imaging and Radiation Sciences*, 52.4: S45–50, https://doi.org/10.1016/j.jmir.2021.08.012

Porter, Judi, and Anita Wilton. 2019. 'Professional identity of allied health staff', *Journal of Allied Health*, 48.1: 11–17.

Richard, Amélie, Mathieu Gagnon, and Emmanuelle Careau. 2018. 'Using Reflective Practice in Interprofessional Education and Practice: A Realist Review of Its Characteristics and Effectiveness', *Journal of Interprofessional Care*, 33.5: 424–36, https://doi.org/10.1080/13561820.2018.1551867

Rycroft-Malone, Jo. 2005. 'Getting Evidence into Practice: A Contact Sport', *Worldviews Evidence Based Nursing*, 2.1: 1–3, https://doi.org/10.1111/j.1524-475x.2005.04090.x

Rycroft-Malone, Jo. 2008. 'Evidence-Informed Practice: From Individual to Context', *Journal of Nursing Management*, 16.4: 404–8, https://doi.org/10.1111/j.1365-2834.2008.00859.x

Sackett, David L, et al. 1996. 'Evidence Based Medicine: What It Is and What It Isn't', *BMJ*, 312.7023: 71–72, https://doi.org/10.1136/bmj.312.7023.71

Schön, Donald. 1991. *The Reflective Turn: Case Studies in and on Educational Practice* (New York: Teachers College Press).

Szajna, Amy, and Julia Ward. 2014. 'Access to Health Care by Refugees: A Dimensional Analysis', *Nursing Forum*, 50.2: 83–89, https://doi.org/10.1111/nuf.12051

Taylor, Clare M. 2007. *Evidence-based Practice for Occupational Therapists*, 2nd edn (Oxford: Blackwell Publishing).

Tickle-Degnen, Linda, and Gary Bedell. 2003. 'Heterarchy and Hierarchy: A Critical Appraisal of the "Levels of Evidence" as a Tool for Clinical Decision Making', *American Journal of Occupational Therapy*, 57.2: 234–37, https://doi.org/10.5014/ajot.57.2.234

Wald, Hedy S. 2015. 'Refining a Definition of Reflection for the Being as Well as Doing the Work of a Physician', *Medical Teacher*, 37.7: 696–99, https://doi.org/10.3109/0142159x.2015.1029897

World Health Organization. 2010. *Framework for Action on Interprofessional Education & Collaborative Practice* (Geneva, Switzerland: WHO), https://www.who.int/publications/i/item/framework-for-action-on-interprofessional-education-collaborative-practice

8. Engagement and Disengagement: Reflecting on the Challenges for Professionals in Supporting Those Seeking Refuge

Fintan Sheerin

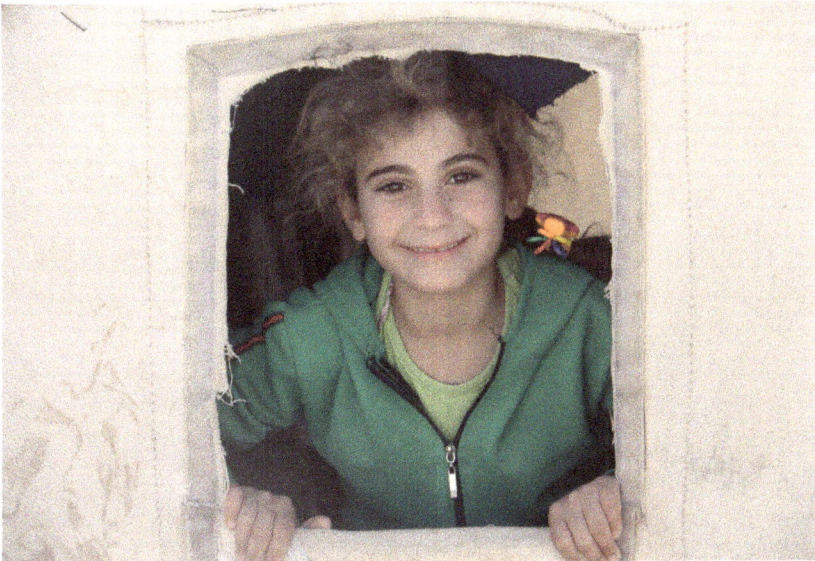

© Independent Doctors Association, CC BY.

  https://doi.org/10.11647/OBP.0479.08

Introduction

Human engagement is fundamental to the knowing of others and to providing a basis for true solidarity. Paulo Freire (1993) in his famous book, *Pedagogy of the Oppressed*, noted that such engagement supports one to enter into the reality of the other person, the revelation of which compels the two individuals to work together in social action to achieve real change.

Throughout my 40 years as a health professional, I too have come to understand human engagement as being key to the achievement of de-marginalisation and to building the important links upon which community and community action are premised. In this chapter I will explore human engagement, drawing from my own experiences of working with people across diverse settings, and reflect on what I have gleaned from the writings of others. I will consider the factors that cause distance between people and thus contribute to disengagement, particularly in the context of professional practice, and I will explore how these may contribute to the attitudinal and, ultimately, physical displacement of devalued people. Moreover, I will contextualize the relationship between disengagement and displacement as an oppressive one and propose an approach to achieving true engagement.

Background

Social interactions are, by their very essence, formative and play a significant part in how we become the people we are. This was alluded to Imogene King's General Systems Model—an early theoretical model of nursing (Aggleton & Chalmers 2000)—in which she described the importance of the interactions that take place between individuals' personal systems. Hildegard Peplau developed this further, proposing that our self-systems develop through interactions with others, and that the nature of these interactions, whether positive or negative, can significantly influence our emotional growth (ibid). Professional development is not immune to this and perhaps incorporates even more structured and formative processes, which are designed to ensure that new initiates are properly socialized and moulded into the idealized professional personage. This process involves control, training, internalisation of social mores, transfer of the formal professional knowledge, redefinition of one's self-identity, and development of a sense of belonging (Freidson 1975: 1986). So, from a professional context, distance and displacement appear to be embedded in the modelling process that is central to professional development and identity. When considering this, I like to reflect on my own professional development.

My background has exposed me to some strongly formative processes. Having finished secondary school in 1982, I embarked on the crucial years of my young adulthood by entering a Roman Catholic seminary. I visualized myself, dressed in the uniform of the priesthood, travelling as a missionary to countries in Africa, Asia, and South America. As a novice, I had to leave my family and be 'adopted' into my new religious one. From the outset, the day was structured around religious services and prayer, with educational sessions focused on the history of the religious order and Christian spirituality. Contact with others from outside that way of life was very limited, particularly with family, and was largely by way of written letters, with no home visits permitted. It was a hugely significant time for me, an impressionable young person, yet a period that I look back on fondly. Over the 18 months or so that I spent in the seminary, I became aware of forces that were starting to mould me into a religious student and, through that, a priest. Religious orders call this process 'formation'. It is mediated through the use of controlled environments, development of a sense of belonging and uniformity, a rules-based pattern of life, and the instilling of associated mores. Bit by bit, my group of theretofore fun-loving young men started to walk, talk, and act like priests. It was fascinating! In many ways, I counted myself lucky to get out before any such changes happened to me, though, interestingly, despite this being more than 40 years ago, people still tell me that I remind them of a priest. Despite my reticence towards being formed, it is interesting that I quickly drifted into another career where I did undergo formation, this time as an intellectual disability nurse. I learned to walk, talk, and act as a nurse. I even wore the uniform!

The formation of professionals such as nurses, primary teachers and clerics is particularly stringent. It is based on the inculcation of a very particular body of knowledge which is carefully bounded such that it affirms the role, position, and activities of the professional (Illich et al.

1977). I have elsewhere referred to the function of "subjectivised" and "objectivised formation" in this regard (Sheerin 2019). Professional formation develops the initiate's self-image as a professional in their relationship with others, through the use of associated symbols and uniforms. These, in turn, help to mould other people's expectations and beliefs about the individual as a professional, contextualizing instances of interaction between professionals and those who are the focus of their expertise. In doing so, formation creates the development of distance between professionals and other people, particularly those who are the recipients of their service. Engagement is, therefore, limited and is for the purpose of providing a service; in this it protects the identity and privileged position of the profession. This result has a number of potential implications for how we see those whom we serve (Figure 8.1).

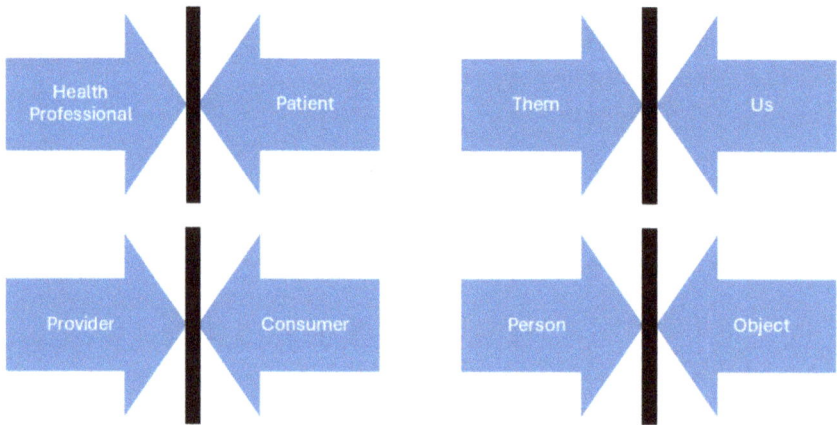

Fig. 8.1 Creating distance.

Breaking Out of the Mould

I worked in nursing clinical practice for about 20 years before I started to realize the role that formation had played in my professional and personal life. As is the case for many people, work, mortgage, and other responsibilities increase through early adulthood and into middle age. I pursued further education for many years, whilst working full-time and seeing our family grow. It was only when I started to broaden my own understanding through exposure to critical theory that I started to understand how the above processes had potentially left me uncritical and supportive of a status quo that was inherently oppressive to those who were in receipt of my service. There have been a number of key theorists who have provided me with diverse lenses through which I have examined my role. These include Paulo Freire (1993), Albert Memmi (1990), Ivan Illich (1977), Franz Fanon (2008), Jon Sobrino (2008), Iris Young (1990), amongst others. As I read these, I wondered if I could have been one of Friere's (1993) "unwitting oppressors", Young's (1990) "well-meaning people", Memmi's (1990) "colonialists" or a provider of charity (Sobrino 2008), absolving society of its responsibilities. Moments such as these are terribly unsettling and whilst they do not present truth in its fulness, they do provide new perspectives on what may in fact be true. For me, it meant that I needed to seek further perspectives on oppression, including those from outside of my professional area. As part of this ongoing journey, I have had the opportunity to travel to parts of sub-Saharan Africa to work with people living in rural communities and have spent time assisting in refugee camps across Europe. These have afforded me insights into the realities of inequity and inequality and have particularly highlighted for me the importance of redressing the distance that typically exists between the providers and recipients of human service. They have reinforced for me a belief that dehumanisation and oppression are key mediators of disengagement in the realities of many devalued people across the world, and that these must be addressed if there is to be any hope of their material realities changing

In the remainder of this chapter, I will focus particularly on my experiences in refugee camps and how that has informed my understanding of human engagement.

Human Displacement in Situations of Migration

For a number of years, I had been travelling to Malawi as part of a Canadian Irish initiative to work collaboratively with a rural community and to support their efforts to develop sustainable health and educational resources. While this work was happening throughout the year, I travelled for about six weeks each summer to spend time living with the community. The poverty experienced there meant that many people had travelled to South Africa to try and find work so that they could send money back to their families. This was typical of the migration that is evident across many parts of sub-Saharan Africa. It is also typical of the realities of migration across the world, and there are many major routes along which people travel, seeking to escape from war, persecution, and poverty. These routes are not new, and others are often oblivious to this migration unless specific drivers lead to an increase in activity along these paths.

Around 2015, events along part of the Eastern Mediterranean Sea route made their way onto news channels and into the consciousness of Europeans. The news item related to the tragic drownings of people who had attempted to cross the Aegean Sea from Turkey to the Greek islands. An image was shown of the body of a three-year old child, washed up on a Turkish beach. For some reason this awoke people to the events that were happening on Europe's doorstep, whereby large numbers of people were making treacherous journeys, with many dying along the way. We also became aware of the fact that those who had safely reached Europe often ended up spending extended periods in makeshift refugee camps, on the Italian or Greek islands, along the Balkan route, or along the northern coasts of France and Belgium. In response to this, volunteer groups from across the European region became active in seeking to meet the needs of these people, needs that were not being met by governments or other agencies. This also happened in Ireland, leading to a convoy of aid and volunteers travelling to Calais to offer support. This was my first encounter with this issue, and I led the health team during their week-long action. Thereafter, I travelled to Lesbos to assist there and throughout the following year I spent a week, almost every month, in Calais working to provide human engagement and healthcare to the many people who were living there. Most recently, in 2023 and 2025, I spent some time working with a non-governmental organisation in Dunkerque, France.

In Chapter 2, we read about the effects of displacement on the health and wellbeing of those seeking refuge and asylum. During my time working in camps, I too witnessed these playing out in the lives of displaced people. This trauma is mediated via a number of oppressive processes which I first proposed in my paper, 'The Cloaked Self.

Professional De-Cloaking and its Implications for Human Engagement in Nursing' (Sheerin 2019). In these, people are: 1) cast as deviants through the use of negatively loaded and stigmatizing language or narratives; 2) forced to exist in marginalized spaces that are distant from those of valued society; 3) congregated together based on their stereotyped deviancy; 4) controlled in all areas of their lives through regulations, which are enforced by police and by the creation of perpetual jeopardy; 5) exposed to violence through the denial of citizen and human rights, dehumanisation, lack of health intervention, heavy-handed control (including physical violence), and denial of security of the person in the face of anti-immigrant aggression; 6) isolated from engagement with others who might offer support and solidarity; and 7) made passive and obedient through the denial of voice and imposed vulnerability (Wolfensberger 1972; Young 1990; Memmi 1990; Kurtz et al. 2008).

It can only be imagined how these processes play out for individuals, but I can still see the faces of particular people which give insight. During my time in Lesbos, I recall sitting with an older woman who had just been assisted from an over-filled inflatable dingy, her terrible night-time journey across the Aegean Sea over. She sat on a rock, looking back forlornly towards Turkey and beyond to her homeland. My reading of the look on her face was one of loss; her life was back there and not in the direction of Europe. This was unlike those of the younger people, who, bolstered by their success in crossing mountains and the sea, could now look forward with energy and enthusiasm to the final part of their journey, with the hope of a new life.

Unfortunately, the realities of camps such as the Calais Jungle lay ahead. The journey would also involve further exposure to individuals who would seek to make a profit from their misfortune and others who would prey on them out of racism and hatred. Practically every person I met in the camps had experienced this and some had been badly beaten by gangs, whereas others had received head injuries and broken bones at the hands of those who are supposed to protect us from harm, the police. It was clear that these people were, however, non-people, non-citizens, and not privy to the protection or services normally afforded human beings in Europe. I witnessed this in the refusal of hospitals to treat people from the camps and the lack of interest of social services in the sexual abuse of displaced children which we reported to them. Instead, it was begrudgingly left to volunteers such as me to treat wounds using donated supplies and offer whatever humanizing engagement I could. One gentleman in the Calais camp presented himself at our caravan and asked to see me alone. He had travelled from Afghanistan and was feeble and emaciated. He spoke no English and I spoke neither Dari nor Pashto. As he removed his shirt, I noticed the stains of infected wounds on his vest. I gently removed this to reveal eight circular burn wounds on his back, systematically applied in two rows of four. As a nurse, I was able to clean and dress the wounds, but I do not have the skills needed to support someone who has experienced torture. All we could do was sit together, hold each other, and cry. There was no service for this man whose physical wounds were likely nothing compared to his emotional and psychological ones. More recently, in Dunkerque, I supported a man who clearly had mental health concerns and was expressing suicidal ideation. Both I and the volunteering doctor agreed that he desperately needed skilled support. We referred him to the local emergency department where he was prescribed paracetamol and send back to the 'camp' located among the bushes in the industrial wasteland near the coast.

Stepping into the Breach

I could recount many more instances such as those above, but I would prefer to focus now on what I have learned about human engagement and to consider its potential as part of the response to such oppressive realities. Throughout my career as a nurse, I have been present with people during life-changing situations. During six years of work in a spinal injury unit, I sat with many (particularly young) people who were coming to terms with the fact that they had just lost significant physical function through paralysis. I have learned the importance of "being present" with people (Fahlberg & Roush 2016) and so, have often cried with my patients. This is a recognized nursing intervention but is often not given the importance it deserves. It was this that informed me in my response to the gentleman with the torture wounds. I have also been present with many people as they have approached death and have tried to support them along what, for many people, is a journey to another reality. The death of another person is a moment of intense meaning and should, wherever possible, be marked by humanizing presence and sensitivity. While these clinical situations may seem markedly different to the realities outlined earlier in this chapter, they are all hugely significant parts of the human journey and amenable to the benefit of human engagement. It may be useful, at this point, to provide a definition of what I mean by 'human engagement'.

I understand human engagement in these contexts to refer to the coming together of two human beings such that each has the potential to know the other person, their happiness, their pain, their hopes and their fears. Willis et al. (2008) allude to this as they describe humanisation as a function of engaging in the knowing of each other's experiences. For such knowing to take place, it is necessary to recognize the things that create distance and to cast these aside. Thus, we need to understand that professional roles, power relationships, and the like, get in the way of human engagement and must be divested. Freire (1993) considers that this level of knowing is such that one becomes aware of the other person's reality and in doing so creates the potential for the two individuals to be solidary together. He continues that solidarity, if valid, must lead to the compulsion to work with the other person to see their reality change for the better. Sobrino (1988) describes this as seeing things as they really are. When I referred to my own awakening in the light of critical literature and the ensuing change, there was, as I noted, an awareness of having played a role, through passivity, in maintaining the realities of people with intellectual disabilities. Part of seeing things as they really are requires one to examine one's own role in the other person's reality. This may be particularly pertinent in respect of our action or inaction with regard to people who have been displaced. Young (1990) notes how oppression is often the result of well-intentioned, liberal people, going through their everyday existence, simply doing their jobs or living their lives, often unconscious and unquestioning, blinkered to the realities of how their indifference and choices affect the lives of others. The knowing of the other person brings with it a knowing of ourselves and should drive us to move away from the negative rhetoric about, and demonization of displaced people and instead focus on their innate humanity.

Sobrino (1988) and Freire (1993) propose that solidarity must lead to solidary or participatory action whereby people stand together and fight for justice and rights. This does not entail speaking for the other person but ensuring that their valid voice is heard and that this becomes the main factor in directing and changing the course of their lives (Figure 8.3). My experience of such participatory action is that the resultant change is usually not confined to one person but instead often leads to pervasive change in the realities of both people, something alluded to in the words of the murdered Jesuit philosopher, Ignacio Ellacuría (1989), who asserted that we can "...reverse history, subvert it, and move it in a difference direction."

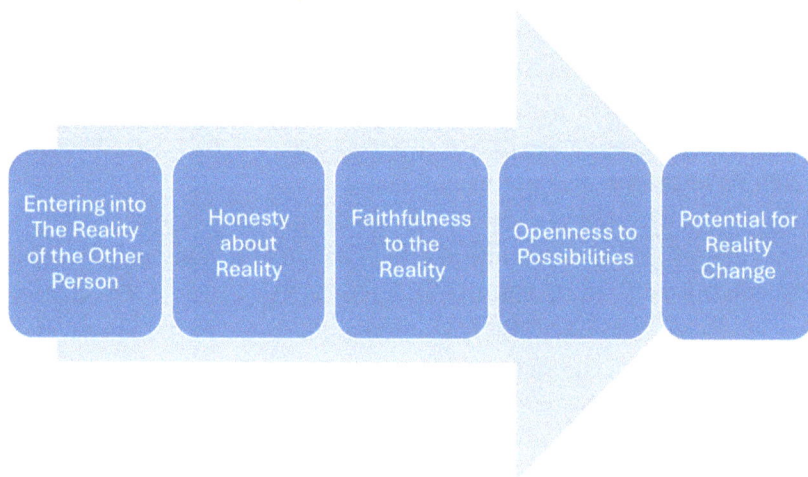

Fig. 8.2 Dialogic engagement and change.

To summarise, I argue that we need to move away from titles and constructions of power and to divest ourselves of positions that create distance between us and our fellow human beings. In situations such as those presented by the realities of human displacement, we must enter into engagement as humans, as citizens of diversity, ready to work alongside our fellow humans both within and towards the dissolution of the margin that displaced people find themselves in, but also within and towards the removal of the (particularly Global North–Global South) inequity upon which many of the reasons for human displacement are premised.

Conclusion

Oppression is highly institutionalized and embedded in the formal and informal processes and protocols that govern our interactions with other human beings, particularly those who have been pre-contextualized in terms of their perceived value and situation of powerlessness. Young (1990: 41) suggests that the pervading manifestation of oppression in recent decades has been that which has become structured in the "unconscious assumptions and reactions of well-meaning people in ordinary interactions". This has the potential to stymie critical reflection and questioning, something that in turn maintains inequality and exclusion. Illich et al. (1977) would propose that this is inherently advantageous in the context of professional practice, in sustaining the privileged position of power held by professional people. In this chapter, I have explored these processes in the context of my own professional and human engagements with people who have found themselves displaced as they seek refuge from varying situations. It is my contention that the disengagement and distancing experienced by these people, and by other marginalized groups, can be subverted by engagement activities that are grounded in humanisation, solidarity, and inclusion.

References

Aggleton, Peter and Helen Chalmers. 2000. *Nursing Models and Nursing Practice, 2nd edn* (London: Macmillan Press Ltd).

Ellacuría, Ignacio. 1989. 'El desafío de las mayorías pobres', *Estudios Centroamericanos*, 493-494.

Fahlberg Beth and Tom Roush. 2016. 'Mindful presence: Being "with" in our nursing care', *Nursing*, 46.3: 14–15, https://doi.org/10.1097/01.NURSE.0000480605.60511.09

Fanon, Frantz. 2008. *Black Skin, White Masks* (London: Pluto Press).

Freidson, Eliot. 1975. *Doctoring Together* (Chicago: University of Chicago Press).

Freidson, Eliot. 1986. *Professional Powers* (Chicago: Chicago University Press).

Freire, Paulo. 1993. *Pedagogy of the Oppressed* (London: Penguin Books).

Illich, Ivan et al. 1977. *Disabling Professions* (London: Marion Boyars), pp. 11–40.

Kurtz, Donna et al. 2008. 'Silencing of voice: an act of structural violence', *Journal of Aboriginal Health,* 4.1: 53–63, https://doi.org/10.18357/ijih41200812315

Memmi, Albert (1990) *The Colonizer and the Colonized* (London: Earthscan Publications).

Sheerin, Fintan. 2019. 'The Cloaked Self: Professional de-cloaking and its implications for human engagement in nursing', *International Journal of Nursing Knowledge,* 30.2: 99–105, https://doi.org/10.1111/2047-3095.12211

Sobrino, Jon. 2008. *The Eye of the Needle: No Salvation Outside the Poor* (London: Darton, Longman and Todd).

Willis, Danny G., Pamela J. Grace and Callista Roy. 2008. 'A central unifying focus for the discipline: facilitating humanization, meaning, choice, quality of life, and healing in living and dying', *Advances in Nursing Science,* 31.1: E28–E40, https://doi.org/10.1097/01.ANS.0000311534.04059.d9

Wolfensberger, Wolf. 1972. *The Principle of Normalization in Human Services* (Toronto: NIMR).

Young, Iris M. 1990. *'Five Faces of Oppression', Justice and the Politics of Difference* (Princeton: Princeton University Press), pp. 39–65, https://doi.org/10.2307/j.ctvcm4g4q

9. Ethical Practice and Personal Conduct in Refugee Health

Sandra Schiller

This chapter explores the principles and values that underpin ethical practice and personal conduct in interprofessional health and social care, particularly in relation to refugee health. The importance of a shared ethical framework for effective interprofessional collaboration is emphasized and the ethical dimensions of refugee health are discussed by looking at the social determinants of health, the role of critical awareness, and a human-rights-based approach. This chapter addresses the healthcare needs of persons with refugee experience and the problems they face within the scope of an ethical framework. It also discusses a capabilities approach to refugee health from an ethical perspective and explores ethical principles relevant in research involving persons with refugee experience. The final section considers how individual behaviour and professionalism contribute to effective teamwork and overall ethical practice in refugee health.

Values and Ethics in Interprofessional Health and Social Care

In a pluralistic society, recognizing different perspectives and values when working with people and considering these in therapeutic decisions is crucial. When patients and health and social care professionals come from diverse backgrounds and might not agree on a common set of values (Black & Wells 2007), the challenge is to engage in a collaborative development process. This requires an attitude of recognizing both

 https://doi.org/10.11647/OBP.0479.09

differences and similarities between healthcare professional and patient. Respect for diversity particularly involves: being sensitive to one's own knowledge gaps and avoiding assumptions based on one's own personal attitudes and behaviour; being willing to explore the other person's perspective first; and being capable of recognizing and resolving value conflicts collaboratively (Schiller 2018).

While adherence to ethical standards has traditionally been viewed as a characteristic of individual health and social care professions, the rise of team-based approaches in 21st-century healthcare delivery necessitates interprofessional discussions on values and ethics among the diverse professions that have many different roles and responsibilities in this field (Thistlethwaite 2012). This involves paying attention to and understanding the values of both patients and colleagues, which stem from their individual professional identity, cultural background, and/or personal experiences, in order to minimize the likelihood of miscommunication. In the context of refugee health, professionals from diverse cultural backgrounds can facilitate culturally sensitive care (Thistlethwaite 2012). However, it remains essential for professionals and institutions to be mindful of not stereotyping individuals. McAuliffe (2022: 22) warns of the dangers of ethically illiterate teams or team members jeopardizing the provision of quality care to vulnerable people: "If a group of people working together do not understand client rights, informed consent, implications of privacy and confidentiality, how to treat people with respect and encourage self-determination and autonomy, or if there are unclear boundaries around professional relationships, harm can be caused".

The assertion of health and social care professionals as a moral community is based on the notion that they have a joint obligation to work collaboratively, aiming to reach a shared understanding of how to collectively maximize health outcomes for their patients. Efforts to establish a collaborative value structure as a foundation for cohesive healthcare teams rely on the following key approaches to interprofessional healthcare ethics: virtues shared by different professions, cooperation to uphold healthcare as a right, and relationships rooted in values (Corr 2019). In this context, the impact of organisational structures and culture on professional relationships also needs to be taken into consideration. Values-based health and social care practice, which attempts to take into account the perspectives of all involved parties, has been developed as a complementary approach to evidence-based practice (discussed in Chapter 7)—taken together, both approaches lead to learning about the values and facts relevant to a situation (Seedhouse 2005). Using the principles of values and values-based practice in interprofessional education has been considered a useful way to contribute to person centred collaborative care (Merriman et al. 2020).

The concepts of human rights and social justice have gained increasing attention in health and social care in recent decades, providing a specific focus for interprofessional ethics—particularly in refugee health. Human-rights-based approaches focus on the rights of the individual and/or group in healthcare, which means that professionals need to know what these rights entail and need to be willing to support people fighting for them (McAuliffe 2022). The Human Rights Act 1998 that came into force in October 2000 incorporates most of the rights protected under the European Convention on Human Rights (ECHR). According to Curtice & Exworthy (2010), the development of "a bottom-up human rights-based approach" available to organisations and the professionals working within them to support their everyday practice, was seen as a useful way of addressing the widespread lack of knowledge and understanding of the relevance of this legislation among patient and carer groups, health professionals, and health management. In essence, the idea is to protect human rights in clinical and organisational practice by adhering to the underlying core values of fairness, respect, equality, dignity, and autonomy (FREDA) as the basics of good clinical care already provided by clinicians on a daily basis.

Self-reflection exercise:

Watch the following video by the Health Information and Quality Authority of the Republic of Ireland as an introduction to FREDA: HIQA: Human Rights in Health and Social Care Services. Available at: https://www.youtube.com/watch?v=9noiJnloIKc

1. Which factors in your own workplace allow you to adhere to these human-rights-based core values? Which factors make this difficult?

2. Is this a bigger challenge when you work with persons with refugee experience?

Working Towards Health Equity and Social Justice: An Ethical Framework for Refugee Health

To emphasize the pursuit of health equity and social justice, an ethical framework for refugee health must be grounded in a comprehensive understanding of the social determinants of health and their impact on individual well-being and illness. This framework necessitates recognizing the design and accessibility of health services for persons with refugee experiences as an imperative of social justice. It also requires healthcare professionals to cultivate critical consciousness and develop the ability to implement a human-rights-based approach in their practice. Additionally, it demands awareness of the unique vulnerabilities faced by persons with refugee experience living in precarious conditions, thereby calling for a tailored ethical framework for healthcare services aimed at this population. Moreover, the potential applicability of a capabilities approach to refugee health should be considered, along with rigorous ethical considerations specific to research in refugee health contexts.

Social Determinants of Health in Migrants and Persons with Refugee Experience

The World Health Organization (2022) emphasizes that persons with refugee experience have a diverse range of physical and mental health needs, originating from experiences in their country of origin, their migration journey, their host country's entry and integration policies, as well as their current living and working conditions. For example, a scoping literature review using the social ecological model (SEM), which considers the individual, interpersonal, organizational, and community levels, showed that refugee women are particularly vulnerable to violence during forced migration leading to a high incidence of post-traumatic stress disorder (Hawkins et al. 2021). It also highlighted concerns about secondary victimization by providers post-resettlement. Social support, often contingent on language skills and difficult to sustain, was identified as crucial in reducing isolation, improving access to healthcare, and enhancing mental health outcomes.

Persons with refugee experience are faced with enormous stressors related to social determinants of health, as they are widely excluded from access to fundamental human rights in a number of essential domains, such as healthcare, housing, education, employment and freedom of movement (WHO 2019). Additionally, migrants and refugees are increasingly exposed to violence and prejudice. In fact, discrimination has been identified as a major stressor and influence on the health of migrants in general and persons with refugee experience in particular. Healthcare systems, institutions, and professionals are strongly influenced by historical, sociopolitical, economic, and legal contexts that facilitate the occurrence of discrimination and racism towards diverse groups of migrants and refugees. International research studies that address the question of how refugees and asylum seekers experience health services have reflected this. For example, respondents expressed the hope of not being disadvantaged because of their background and to be treated equally (Hahn et al. 2020). They emphasized the importance of a friendly and respectful attitude on the part of health professionals, as trust cannot develop without a sense of acceptance (Van Loenen et al. 2018). In particular the fear of stigma makes people with refugee experience afraid to accept medical care (Bahita & Wallace 2007; van Loenen 2018). This is illustrated, for example, by the following quote from the research by Bahtia and Wallace (2007): "Being an asylum seeker... you feel people look at you as if you're not a human being [but] you're something different." It is clear that there is an urgent need for a change in attitude, not only in the health system, but in society as a whole, towards the situation of people with refugee experience.

Key resources:

Professor Melissa Siegel, head of Migration Studies and head of the Migration and Development research section at UNU-MERIT & Maastricht University, has created a refresher overview on the effects of migration on healthcare access and outcomes in destination countries with a particular focus on the migrant themselves: https://www.youtube.com/watch?v=bNY2zGhJ2mQ

To enhance familiarity with the social determinants of health, the video 'What Makes Us Healthy? Understanding the Social Determinants of Health' provides a basic introduction to the topic: https://www.youtube.com/watch?v=8PH4JYfF4Ns

Health Services for Persons with Refugee Experience as a Matter of Social Justice

Culturally responsive interprofessional practice in Refugee Health needs to be seen as a contribution to social justice. The complex circumstances of persons with refugee experience in particular place high demands on professional conduct and necessitate the ability to critically reflect. Critical consciousness and critical reflexivity have become a fundamental ethical guiding principle and a cornerstone of professionalism in health and social care (Campesino 2008; Kinsella & Durocher 2016). Kumagai and Lypson (2009) promote the development of critical consciousness as a framework that situates the health professions in a specific social, cultural, and historical context and thus can help to achieve the provision of high quality, diversity-sensitive health services based on the recognition of the dignity and autonomy of all members of society. Their description of critical consciousness does not only demonstrate the move away from outdated understandings of 'cultural competency' in healthcare, but also illustrates the role of ethics in this context:

> Critical consciousness plays an essential role in these areas of medical education. From a pedagogic perspective, development of true fluency (and not just "competence") in these areas requires critical self-reflection and discourse and anchors a reflective self with others in social and societal interactions. By 'critical self-reflection', we do not mean a singular focus on the self, but a stepping back to understand one's own assumptions, biases, and values, and a shifting of one's gaze from self to others and conditions of injustice in the world. This process, coupled with resultant action, is at the core of the idea of critical consciousness (Kumagai & Lypson 2009).

A (self-)critical, diversity-sensitive professional attitude develops when cultural and diversity dimensions are acknowledged in relation to the lifeworld and habitus of both patients and professionals. Following Freire's (2017) critical education theory as a framework for developing a critical social justice agenda, reflection on action and critical thinking are key aspects of authentic praxis. Critically reflective ethical reasoning, as a contribution to a transformative agenda in refugee health, involves reflecting on how everyday professional actions and interactions maintain or change existing social structures and power relations (e.g., structural racism), and the professional responsibilities that arise from this. Research in higher education pedagogy that develops methodologies to foster such critical attitudes in health and social care professionals is highly relevant to the field of refugee health. The research by Norton and Sliep (2018; 2020), for example, has explored how working reflexively with life stories enhances critical thinking, identity, belonging, and agency. Adopting this approach in refugee health education could facilitate exchanges between students with and without personal experience of forced displacement through iterative processes of deconstructing power in the collective, mapping values and identity, negotiating agency, and rendering accountable performance (Norton & Sliep 2018).

Self-reflection exercise:

1. How has critical consciousness played a role in your own education and professional work?

Human-Rights-Based Approach: A Self-Assessment Tool

Social justice means that everyone's human rights are respected, protected, and promoted. Rights-based care in particular means recognizing the human rights of persons with refugee experience, promoting their dignity, and advocating for their health and wellbeing. The ability for health professionals to work across disciplines is seen as a critical step in promoting health equity based on the principles of diversity and inclusion (Worabo et al. 2022). Collaborating across professions can help to identify and address systemic barriers to care that may be impacting refugees' health and wellbeing, and advocate for policies and programs that support their needs.

The 'Human-Rights-Based Approach: A Self-Assessment Tool' developed by the Scottish Human Rights Commission in 2018 serves as a pioneering guide for organisations seeking to integrate human rights principles into their work. This tool is based on the PANEL principles—participation, accountability, non-discrimination, empowerment, and legality—which together underpin a human-rights-based approach. The primary objective of the tool is to help organisations assess their practices and identify areas for improvement in order to more effectively embed a human-rights-based framework.

A noteworthy aspect of this tool is its diagnostic capability. Organisations are likely to find that some of their practices are already aligned closely with these principles, building on existing strengths. However, the tool also helps to identify gaps, enabling organisations to set priorities and take targeted action. As a dynamic reference point, it allows for continuous monitoring of improvements across different dimensions of the organisation's work. It is essential to recognize that implementing a human-rights-based approach is an ongoing process. The ultimate goal is to achieve full compliance with all the PANEL principles, although it is acknowledged that this is a gradual process. It is available at: www.scottishhumanrights.com

Self-reflection exercise:

1. What does a human-rights-based approach mean for how healthcare institutions are organized and how health professionals need to act in their professional practice?

2. Thinking about the institution where you work or have worked, what actions would be urgently needed to address people with refugee experience?

3. If you work for an institution that is concerned with providing health services to persons with refugee experience, use this tool to check where a human-rights-based approach has already been implemented. How can you embed it more vigorously?

An Ethics Framework for Healthcare Services Provided to Refugees

The health needs of persons with refugee experience and the challenges they encounter with healthcare services need to be addressed within an ethical framework. An example of this is provided by Özdinç (2022). Persons with refugee experience are entitled to the rights and freedoms enshrined in international human rights instruments. At the same time, health professionals need to be aware of the fact that the legal rights and opportunities of people who flee across borders are not the same as those of the citizens of a country. They therefore have an ethical obligation to consider carefully the precarious legal status of these individuals. The situation of displaced persons is often characterized by unequal power relations, as they are dependent on the government, humanitarian donors, and/or service providers for their survival and/or legal status. This extreme dependency can affect their access to healthcare. A number of international ethical frameworks define the assistance provided to persons with refugee experience and guide its implementation. Özdinç (2022) discusses the philosophical foundations of refugee healthcare, including the concepts of rights and human rights, as well as the ethical rules for health aid as defined by the Sphere Project (CHS Alliance et al. 2024), The People in Aid Code of Good Practice (2003), the International Federation of Red Cross and Red Crescent Societies code of conduct (1994), the Core Humanitarian Standard on Quality and Accountability (CHS), and the principles of biomedical ethics (Beauchamp & Childress 2019). The ethical framework that emerges from these foundations leads to the conclusion that when resources are limited, "ethical evaluation should be in reference to health service utilization, regardless of the characteristics of the recipient" (Özdinç 2022: 15). In addition, the principle of justice should be at the forefront of this assessment in order to make ethically justifiable decisions.

Self-reflection exercise:

1. How familiar were you already with the main foundations of an ethical framework for healthcare services provided to refugees? How well do they relate to your own professional ethical framework?

2. Which ethical tensions (e.g., regarding resource allocation) does the article outline?

3. How would you develop an ethical position to substantiate your own professional praxis with the help of this framework?

A Capabilities Approach to Refugee Health

The "capabilities approach" was developed in the 1980s and 1990s by economist Amartya Sen and philosopher Martha Nussbaum, and initially refers to a general theory of social justice. Sen defines the core of the approach as "the possibilities or comprehensive capabilities of people to live a life that they can choose for good reasons and that does not challenge the foundations of their self-respect" (Sen 2000). It is therefore primarily a matter of determining what people need in terms of real freedoms, material, and cultural resources in order to be able to develop an autonomous life plan in a well-founded way and to be empowered to implement this life plan in practice.

Applying this approach to refugee health involves paying attention to the skills and freedoms refugees have or can develop to lead a healthy and dignified life. Professor of Family and Community Medicine, Julie M. Aultman (2019), outlines how the capabilities framework can serve as an ethical basis for understanding and evaluating how the multiple, often interrelated social determinants of health—such as living conditions, education, work status, and social support—affect persons with refugee experience.

Self-reflection exercise:

1. In her commentary on the case narrative, Julie Aultman looks at the general health conditions of resettled refugees and how this is influenced by the social determinants of health they experience. She also considers the recognition or violation of the refugees' rights (pp. 225–226). Can you transfer this analysis to a case of your own and to the healthcare system you work in?

2. According to Aultman (2019): "Part of a social justice analysis also includes identifying avoidable social determinants of health (SDH) that create unfortunate constraints on human capabilities." How is this illustrated in the commentary (pp. 227–228)? Can you apply this to your own case/your own healthcare system?

3. "To contribute to the change that is needed to promote human capabilities and overall patient health, healthcare professionals and organizations need to be advocates for their refugee patients by identifying barriers to care that compromise capabilities such as lack of transportation, health illiteracy, the inability to take time off work, and the high costs of quality care [...]" (Aultman 2019: 228). Can you link this statement to a call for interprofessional collaboration in refugee health?

4. Aultman (2019) sees a general ethical obligation of healthcare professionals and institutions to the community and to society at large and quotes the relevant ethical principles of her own professional association, the American Medical Association (AMA). How do the ethical guidelines of your own profession address this issue?

Research Ethics in Refugee Health

The underlying concern in ethical discourse regarding research in refugee health revolves around the inherent power imbalance that invariably exists between researchers and refugees. This power disparity emerges from the vulnerable position of refugees juxtaposed with the privileged position of researchers. For refugee research participants, this vulnerability often stems from a combination of factors, including restricted mobility, diminished autonomy as they are reliant upon non-governmental organizations, linguistic barriers, uncertain legal status both in the present and future (which increasingly involves potential criminalization), as well as the enduring impact of past and ongoing traumatic experiences. As a consequence, the researcher's approach in terms of planning, preparation, and practical implementation should be shaped in recognition of this power asymmetry and in an attempt to minimize its effects (Deps et al. 2022). Excluding persons with refugee experience from research or public health investigations based on their (perceived) vulnerability is not an option, as it contravenes principles of justice and fairness (Seagle et al. 2020). Research that elevates the voices of persons with refugee experience, rather than excluding them, is urgently needed to inform targeted interventions, validate models of health service delivery, and ultimately contribute to the well-being of individuals affected by displacement (Seagle et al. 2020).

For researchers who participate in European research collaborations in refugee health, it is important to know that there are guidelines available to them. The European Commission published a Guidance Note: Research on Refugees, Asylum Seekers and Migrants in 2021. This document is available at: https://ec.europa.eu/info/funding-tenders/opportunities/docs/2021-2027/horizon/guidance/guidance-note-research-on-refugees-asylum-seekers-migrants_he_en.pdf

Furthermore, there exist frameworks that offer researchers guidance for designing and conducting studies involving persons with refugee experience in a manner that is both respectful and sensitive to the unique challenges these participants often face. For example, the Valuing All Voices Framework, as proposed by Roche et al. (2020), is "a trauma-informed, intersectional and critically reflexive approach to patient and public involvement in health research". It aims to provide a social justice and health equity lens so that research teams can engage patients in health research in a way that enhances safety and inclusivity. The key components of this framework are trust, self-awareness, empathy, and relationship building.

In his critical self-reflexive account of privileged researchers working in refugee camps, social work ethics researcher Neil Bilotta (2021) emphasizes that researchers in forced migration contexts must go beyond procedural research ethics to include relational ethics. While research ethics boards may formally approve research conducted in refugee camps, this alone is insufficient and fails to prepare researchers for the complexities of situational and relational ethics. Furthermore, definitions of 'respect' and 'reciprocity' should be collaboratively determined by researchers and research participants. Following Probst (2015) that reflexivity primarily focuses on the researcher, Bilotta (2021) emphasizes that reflexivity offers limited insight into how research participants perceive power and privilege in a refugee camp. Future empirical research should therefore investigate how respect and reciprocity are understood and implemented from the perspectives of participants with refugee experience. Similarly, Clark-Kazak (2023) highlights the importance of radical care ethics for forced migration research: a radical ethics of care emphasizes reciprocal relationships and requires researchers to critically consider their positionality within power asymmetries. Researchers should shift focus from their own careers to caring *with others* by "amplifying, uplifting and working in solidarity" (Clark-Kazak 2023: 1153), recognizing the interdependence of relationships even in unequal power dynamics. Radical care ethics adopts a "proactive approach to preventing harm" (Clark-Kazak 2023: 1153) by intentionally dismantling harmful power structures within research design, contrasting with the dominant procedural ethics that merely seek to minimize harm. This approach includes integrating (self-) care mechanisms and addressing the differential impacts of research on various participants, such as peer researchers, interpreters, and contract researchers, who often lack secure employment and/or health insurance. Radical care ethics rejects any positivist notion of objectivity and instead values the productive work of emotions performed by all participants in the research process, including gatekeepers, translators/interpreters, and research assistants.

The Importance of Personal Conduct in Interprofessional Refugee Health

The concept of personal conduct—namely, the ethical responsibilities and behaviours of individual health professionals—has its roots in healthcare ethics, serving as a framework and guideline for navigating complex ethical issues by engaging in a process of ethical reasoning and decision-making. Personal conduct influences this process, as health professionals with a strong ethical foundation are more likely to consider the values and rights of patients, respect diversity, and adhere to professional codes of conduct when facing difficult choices (Louw 2016). Consequently, personal conduct is regarded as playing a crucial role in establishing and maintaining patient-provider relationships that are based on prioritizing the patients' needs and dignity. This involves capabilities such as effective communication, active listening, mutual respect, and empathy. Ethical behaviour—including honesty, integrity, and accountability—contributes to building and sustaining trust between health professionals and patients, as well as among members of the interprofessional health and social care team, which has a positive effect on the dynamics of teamwork and the delivery of high-quality care (McAuliffe 2022). Personal conduct and ethically reflected professional practice can also have a positive effect on the behaviour and attitudes of others: Professionals who demonstrate ethical conduct set positive examples can inspire others (students, colleagues, and other health professionals) to uphold high standards of ethics in their professional practice. This is particularly important in the area of refugee health, which requires a professional, empathetic way of dealing with complex situations that can easily lead to the experience of moral distress (Jawed et al. 2021).

Personal conduct is one of the five domains highlighted in the WHO's *Global Competency Standards for Health Workers in Relation to Refugee and Migrant Health* (WHO 2021). This domain encompasses two competency standards: Firstly, it pertains to the individual health professional's commitment to lifelong learning and reflective practice aimed at promoting the health of persons with refugee experience. Secondly, it addresses the responsibility of both organizations and the individual health professionals within them to foster a culture of self-care and mutual support in the context of refugee health (WHO 2021).

Regarding the first competence —commitment to lifelong learning and reflective practice—personal conduct is an essential aspect of culturally sensitive refugee health. Health professionals must recognize their own implicit biases, beliefs, and values, and understand how these may influence healthcare services. They should maintain confidentiality, strive to approach patients with cultural humility and respect, and engage in effective communication to understand patients' experiences and perspectives (Nowak & Hornberg 2023). Health professionals can only contribute to equal healthcare, as advocated by the WHO's call for "health for all", if they adequately recognize patients' needs. Reflective practice is, therefore, a central element of personal conduct.

According to the WHO's (2021: 11) competency standards, such reflective practice includes addressing "the impact of own culture, beliefs, values and biases as well as institutional discrimination on interactions in health-care settings, including by continually adapting practice to respond to the needs of relevant communities". Health professionals are thus encouraged to "contribute to introducing or improving cultural sensitivity in existing practices by modelling appropriate behaviour and avoiding culturally insensitive practices". This necessitates a power-critical and discrimination-sensitive perspective on one's own actions. Professionals must be aware of the power dynamics and the resulting disadvantages and experiences of discrimination for others. The WHO (2021: 11) emphasizes the importance of health professionals demonstrating "awareness of institutional discrimination experienced by refugees and migrants, in particular its impacts on health status". This requires a critical understanding of the "intersections of systems, structures and patterns of power that determine a person's position of disadvantage and impact their access to, and experience of, healthcare" (WHO 2021: 11). To actively counteract discrimination, it is essential to reflect on and, if necessary, consciously unlearn one's own values and beliefs. Health professionals must recognize how they are influenced by their environment, including societal beliefs, institutional practices within the healthcare system or workplace, and beliefs embedded in professional thinking. At the same time, it is important to understand how the patients are shaped by their individual lifeworlds, as this is the basis for a safe relationship and shared decision-making.

However, if the structures of the healthcare system are not adequately established, ethically appropriate and culturally sensitive patient care depends on isolated individual measures. This situation makes it difficult, or even impossible, for health professionals to effectively apply their skills (Peters et al. 2014). Given the increasing prejudices and hostility towards persons with refugee experience across European countries that are fanned and exploited by right-wing and far-right parties and groups, institutional structures should include anti-racist measures. These measures should include mandatory, funded, implicit-bias training for health professionals and the establishment of mandatory reporting channels for experienced or witnessed discrimination, and policies to ensure that perpetrators are held accountable (Stevens et al. 2024).

Personal conduct, as a reflection of the professionalism and integrity of health professionals and the institutions they represent, is particularly important when collaborating with refugee organisations. These organisations are more willing to engage in joint initiatives to address the healthcare needs of persons with refugee experience if they feel confident that health professionals are committed to learning from their expertise.

For the WHO (2021), the domain of "personal conduct" also includes another area of competency: the responsibility of organizations and individual professionals to contribute to a culture of self-care and mutual support in the context of refugee health. Health professionals providing care to persons with refugee experience may be confronted with second-hand exposure to stressful and potentially traumatic events, such as the uncertainty of residence, bureaucratic hurdles, restrictive regulations, and traumatic experiences. Added to this is the great responsibility in this area of work, the high caseload, and the making do with limited resources. As an important competency in personal conduct, health and social care professionals need to be able to recognize and reflect on their own feelings, as working with traumatized people can also lead to the (re)emergence of private issues that need to be addressed separately or situationally (e.g., in supervision, counselling, therapy) (BAfF 2020: 47). Just like trauma workers, health and social care professionals in general who work with persons with refugee experience are susceptible to secondary or vicarious traumatisation and should be attentive to potential signs of stress, which may manifest as feelings of helplessness and hopelessness, changes in beliefs, and distrust of the world as a safe place, but which may also manifest somatically, e.g., as nausea and numbness (Cohen & Collens 2013).

Self-care describes being loving, appreciative, attentive, and compassionate to oneself and taking one's needs seriously (Reddemann 2005). Five primary domains of self-care practice are recognized in the literature: physical, psychological, emotional, spiritual, and professional self-care (Saakvitne & Pearlman 1996). Furthermore, to avoid burnout or secondary traumatisation, health and social care professionals need to consider not only personal factors, i.e., their own ability to cope with stress, but also environmental factors. This means insisting on supportive structural conditions that allow them to do their work as well as possible and to expose and criticize insufficient working environments (BAfF 2020). At the organizational level, the ability to "contribute to a safe and supportive team environment where the emotional and social aspects of providing healthcare to refugees and migrants can be discussed among colleagues" is crucial (WHO 2021: 27). Furthermore, the WHO (2021: 26) points out the potential positive effect that experiences of "professional or personal development and growth can also occur as a result of working with survivors of torture and other traumatic events. Health workers may feel empowered and personally motivated from working alongside refugees and migrants, drawing lessons from their perseverance and determination."

Self-reflection exercise:

1. What are essential elements of personal conduct in your own profession? How did you learn about them?

2. Can you give examples of shared understandings of good personal conduct in specific team settings? How was this understanding reached or how was it communicated to new team members?

3. Which elements of personal conduct required in the area of refugee health do you still need to develop because they have not (yet) received sufficient attention in your own profession?

Conclusion

The realisation that individuals with refugee experience are fundamentally like any other human being, yet have undergone experiences significantly different from those who have not encountered forced migration, underscores an inherent tension. It necessitates a professional approach that counters tendencies of 'othering' in healthcare while remaining compassionate and attentive to the specific needs of persons with refugee backgrounds. This highlights the critical importance of ethical practice and personal conduct in the field of refugee health. Furthermore, interprofessional teams in refugee health often comprise professionals from diverse healthcare backgrounds, including medicine, nursing, social work, allied health, and psychology. In this context, interprofessional values and ethics provide common ground and help to integrate diverse professional perspectives respectfully and collaboratively, promoting holistic and person-centred care for individuals with refugee experience.

Ethical practice and personal conduct should reflect an awareness of the social determinants of health that disproportionately affect persons with refugee experience, who often face complex health and social challenges, including trauma, legal issues, discrimination, lack of participation, and unstable living conditions. It involves striving for equity in access to services and advocating for the rights and needs of persons with refugee experience within healthcare systems. Ultimately, ethical practice and personal conduct in refugee health, focused on human rights and social justice, require continuous education and reflection to foster an environment where individuals with refugee experience feel safe, respected, and supported as they navigate healthcare systems that they often experience as alien and hostile.

References

Aultman, Julie M. 2019. 'How Should Health Care Professionals Address Social Determinants of Refugee Health?', *AMA J Ethics*, 21.3: E223 Justice and the Politics of Difference (Princeton: Princeton University Press), 231, https://doi.org/10.1001/amajethics.2019.223

BAfF (Bundesweite Arbeitsgemeinschaft der psychosozialen Zentren für Flüchtlinge und Folteropfer) [German Association of Psychosocial Centres for Refugees and Victims of Torture]). 2020. e.V., *F.A.Q.: Häufig gestellte Fragen zu Trauma, Flucht und psychosozialer Beratung bzw. Therapie: August 2020* [F.A.Q.: Frequently Asked Questions about Trauma, Flight and Psychosocial Counselling or Therapy: August 2020] (Berlin: Bundesweite Arbeitsgemeinschaft der psychosozialen Zentren für Flüchtlinge und Folteropfer – BafF e.V.), https://www.baff-zentren.org/wp-content/uploads/2020/10/BAfF_FAQ_2020.pdf

Beauchamp, Tom L., and James F. Childress. 2019. *Principles of Biomedical Ethics.* 8th edn (New York, Oxford: Oxford University Press).

Bhatia, Ravi, and Paul Wallace. 2007. 'Experiences of Refugees and Asylum Seekers in General Practice: A Qualitative Study', *BMC Family Practice*, 8.48, https://doi.org/10.1186/1471-2296-8-48

Bilotta, Neil. 2021. 'A Critical Self-Reflexive Account of a Privileged Researcher in a Complicated Setting: Kakuma Refugee Camp', *Research Ethics*, 17.4: 435–447, https://doi.org/10.1177/17470161211037386

Black, Roxie M., and Shirley A. Wells. 2007. *Culture and Occupation: A Model for Empowerment in Occupational Therapy* (Bethesda, Md.: AOTA Press).

Broussard, Grant, et al. 2019. 'Challenges to Ethical Obligations and Humanitarian Principles in Conflict Settings: A Systematic Review', *International Journal of Humanitarian Action*, 4.15, https://doi.org/10.1186/s41018-019-0063-x

Campesino, Maureen. 2008. 'Beyond Transculturalism: Critiques of Cultural Education in Nursing', *Journal of Nursing Education*, 47.7: 298–304, https://doi.org/10.3928/01484834-20080701-02

CHS Alliance, Groupe URD and Sphere Association (2024). *Core Humanitarian Standard on Quality and Accountability (CHS)*. 2nd edn, https://www.corehumanitarianstandard.org/

Clark-Kazak, Christina. 2023. '"Why Care Now" in Forced Migration Research?: Imagining a Radical Feminist Ethics of Care', *ACME: An International Journal for Critical Geographies*, 22.4: 1151–1173, https://doi.org/10.14288/acme.v22i4.2210

Cohen, Keren, and Paula Collens. 2013. 'The Impact of Trauma Work on Trauma Workers: A Metasynthesis on Vicarious trauma and Vicarious Posttraumatic Growth', *Psychological Trauma: Theory, Research, and Policy*, 5.6: 570–80, https://psycnet.apa.org/doi/10.1037/a0030388

Corr, Matthew. 2019. *A Rhetoric and Philosophy of Interprofessional Healthcare Education: Communication Ethics in Action* (Doctoral dissertation, Duquesne University), https://dsc.duq.edu/etd/1759

Curtice, Martin J. and Tim Exworthy. 2010. 'FREDA: A human rights-based approach to healthcare', *The Psychiatrist*, 34.4: 150–156, https://doi.org/10.1192/pb.bp.108.024083

Deps, Patricia D., et al. 2022. 'Ethical Issues in Research with Refugees', *Ethics, Medicine and Public Health*, 24: 100813, https://doi.org/10.1016/j.jemep.2022.100813

European Commission/Directorate-General for Research and Innovation. 2021. *Guidance Note: Research on Refugees, Asylum Seekers and Migrants* (European Commission), https://ec.europa.eu/info/funding-tenders/opportunities/docs/2021-2027/horizon/guidance/guidance-note-research-on-refugees-asylum-seekers-migrants_he_en.pdf

Freire, Paulo. 2017. *Pedagogy of the Oppressed* (London: Penguin Random House).

Hahn, Karoline, Jost Steinhäuser, and Katja Goetz. 2020. 'Equity in Health Care: A Qualitative Study with Refugees, Health Care Professionals, and Administrators in One Region in Germany', *Biomed Research International*, 2020.1: 4647389, https://doi.org/10.1155/2020/4647389

Hawkins, Maren M., et al. 2021. 'Promoting the Health of Refugee Women: A Scoping Literature Review Incorporating the Social Ecological Model', *International Journal for Equity in Health*, 20.45, https://doi.org/10.1186/s12939-021-01387-5

International Federation of Red Cross and Red Crescent Societies. 1994. *Code of Conduct for the International Red Cross and Red Crescent Movement and Non-Governmental Organisations (NGOs) in Disaster Relief* (Geneva: International Federation of Red Cross and Red Crescent Societies), https://www.ifrc.org/document/code-conduct-international-red-cross-and-red-crescent-movement-and-ngos-disaster-relief

Kinsella, Elizabeth A., and Evelyne Durocher. 2016. 'Occupational Justice: Moral Imagination, Critical Reflection, and Political Praxis', *OTJR: Occupation, Participation and Health*, 36.4: 163–166, https://doi.org/10.1177/1539449216669458

Kumagai, Arno K., and Monica L. Lypson. 2009. 'Beyond Cultural Competence: Critical Consciousness, Social Justice, and Multicultural Education', *Academic Medicine*, 84.6: 782–787, https://doi.org/10.1097/ACM.0b013e3181a42398

Jawed, Areeba, et al. 2021. 'High Moral Distress in Clinicians Involved in the Care of Undocumented Immigrants Needing Dialysis in the United States', *Health Equity*, 5.1: 484–492, https://doi.org/10.1089/heq.2020.0114

Louw, Brenda. 2016. 'Cultural Competence and Ethical Decision Making for Health Care Professionals', *Humanities and Social Sciences*, 4.2: 41–52, https://doi.org/10.11648/j.hss.s.2016040201.17

MacFarlane, Anne, et al. 2024. 'Normalising Participatory Health Research Approaches in the WHO European Region for Refugee and Migrant Health: A Paradigm Shift', *The Lancet Regional Health – Europe*, 41: 100837, https://doi.org/10.1016/j.lanepe.2024.100837

McAuliffe, Donna. 2022. *Interprofessional Ethics: Collaboration in the Social, Health and Human Services.* 2nd edn (Cambridge etc.: Cambridge University Press).

Merriman, Clair, et al. 2020. 'Values-based Interprofessional Education: How Interprofessional Education and Values- based Practice Interrelate and Are Vehicles for the Benefit of Patients and Health and Social Care Professionals', *Journal of Interprofessional Care*, 34.4: 569–571, https://doi.org/10.1080/13561820.2020.1713065

Norton, Lynn, and Yvonne Sliep. 2018. 'A Critical Reflexive Model: Working With Life Stories in Health Promotion Education', *South African Journal of Higher Education*, 32.3: 45–63, https://hdl.handle.net/10520/EJC-10047ba5d2

Norton, Lynn and Yvonne Sliep. 2020. 'Performing Life Stories: Hindsight and Foresight for Better Insight', *LEARNing Landscapes Journal*, 13.1: 173–188, https://doi.org/10.36510/learnland.v13i1.1013

Nowak, Anna C., and Claudia Hornberg. 2023. 'Erfahrungen von Menschen mit Fluchtgeschichte bei der Inanspruchnahme der Gesundheitsversorgung in Deutschland: Erkenntnisse einer qualitativen Studie [Experiences of People with Refugee Backgrounds in Utilising Healthcare in Germany: Findings from a Qualitative Study]', *Bundesgesundheitsblatt*, 66: 1117–1125, https://doi.org/10.1007/s00103-022-03614-y

Özdinç, Ahmet. 2022. 'An Ethics Framework for Healthcare Services Provided to Refugees', *TRC Journal of Humanitarian Action*, 1.1: 7–12, https://doi.org/10.55280/trcjha.2022.1.1.0002

People in Aid. 2003. *People in Aid Code of Good Practice in the Management and Support of Aid Personnel* (London: People in Aid, 2003), https://reliefweb.int/report/world/people-aid-code-good-practice-management-and-support-aid-personnel

Probst, Barbara. 2015. 'The Eye Regards Itself: Benefits and Challenges of Reflexivity in Qualitative Social Work Research', *Social Work Research*, 39: 37–48, https://doi.org/10.1093/swr/svu028

Reddemann, Luise, 'Selbstfürsorge' [Self-care] in *Wir: Psychotherapeuten über sich und ihren 'unmöglichen' Beruf* [*We: Psychotherapists about Themselves and Their 'Impossible' Profession*], ed. by Kernberg, Otto F., Birger Dulz, and Jochen Eckert (Stuttgart, New York: Schattauer), pp. 92–101.

Roche, Patricia, et al. 'Valuing All Voices: Refining a Trauma-informed, Intersectional and Critical Reflexive Framework for Patient Engagement in Health Research Using a Qualitative Descriptive Approach', *Research Involvement and Engagement*, 6.42, https://doi.org/10.1186/s40900-020-00217-2

Saakvitne, Karen W., and Laurie A. Pearlman. 1996. *Transforming the Pain* (New York: Norton).

Schiller, Sandra. 2018. 'Ethisches Reasoning und diversitätssensibles Handeln in der Sprachtherapie [Ethical Reasoning and Diversity-sensitive Professional Behaviour in Speech Therapy]', *Sprache–Stimme–Gehör,* 42.03: 127–132, https://doi.org/10.1055/a-0625-5847

Scottish Human Rights Commission (SHRC). 2018. *Human Rights Based Approach: A Self-Assessment Tool* (Edinburgh: Scottish Human Rights Commission), https://www.scottishhumanrights.com/media/1814/shrc_panel_self-assessment_tool_vfinal.pdf

Seagle, Emma E., et al. 2020. 'Research Ethics and Refugee Health: A Review of Reported Considerations and Applications in Published Refugee Health Literature, 2015–2018', *Conflict and Health,* 14.39, https://doi.org/10.1186/s13031-020-00283-z

Seedhouse, David. 2005. *Values-based Decision Making for the Caring Professions* (Chichester: John Wiley & Sons).

Sen, Amartya. 2000. *Development as Freedom* (New York: Anchor Books).

Stevens, Amy J., et al. 2024. 'Discriminatory, Racist and Xenophobic Policies and Practice against Child Refugees, Asylum Seekers and Undocumented Migrants in European Health Systems', *The Lancet,* 41: 100834, https://doi.org/10.1016/j.lanepe.2023.100834

Thistlethwaite, Jill E. 2012. *Values-Based Interprofessional Collaborative Practice: Working Together in Health Care* (Cambridge etc.: Cambridge University Press)

Van Loenen, Tessa, et al. 2018. 'Primary Care for Refugees and Newly Arrived Migrants in Europe: A Qualitative Study on Health Needs, Barriers and Wishes', *European Journal of Public Health,* 28.1: 82–87, https://doi.org/10.1093/eurpub/ckx210

Worabo, Heidi J., et al. 2023. 'Promoting Social Justice through Experiential Learning at an Interprofessional Refugee Clinic', *Nurse Education Today,* 121: 105699, https://doi.org/10.1016/j.nedt.2022.105699

World Health Organization. 2019. *Global action plan on promoting the health of refugees and migrants, 2019–2023: Annex 5 of 72nd World Health Assembly,* Geneva, 20–28 May 2019: Resolutions and Decisions; Annexes, https://www.who.int/publications/i/item/WHA72-2019-REC-1

World Health Organization. 2021. *Refugee and Migrant Health: Global Competency Standards for Health Workers; 2021* (Geneva: World Health Organization), https://www.who.int/publications/i/item/9789240030626

World Health Organization. 2022. 'Refugee and migrant health (Fact Sheet)', https://www.who.int/news-room/fact-sheets/detail/refugee-and-migrant-health

IV. Diversity in Society and in Healthcare

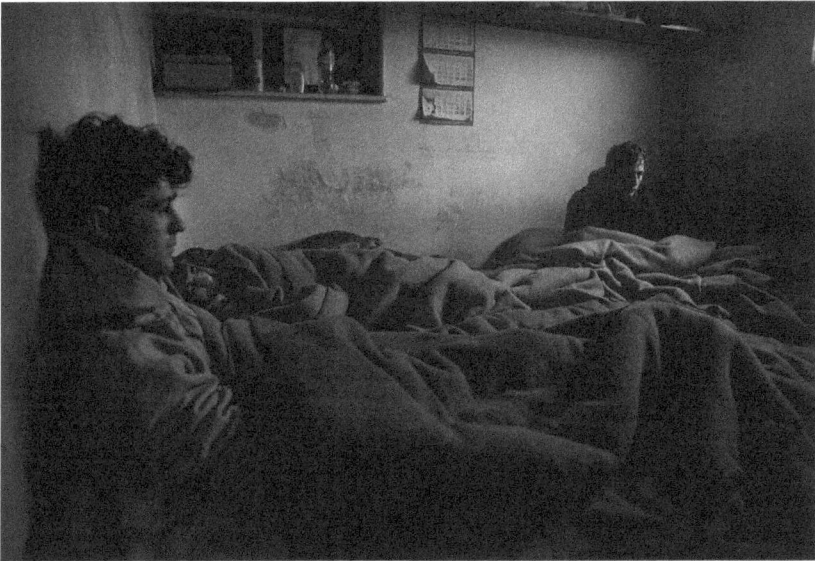

10. Culturally Responsive Practice in Refugee Health

Sandra Schiller with Angelika Roschka and Kathrin Weiß

The health of persons with refugee experience is a multifaceted issue, strongly influenced by culture, diversity, and the principles of health equity. This chapter explores these dimensions by introducing key concepts and providing examples of practical applications in the context of refugee health. The first section introduces the constructivist understanding of culture and shifts the focus from merely understanding cultural nuances to appreciating diversity as a critical component of health equity in a diverse society. To illustrate the practical relevance of this approach, in the following section Angelika Roschka describes the role of occupational therapists in facilitating social inclusion Another important issue is the influence of the cultural backgrounds of both patients and health practitioners on their perceptions and interpretations of illness and pain, which is discussed in the third section of this chapter. Last but not least, the final section integrates international case stories of individuals with refugee experience and case studies on interprofessional practice. This section emphasizes the collaborative efforts required in culturally responsive interprofessional practice to effectively address the health needs of persons with refugee experience. Overall, the chapter aims to outline prerequisites for culturally responsive practice as an essential contribution to a more inclusive and equitable healthcare environment for all.

   https://doi.org/10.11647/OBP.0479.10

Understanding Relevant Concepts: Culture, Diversity and Health Equity

International literature reports that healthcare practitioners sometimes struggle to understand the meaning of culturally responsive practice "due to the perceived complexity and indeterminate nature of the concept of culture" (Minnican & O'Toole 2020). Although culture is a word that is regularly used in everyday language, its exact meaning can be difficult to grasp. Since the term 'culture' is understood very differently in academia depending on the epistemological interests of the authors using it, this chapter starts with an introduction of the constructivist understanding of culture (that originated in the humanities) and the related concepts of diversity and health equity in relation to interprofessional refugee health.

People as Products and Creators of Culture: The Constructivist Understanding of Culture

The outdated positivist (or ethicised) understanding of culture and cultural groups typically equates origin with culture and thus defines people in terms of their (presumed) ethnic, national, or religious origin and affiliation. In this view, cultures are supposedly given entities that can be observed and described, that have clear boundaries to other cultures and that change only slowly. The basic assumption that members of a group share certain characteristics leads to a simplistic description of expected ways that people will think and behave, which hinders the perception of real-life heterogeneity and ambiguities and encourages stereotyping. It also disregards the dynamic processes of human action.

In constructivist theory, cultures are no longer understood as entities to be found in reality, but rather, the 'reality' of culture that we believe we can see and describe in the real world is always also a consequence of how we understand culture. This reflects the epistemological basis of cognitive theory: we socially and culturally, i.e., collectively, generate our reality (see e.g., Williams 1983; Grossberg 1997; Barker & Jane 2016). Such an open, process-, meaning- and practice-oriented concept of culture is interested in the learned patterns of how individuals and groups perceive and interpret the world and how they adapt to it. Worldwide social, political, and economic upheavals and, not least, global migration processes have fundamentally challenged the idea that the world is a mosaic of separate and unchangeable cultures. Current academic debates consequently conceptualize culture within complex, increasingly differentiated and thus highly heterogeneous social contexts.

In health research, a stronger orientation towards the humanities and social sciences, particularly in public health and in the medical and health humanities, has contributed to the realisation that health and illness are not only biological phenomena, but also social constructs that are closely linked to cultural, political, and economic factors and influenced by a specific historical context. In this context, the constructivist understanding of culture refers to a system of beliefs, values, practices, and rules shared by a group and used to interpret experiences as well as behavioural patterns. Culture can thus be described at different levels, including the organizational and group level, e.g., in the context of interprofessional teamwork. According to the constructivist view, culture is something learned, not innate, and, though it may seem persistent, culture is always changing. Since we are all members of different groups, we are all influenced in a unique way by a diversity of cultural backgrounds. Cultures and the people who belong to them are heterogeneous; belonging to a culture does not define the whole person. We all learn culture from many different sources, e.g., parents and other family members, friends and peers, neighbourhood and community members, educational institutions, social institutions, religious affiliations, the media, shared experiences of events, historical traditions, and stories. Consequently, the way in which individuals understand health and illness, and the health/illness behaviour they exhibit as a result, is not only shaped by their language, cultural beliefs, and everyday practices, but also by a range of social and economic factors, by the specific organisation of a healthcare system, and by a person's health literacy, i.e., the ability to understand health and use health services.

From Culture to Diversity: Health Equity in a Diverse Society

Interdisciplinary research on diversity and intersectionality in health has developed, on the one hand, as a response to the effects of transnational migration and globalisation processes. On the other hand, it is the result of human rights concerns raised by social movements such as the Black anti-racism and civil rights movement, the women's and LGBTIQ+ movements, or the disability rights movement, which advocated for the recognition of rights and equal opportunities for various groups within a pluralistic society. This research integrates multiple disciplines, including sociology, psychology, anthropology, medicine, and public health, to analyse the complex interactions between diversity, social structures, and discrimination.

The concept of diversity is an approach to understanding the impact of social categories of difference on the life situations and related experiences of individuals (Pincus & Ellis 2021). These categories may include gender, sexual orientation, ethnicity/'race', religion, socio-economic status, disability, and age. The analysis focuses on the relationships between categories of diversity, social hierarchies of difference, and experiences of discrimination.

Research from a diversity perspective postulates that differences are not inherently given but result from social practices of distinction. Consequently, it aims to explore how certain social categories become categories of difference within existing social power relations influenced, for example, by racism, ethnocentrism (hetero)sexism, classism, and ableism, upon which power hierarchies are built (Mecheril 2008).

The concept of intersectionality (Crenshaw 1989) complements the concept of diversity by highlighting the complex interactions between categories of difference that generate inequality, which can influence and mutually reinforce or alleviate each other (Winker & Degele 2010; Collins & Bilge 2020). For example, a migrant woman with a disability may be subject to multiple forms of discrimination.

Typically, categories of difference are created through binary opposition, i.e., the understanding of a person's social identity and position in society is created through demarcation from the perceived other. In social psychology, social identity develops in "fluid processes of identification with personal characteristics and social groups in the context of normative social and societal power relations" (Lerch 2019: 54). As social power relations are firmly rooted in socialisation processes, they are often taken for granted by members of the socially dominant groups and thus become invisible. For example, "the description and categorisation of people, as it occurs in cross-cultural nursing research and practice, most often takes place from within a White dominant perspective, presented to White audiences, and focuses on description of a non-White or a non-Western group" (Campesino 2008). The term 'othering' refers to the socio-psychological mechanisms by which subjects are constructed, classified, and made visible as others or strangers, while the subject positions of members of dominant social groups remain unexamined and unmarked (Rohleder 2014).

Categories of difference are accompanied by norms, stereotypes, and prejudices. They determine which groups are privileged and which are discriminated against. According to Scherr (2008: 2009), discrimination can be understood as disadvantages that "affect social 'groups' or individuals on the basis of their actual or perceived membership of a social 'group'." Experiences of discrimination occur when people are not only individually affected by a violation of their interests or rights, but are also disadvantaged, excluded, or treated unfairly because of their group affiliation(s). Discrimination is also a frequently discussed, "philosophically challenging" concept in healthcare ethics (Hädicke & Wiesemann 2021). The experience of discrimination in society negatively impacts the health of those affected (Yeboah 2017; Williams et al. 2019; Kluge et al. 2020; Abubakar et al. 2022) and is therefore considered to be one of the social determinants of health. Against this background, it becomes clear that solely focusing on a patient's (presumed) ethnic-cultural background as the only explanatory variable, while neglecting other factors, amounts to culturalization—i.e., a culturalist interpretation of social interactions associated with stereotypes and prejudices. The German Association of Psychosocial Centres for Refugees and Victims of Torture (BAfF) describes the impact of racism on the lives of persons with refugee experience in Germany and warns health and social care professionals against the temptation of racist and culturalizing explanations in the following way:

> In the context of discourse in society as a whole and also specifically in psychosocial work on displacement, trauma and violence, culturalising and racialising assumptions about the situation of refugees are the normal state of affairs. Racism is a solution to many social challenges that has been tried and tested for centuries, since colonialism. It is a

transgenerational body of knowledge that is readily available and can be accessed. It is therefore not surprising that racist and culturalising explanatory patterns are used to explain and categorise complex and overwhelming situations. Often, the solution to these problems lies outside the sphere of influence of individual professions and structures, even though they are active in the context of displacement, trauma and violence, which can reinforce the dynamic of arguing in a racist and culturalising way in order to cover up the powerlessness in the face of structural hurdles and to shift the responsibility to the person. (BAfF and Teigler 2022 – own translation into English)

From a diversity perspective, the situation of persons with refugee experience instead needs to be understood as a complex intersection of various factors such as cultural, ethnic, religious, and linguistic backgrounds, as well as socioeconomic status, political context, and past experiences of displacement and trauma. Health professionals should, for example, be aware of the importance of residence status on a person's life situation—as it influences access to health services, to the education system, to the labour market, possibilities to participate in cultural activities, the right or denial to choose one's own residence, as well as a person's overall future prospects and associated potential psychosocial burdens.

In this context, the human right to health plays a central role, because it expresses the normative conviction that people must not be disadvantaged based on categories or attributions such as social origin, ethno-culturally coded or racialized affiliation, gender or sexual orientation, age, or physical or mental condition. From a social justice perspective, diversity in society and healthcare calls for a commitment to promoting equity and reducing health disparities across diverse communities to improve health outcomes for all individuals, particularly those from marginalized communities. This perspective emphasizes the importance of recognizing and addressing the systemic barriers and social determinants of health that impact individuals and communities from diverse backgrounds, such as poverty, racism, and discrimination (Yeboah 2017; Kluge et al. 2020). This includes an understanding of the significance of socially produced and communicated cultural stereotypes and prejudices, and a critically reflective way of dealing with them.

Self-reflection exercise:

1. Focusing on the context of interprofessional collaborative healthcare practice and racism in the United States, Cahn (2020) explores the possibilities for dismantling structural racism in interprofessional collaborative practice. In this article, the author criticizes the "artificial separation between interprofessional collaborative practice and anti-racism". It is worth engaging with the arguments he brings forward to substantiate this view. Furthermore, the text characterizes "structural competency".

2. Do you see parallels between interprofessional collaborative healthcare practice and the situation of persons with refugee experience in your own country? What can you learn from this text regarding culturally responsive interprofessional practice in refugee health?

From the foregoing, it can be concluded that diversity-responsive practice in healthcare is invariably linked to social justice. In 2015, American occupational therapists Pamela Talero, Stephen B. Kern, and Debra A. Tupé developed a model for "Culturally Responsive Care in Occupational Therapy Service-Learning", which places diversity at its core and relates it to issues of equity and social inclusion. An essential element of diversity-sensitive healthcare education is, therefore, not to separate issues of socio-economic status from so-called 'cultural' issues, but to systematically include them in the discussion: "because health care disparities are largely based upon socioeconomic status (SES), socioeconomic status is an effective alternative strategy for addressing diversity issues in health care education" (Gordon 2005: 23).

The reference to human rights is all the more important in an era when dichotomizing social discourses, which tend towards populist argumentation patterns, dominate the topic of culture and cultural identity, so that the demand for the recognition of equal rights is no longer derived from the identification of (alleged) differences.

The discussion in this section has highlighted that health professionals who view culturally responsive practice primarily as a human rights issue, emphasizing social participation, appreciate the opportunities offered by an intersectoral approach in their field. The concept of occupational justice has empowered occupational therapists to adopt a rights-based focus on enabling persons with refugee experience to participate in everyday activities and occupations. This will be explored from a practical perspective in the next section.

Practice Experience: The Role of Occupational Therapists in Supporting Persons with Refugee Experience in Germany

Angelika Roschka, M.Sc., is an occupational therapist and a lecturer in the Occupational Therapy programme at Ernst-Abbe-Hochschule Jena, University of Applied Sciences, and a trainer and coach for transculture, anti-bias, and democracy. Angelika has years of experience working with refugees in a small town in Germany. Prior to this, she worked as a community occupational therapist in Kathmandu, Nepal, and then in Cairo, Egypt, conducting and supervising the training of teachers in therapeutic assessment and intervention for children with special needs. The following interview was originally conducted by Bettina M. Heinrich, an occupational therapist working for the editorial team of the German occupational therapy journal *ergopraxis* in 2016. Angelika Roschka received permission to update and significantly expand the original interview as a section for this chapter. It was translated into English by Angelika Roschka and Sandra Schiller.

Q: Occupational therapists' education already provides the therapists with transcultural competences, doesn't it?

Theoretically, you could see it that way, insofar as the education provides understanding and teaches diversity as a cross-cutting theme through all modules. From my practical experience, transcultural competence is multi-faceted, highly complex, and a lifelong learning process. Somewhere I once read the sentence: "No one can know everything about everything at any one time". For me, this describes very aptly the learning mission that transcultural action implies. I don't like the term 'competence' so much, because a competence would be measurable at some point. In my understanding, however, there can be no such thing as a certificate for being 'transculturally competent', because there are no blanket recipes, no 'do' and 'don't' lists, no matter how much we may long for them in our dealings with diverse clientele. Rather, I find the term 'transcultural learning' more appropriate. Every encounter with people—including those who seem 'foreign' to us because of our own conditioning—offers an opportunity for learning. Every person has a 'universe of cultures' within them that changes over time and can sometimes be contradictory. This includes e.g., symbols, rituals, value assumptions, and beliefs, as well as all routines and habits of activity in everyday life. In a transcultural encounter, two universes meet. There is communication (verbal, and crucially also nonverbal) and it is almost impossible for this not to be a learning task. We cannot know exactly why our counterpart thinks, feels, and acts the way she/he does.

Q: So, does transcultural competence mean the willingness to open up to cultural differences?

Besides differences, there are always similarities that I notice when I look closely. And it means having the openness to embrace the uncertain. It implies the willingness to let one's own world view 'collapse'—if necessary several times a day. And that means triggering the process of transcultural learning within oneself and reducing that diffuse fear of losing control that is so inhibiting.

Q: How do you convey this? How do the participants in your courses learn this?

The process of transcultural learning in an occupational therapy context shows itself in a socially successful interaction with culturally diverse clients. I do not understand culture as something that results purely from a person's national or ethnic origin, but as emerging in relation to different diversity dimensions, such as age, disability, sexual identity, and sexual orientation or socioeconomic background. And when we talk about diversity, it always means at the same time to consciously deal with discrimination, even if this is not easy for us to accept and to speak about. Discrimination (at conscious or unconscious level) always leads to devaluation and exclusion. Thus, in my current educational work, the consideration of power relations in society is in the foreground, which is also a highly relevant context for occupational therapy services. As an occupational therapist, I reflect on this and ask myself, for example, through which cultural glasses I read my client's experiences, with which ear I listen to them and to what extent I (unconsciously) practice attributions. It is the permanent confrontation with client orientation and interactive reasoning that we seem to have internalised. But since we are not free of prejudices, there is a constant danger that we will not do justice to people, in the truest sense of the word, due to societal structures, our own influences, and the socially constructed boxes we are used to thinking in. This is why it is important to be sensitive to the concept of prejudice awareness and to realize the connection between society and its individual members.

In my workshops, I invite the participants to take a look inside themselves in order to deal with the question "Where do I come from?" —not primarily in a geographical sense but from a social point of view. Looking at, becoming aware of, and reflecting on one's own cultural imprints and experiences are an important building block of transcultural learning. For example, the way my parents actively involved me in family decision-making processes in my childhood days still influences my ability to formulate my own wishes today. When people grow up in a more collectivist context, ways of thinking anchored in society in terms of 'we' rather than 'I' categories may be prominent. What does this mean in terms of joint goal formulation with the client? How can the question "What is important to you personally?" affect different people? Does it make sense to them? Do we need alternatives beyond verbal language? In my workshops we discuss such questions and constantly refer to our own diverse cultural backgrounds. These processes of reflection make us sensitive to our own privileges that result from our own cultural background and societal influences, as well as to experiences of discrimination that arise from unequal power relations. It broadens our view for the need to be empathic, e.g., in the everyday life of people with disabilities who—according to an inclusive understanding—are dis-abled by their environment rather than being disabled themselves. The ability to adopt a perspective (without claiming to really understand 'the other') is fundamental.

Q: Where do you see occupational therapy in the context of support for persons with refugee experience?

I definitely see occupational therapists as having a political responsibility to work with persons with refugee experience and other people who are experiencing daily occupational deficits on different levels—from occupational imbalance to occupational apartheid. Occupation is a human right! A large number of persons with refugee experience cannot pursue a self-determined everyday life with activities that are meaningful to them, because they are often accommodated for months or even years in collective accommodation centres—i.e., in an imposed setting with limited privacy. Instead, they experience occupational disruption, marginalisation, and occupational deprivation—as international studies on displaced persons in refugee camps have shown. Theoretical knowledge about occupation, meaningful activities and their impact on quality of life, health, and well-being is researched in the field of Occupational Science. However, in order to allow occupational therapists to truly act in a culturally sensitive way, in-depth research practice is needed that includes all diversity dimensions of people, i.e., occupational therapists' clients, and tries to understand their activities in diverse contexts. In order to achieve occupational therapy services that are diversity-sensitive in the true sense of the word, and thus also discrimination-sensitive, the following is needed: further research on occupational therapy theory formation, specific qualifications for occupational practitioners, as well as an even broader anchoring of diversity topics and the associated discrimination in profession-specific educational curricula. In combination with community-oriented work, this offers enormous future potential for the profession.

Q: How can occupational therapists get involved in this field?

I recommend that occupational therapists who want to make contact with persons with refugee experience for the first time approach social workers working in collective accommodation centres, but also caretakers and security guards, and start a conversation. Social workers are important contacts for occupational therapists, as they are very close to people through the social counselling they offer and are familiar with the problems that affect people's everyday lives in a camp. They work closely with staff in public authority, such as the social welfare office or the foreigners' registration office. It can be helpful to note down names (ideally those of cooperating, friendly persons) of people who can be important in accompanying persons with refugee experience to the authorities. Often there is also useful cooperation to be had with interpreting services and it is valuable to know multilingual people for translation services. Political and church representatives of the municipality are also extremely important to the network for engagement with people with refugee experience. Who are the advocates here with regard to the issues of escape and asylum who honestly and publicly propagate an intercultural opening and support the complex process of the arrival of diverse people in the best possible way, so that the place of arrival can perhaps become a new home? And who are members of civil society who (want to) participate in this challenging process? Are there associations, initiatives, networking meetings, and meeting places for exchange? I would like to encourage occupational therapists to get actively involved in building civil society initiatives. With a handful of people in the community, I was able to set up an initiative for 'New Neighbours' in 2015 and thanks to many great (albeit fluctuating) supporters over the years, the initiative is still operating today and most recently won the Democracy Award (for its persistent commitment).

For a first contact with persons with refugee experience, I recommend occupational therapists not to proceed primarily in a goal-oriented way (as we know it from the Occupational Therapy process), i.e., not necessarily and literally to have a suitcase with materials with them (according to the motto: "We are making Christmas stars today because it is December"), and not to think in advance about what exactly they could do. Some key questions for self-reflection can help, for example: Do I want to do something for persons with refugee experience? In a helping or supporting role? What do I expect from this? Do I want to do something with persons with refugee experience (in the sense of interacting at eye level and with the understanding that everyone has a contribution to make)? It can be helpful to remember that, in the context of escape and asylum, we meet people who are currently stuck in a chronic waiting loop and whose lives are primarily characterized by uncertainty. I do not know their interests, experiences, narratives, but I open myself with awareness of my own prejudices. Accepting the invitation to a cup of tea—as I learned during my work assignments as an occupational therapist in Nepal and Egypt—is a central key to building a relationship. I can offer myself as a listener and a contact person who takes the time to grasp what role meaningful action and meaning-making plays in the lives of persons with refugee experience. I can try to shape their everyday life together with them (within the framework of legal regulations) and gradually fill it with meaningful activities. I can be a bridge-builder who helps them to arrive in the country of arrival and its society, to gain a foothold, to act in a self-determined way and—ideally—to find a new home.

Q: What do persons with refugee experience need?

Persons with refugee experience have a wide range of wishes, needs, and desires. Sometimes a trauma covers up those wishes and longings. In the area of activities of daily living, there are needs that they—due to the current deficit of a common language—are unable to communicate, or often only rudimentarily. Can you imagine being forced to leave your home country and to stay in a totally new place where you don't know anything at all about its culture? Some needs of newly arrived people may seem quite banal to us. It is part of everyday life in a collective accommodation centre that you will meet people who approach you with a letter from the authorities or a health insurance certificate. Gestures are used to articulate that the person does not know what to do at this point. The person doesn't understand the document and may not know what to do next. And they may also need someone to talk to a doctor on the phone and make an appointment. Accompanying them to the authorities or to medical facilities is a great support, especially in the first months of the asylum procedure, when language courses have not yet started or have only just begun. A 'short line' to medical staff who cooperate easily and their willingness to engage—despite the fact that language translation is often lacking—is enormously helpful, especially in acute situations and in the case of chronic illnesses of people who need multiple types of personal assistance and support.

The everyday life of the new arrivals poses countless challenges because it takes place beyond a familiar environment: where can food be bought that caters for a variety of religious backgrounds and related dietary habits? Is there a prayer room in the collective accommodation or somewhere else? What is the imposition of sanitary facilities and communal kitchens shared by many? Where do voluntary language courses or homework supervision for the children take place—beyond the state-subsidized ones? Where can one simply sit down in peace and quiet outside the room shared with many others? Where is access to free Wi-Fi so that you can stay in contact (possibly even undisturbed) with your family in your country of origin? Is there a locality or open space to meet natives and persons who have already settled in the new place who can show places to go for a walk, relax, spend time in a pleasant way?

By visiting the accommodation, the occupational therapist can get an idea of the situation and identify the needs and problems of the people living there that can be addressed. The approach can be 'classic occupational therapy' in the sense of a culturally sensitive and diversity- and discrimination-conscious client orientation: which activities are problematic in the everyday life of the people living in the facility? How important are these activities to them? How satisfied are they with their performance? This is illustrated, for example, by the following words of a woman with refugee experience in a collective accommodation centre:

> Because of the four children, I can't take part in the language course that my husband has been attending for a few months. Soon he will take his first language exam. One of my children has a mental impairment. I have only learned a few German words so far. Yet I worked as a teacher in my home country. I loved it. How can I go on?

Persons with refugee experience face increasing challenges even once they have obtained residence status. When someone with a 'foreign-sounding' name is looking for a flat, it is not uncommon for this person to encounter prejudices and be hindered or prevented from access to the housing market. The same may happen in the application process in the labour market—the hurdles for people who are considered 'foreign' are enormous—despite the fact that some persons with refugee experience have occupational training or university degrees, which are put to the test in lengthy recognition procedures and do not always bring about successful integration into the labour market. Opening a bank account, which is a condition for employment, stands and falls with the attitude of the bank employees.

At all levels of society, it is important to stimulate institutional opening processes so that participation is made equally possible for everyone and—from the occupational therapist's perspective—the claim of occupational justice can be guaranteed. As an occupational therapist who takes on political responsibility, I act as an advocate for occupational rights and demand what people in their diversity are legally entitled to. The prerequisite for this is that I see myself as a member of the majority society, who is privileged simply because I don't face these barriers regarding societal inclusion in many respects.

Q: Do you have a wish regarding your occupational therapy colleagues?

I would like to encourage occupational therapists in Germany to start supporting persons with refugee experience in a way that is sensitive towards culture, diversity, and discrimination. This requires us to become aware of the fact that it matters whether people are read as e.g., 'white' or 'black', as homo-, hetero-, bi-, trans-, inter-, queer-sexual or as a person with a disability and not as a person hindered by environmental conditions. With all the appropriate criticism of westernized occupational therapy's (in)compatibility with the needs of people from all over the world, we can focus on something that connects all people globally and is thus universal common ground: we all have an everyday life with diverse activities, we all shape everyday activities and routines, whether we actively reflect on this or not. We are confronted with specific everyday wishes, needs, and occupational imbalances, even if these may vary strongly between people. What can occupational therapy contribute to ensure that occupational justice does not remain the privilege of parts of society?

If we as occupational therapists become involved as advocates for occupational justice and—even beyond a medical diagnosis—sensitively accompany people with refugee experience or/and persons from other vulnerable groups in their everyday lives and support the process of arriving in a home, which may eventually become a true home for them, then occupational therapy is fulfilling its political responsibility. It helps to shape a pluralistic society with its core competence in supporting occupations, which allows all people to be themselves in their everyday lives, to do something meaningful, to feel they belong and to become the person they want to be in future.

To further engage with this text, consider the following questions:

1. How does Angelika Roschka describe the unique professional perspective, role, and approaches of an occupational therapist supporting persons with refugee experience?

2. Which examples does she provide that illustrate the connection between the concepts of culture, diversity, and health equity described in the introduction?

3. If you are an occupational therapist: would you describe the occupational therapy perspective on working with persons with refugee experience in your own country in a similar way? If you are from another health profession: what unique professional perspectives, roles, and approaches does your own profession bring to interprofessional teams?

4. What kind of interprofessional collaborative practice does Angelika Roschka mention? In addition to that, which other types of culturally responsive interprofessional collaboration in refugee health can you describe?

Throughout the 20th century, occupational therapy was predominantly aligned with the biomedical paradigm and focused on clinical settings. In recent decades, however, the profession has become grounded in a more nuanced understanding of health inequalities shaped by macro-economic, environmental, social, and political factors. As the interview with Angelika Roschka showed, this has broadened the traditional focus of community occupational therapists working with persons with refugee experience from merely addressing medical symptoms to considering a person's entire environment and social context, thereby fostering a comprehensive approach to health and well-being. This can provide an example for other health professions, how the divide between health and social care can be bridged.

Staying more within healthcare, adopting a cross-cultural perspective requires health professionals to critically engage with how culturally mediated perceptions influence our understanding of illness and health, as well as our approaches to illness management and prevention. To what extent do we all possess a unique cultural perspective on health and illness? The following section will focus on how cultural influences can affect the individual experience of pain, including pain perception, description, and management. It is crucial for health professionals to consider how to act sensitively with regard to diversity when dealing with pain experiences and behaviours.

Cultural Influences on Understanding Illness and Pain

Pain is a common symptom of many medical conditions, but for healthcare professionals pain assessment, pain management, and adjustment of pain medication can be challenging. The philosopher Ludwig Wittgenstein's thoughts on pain are also valued by modern pain research. While the tradition of focusing primarily on the individual subject had long prevailed in philosophy, Wittgenstein's philosophy of sensation shifted the focus from the self to a 'we': he regarded human beings as essentially social beings who can only be understood within a linguistic and cultural community. Therefore, pain and other emotions should not be understood as private phenomena known only to oneself (Wittgenstein 2003). Common definitions describe pain as a contextual experience. This context depends on how a person evaluates their pain. Pain originates in the brain and is unique to each individual: it is a highly subjective emotional experience that is culturally influenced and in turn triggers culturally specific behaviours. The culturally determined individual understanding of pain is related to a person's thinking, values, norms, control beliefs, coping strategies, and life experiences (Callister 2003). The culturally transmitted standards for assessing pain, i.e., the individual's experience of pain, develop in childhood and continue to change throughout life. The more experiences are stored in the brain, the more possibilities there are for comparison on how to react to current pain. The experience of pain leads to pain-related behaviours that range from stoically ignoring the pain to wailing and loudly calling for help. The study by Sharma et al. (2016), for example, illustrates the difficulty of describing pain. It compares the words used by people with chronic pain in Nepal to describe their pain with those used by patients in the United States.

Pain is the result of a biochemical process, but can only be experienced "in the isolation of an individual mind" (Morris 1994: 26) and is strongly influenced by the patient's unique socialisation and cultural background (ibid). Living in a diverse society requires healthcare providers to respect and consider the particular cultural backgrounds from which their patients come. Pain is perceived by the patient and can only be reported by the patient. For individual pain assessment, it is important to understand how a patient experiences their pain, what behaviours result, and how cultural perceptions influence this process. Possible cultural differences only become apparent to others when patients disclose their pain. Communication plays a particularly important role in this context. The more the communicating individuals agree in their cultural perspectives, the more likely it is that a healthcare professional will be able to understand the extent of the patient's pain. However, if there is insufficient agreement or if the interpretation is vague, it is important to first understand the patient's individual culture without judgement. On this basis, an accurate representation of the patient's pain can be created by using the patient's narratives to articulate helpful descriptions and explanations.

Self-reflection exercises:

Narajan (2010: 40) provides suggestions for diversity-sensitive approaches to pain experience and behaviour (in terms of pain assessment, helpful/neutral/harmful values and practices). The text includes "self-assessment questions to help nurses determine their cultural norms concerning pain".

The following questions are intended to promote deeper engagement with the topic:

- How do cultural influences and socialisation influence your understanding of illness and health and your approach to illness and prevention? To what extent do you as an individual have a unique cultural perspective?

- What is pain, how is pain relieved? How do cultural influences and socialisation affect your experience of pain (feeling pain, describing pain, dealing with pain)?

- How do cultural influences and socialisation influence the way you as a health professional deal with pain assessment and pain management?

How is pain assessed, quantified, and communicated? How do cultural, institutional, societal, and regulatory influences affect pain assessment and pain management? In a previous project on refugee health, Physiotherapy and Refugee Education Project (PREP), Victoria Zander, PT, PhD created two short presentations about the impact of migration on pain.

The following questions are designed to support active engagement with this content: https://play.mdu.se/media/t/0_iyg9hny1

1. How does Victoria Zander describe the healthcare situation of persons with refugee experience in Sweden? What are typical health concerns and determinants of health for people with refugee experience?

2. How does she explain the influence of (forced) migration on the perception of chronic pain?

3. What could be your own profession's role in this context?

The following questions are designed to support active engagement with this content: https://play.mdu.se/media/t/0_417g24xw

1. How does Victoria Zander describe the connection between culture, health/illness beliefs, perception of pain, and help-seeking behaviour?

2. How does she characterize the challenge provided to health professionals treating migrant or refugee patients with chronic pain? Which solutions does she suggest?

3. What are your own experiences in professional practice with persons with refugee experience?

"The adequate treatment of pain has been highlighted in recent years with emphasis on the need for a multidisciplinary approach" (Pillay et al. 2015). Chronic pain in particular is a multifaceted process arising from the concurrent interplay of pathophysiological, cognitive, affective, behavioural, and sociocultural factors (Pillay et al. 2015). An approach is needed that encompasses the impact of socially constructed concepts such as socioeconomic factors, power dynamics, ethnicity, and racism in pain care and research (McGregor & Walume 2021). Such a perspective takes into account the complexity and distinctions between socioeconomic factors and ethnicity. Narayan (2010) discusses problems complicating pain management, such as language and interpretation issues, which hinder the effective communication that is essential for successful pain management and pain education; nonverbal communication patterns, i.e., facial expressions, body posture, and activity levels, which are likely to be misinterpreted; culturally or linguistically inappropriate pain assessment tools, including numeric, visual analogue, and verbal rating scales; underreporting due to patients' belief that 'good' patients do not complain; and prejudice and discrimination. This contributes to a better understanding of the challenges faced by migrant or refugee patients with (chronic) pain and to developing potential responses to these challenges. Health professionals need to respect the beliefs, experiences, and values of patients, their families, and communities. They need to communicate effectively with them, as well as with other professionals, and within interprofessional teams. Additionally, they must be aware of the potentially positive and negative influences of provider and system factors on effective pain assessment and management, and be able to advocate for patients on individual, systemic, and policy levels. In future, the highly relevant calls for the creation of more opportunities for mutual learning through interprofessional pain education (e.g., Gordon et al. 2018; Garwood et al. 2022; Helms et al. 2023) should be combined with the need for culturally responsive practices in pain management outlined here.

As we deepen our understanding of how cultural influences shape perceptions of illness and pain, it becomes evident that health professionals must engage in continuous self-reflection and learning. This is where the concept of cultural humility becomes pivotal. The final section of this chapter introduces cultural humility as the foundation for exploring an interprofessional understanding of culturally responsive practice in refugee health. This process encourages health professionals to develop an intrinsic therapeutic attitude of humility and modesty. The section will feature case examples from refugee health to facilitate interprofessional exchange, highlighting the value of sharing diverse professional insights. Such exchanges prompt reflection on our practices, biases, and attitudes, enriching our ability to provide culturally sensitive care.

An Interprofessional Perspective on Culturally Responsive Practice in Refugee Health

In a diverse society, healthcare cannot be based on the principle of one-size-fits-all, since patients from diverse social and cultural backgrounds may have unique health needs, expectations, and experiences. Cultural competence has long been seen as an ongoing process of recognising, valuing, and respecting difference (Campinha-Bacote 1999), "through which one develops an understanding of self, while developing the ability to develop responsive, reciprocal, and respectful relationships with others" (Battle 2000). However, as Minnican and O'Toole (2020) point out, the term "culturally responsive practice" has been more strongly favoured in recent years as it "implies the ability to accommodate the cultural needs of the service user rather than being able to function without error in their culture".

Culturally responsive interprofessional practice in refugee health involves a wide range of healthcare professions working together as a team to provide empathetic, respectful, person-centred care that contributes to equal health opportunities. This includes understanding influences on service delivery at micro, meso and macro levels, and how these can be navigated.

Culturally responsive practice is characterized by recognizing the diversity of individual life experiences and cultural or linguistic backgrounds of patients in diagnostics, treatment, and counselling. It is based on an open, appreciative, and empathetic attitude that takes into account the patient's individual needs and perspectives. This also requires sensitivity towards one's own cultural influences and their potential impact on service provision. Culturally responsive practice is characterized by attentiveness to different barriers that could have a negative influence on service delivery or prevent its results from being relevant to the patients' lifeworld, and looks for ways to minimize or overcome these barriers. It also includes avoiding stigmatizing or stereotyping language patterns that could affect a patient's identity or self-image. Beyond the immediate therapy situation, the specific social context of the clients or patients as well as the institutional context of service provision are also considered. This demand for analytical skills on the meso and macro level on the part of the healthcare professionals leads, for example, to a new understanding of therapeutic interaction as collaborative relationship-focused practice (Restall & Egan 2021).

In this context, two diversity concepts in particular have received increased international attention in the healthcare sector: Cultural Safety and Cultural Humility. Cultural Safety is an approach that was originally developed by Maori nurses in New Zealand in response to the ongoing negative effects of colonialism on healthcare and the health status of the Maori (Gray & McPherson 2005; Mortensen 2010). It has since been adopted and further developed in the health literature from countries like New Zealand, Canada, and Australia, i.e., countries where indigenous peoples have demanded their social rights, including health equity within the healthcare system. Within the concept of Cultural Safety, students and professionals must be aware of the influence of the social, economic, and political contexts, as well as historical developments such as racism and colonialism, on the organisation of the healthcare system and its range of services. As power and authority are also embedded in health policies, practices, and protocols, dominant groups and the prevailing health culture need to change and adapt to provide a sense of cultural safety in health services (Ball & Lewis 2011; Peltier 2011).

The approach of Cultural Humility was conceived in 1998 by the physicians Melanie Tervalon and Jann Murray-García as a counter-concept to the widely accepted didactic models for developing cultural competence. They understand cultural differences as an inherent element of the relationship between the equal perspectives of healthcare providers and patients. According to Tervalon and Murray-García (1998: 117), "cultural humility incorporates a lifelong commitment to self-evaluation and self-critique, to redressing the power imbalances in the patient-physician dynamic, and to developing mutually beneficial and non-paternalistic clinical and advocacy partnerships with communities on behalf of individuals and defined populations". With regard to people with refugee experience, this means being continuously in a culturally sensitive, critically reflexive process in order to examine dynamics between healthcare provider and patient, to perceive power imbalances and to consciously counteract them. Power imbalances can arise, for example, because the people involved in the therapeutic process have a different understanding of their roles. This includes paternalistic experiences in the healthcare system. A flexible and humble attitude that develops in a lifelong process of self-reflection enables healthcare professionals to let go of the deceptive feeling of security that arises in a stereotype-based interaction, to assess a situation individually and, if necessary, to admit their ignorance in order to then embark on a search for new resources that can contribute to improving their future professional practice (Tervalon & Murray-García 1998).

The three tenets of cultural humility are described and illustrated by case studies in an article by Lea Ann Miyagawa: 'Practicing Cultural Humility when Serving Immigrant and Refugee Communities.' Available at: https://ethnomed.org/resource/practicing-cultural-humility-when-serving-immigrant-and-refugee-communities/

Self-reflection exercise:

1. Can you relate to these case studies?
2. Have you already been in similar situations?
3. What facilitated or hampered your actions?

The aspects of culturally responsive practice are often difficult to fully grasp for healthcare professionals who have not been in similar situations themselves. Engaging in mental exercises to place oneself in the perspective of the other party can be highly beneficial. Consider attempting the following thought experiment to cultivate cultural humility.

Thought Experiment: Interprofessional Culture Tour

Imagine that you are relocated as health professionals to the country of Utopia, which is completely foreign to all of you.

- What information about this country do you need in order to have a basic understanding of its healthcare system?
- What information do you need to be able to get help with a health problem?
- How would you introduce your profession to strangers in this country so that you could be assigned a meaningful professional role in its healthcare system?
- How does Cultural Humility help you in this process?

Both Cultural Safety and Cultural Humility explicitly address discrimination and racism. This is particularly important given that the generic term 'culture' allows for the avoidance of dealing with the existence and effects of racism and other discriminatory systems of difference in the health sector. This issue is demonstrated by models of cultural competence in which this problem is not addressed (Boutain 2005).

The following three case studies aim to inspire a discussion of culturally responsive practice in the field of refugee health with a focus on interprofessional collaboration. They depict situations that have occurred in the same or a similar way within healthcare facilities. In each instance, interprofessional teams were responsible for the treatment of individuals with a refugee background. The questions accompanying the case studies are designed to stimulate discussions among interprofessional teams about these scenarios, fostering cultural sensitivity and the development of cultural humility. By exchanging ideas, we articulate our thoughts and can build upon each other's insights to further refine our understanding.

If possible, form small groups to discuss the case studies and accompanying questions. For those who wish to explore the topic independently, select a case study and record your reflections on the questions presented.

Narrative 1

Bara'a and her family fled their home in Syria and currently live with her husband and three children in a refugee shelter in Berlin. Bara'a is still traumatized by the birth of her youngest child, Rouba, four years ago. Her hands tremble when she thinks back to that time. Unable to breastfeed her daughter due to psychological exhaustion, Bara'a relied on donations to buy breast milk for Rouba. When the donations ran out after a week, Bara'a had no choice but to feed her newborn with a mixture of sugar and water. Rouba has two older siblings. During Rouba's paediatric examination, the paediatrician notices that Rouba's development is delayed and she tries to talk to Bara'a about the child's situation and the plan for possible therapeutic support by occupational therapy, physiotherapy, and speech therapy. Bara'a barely speaks German and looks at the doctor anxiously, nodding repeatedly in conversation. After a few minutes, Bara'a leaves the room and holds her daughter tightly against her. She does not show up for the first scheduled appointment of the therapy.

(Inspired by https://www.globalgiving.org/learn/ listicle/13-powerful-refugee-stories/)

Narrative 2

David flees from the Gambia with his brother. The brothers' family collects all the money at their disposal to make their escape possible. They flee in a boat across the Mediterranean. David's brother drowns during the crossing. David himself suffers from severe sickle cell anaemia and a shoulder joint restriction. He could not receive adequate treatment in his home country. On the flight, the pain crises worsen. Once in Italy, David receives no health assistance in the refugee camp and continues to flee to Germany. Here he is accepted as an unaccompanied minor refugee in a residential home for young adults and receives support from a counsellor who also helps him to receive good medical care. David then receives psychotherapeutic and physiotherapeutic therapy. David starts a nursing assistant training course. The severe illness leads to repeated hospitalizations and severe pain crises. David fears that he will not be able to complete his assistant training and wants to discontinue it. He is particularly burdened by the recurring pain crises in everyday life, which he cannot hide from others and which are very unpleasant for him. He talks to the doctor about the situation. The doctor asks the supervisor, therapists, and the head of the training program to meet with David for a joint discussion.

Narrative 3

Sergey flees from Ukraine to Germany with his wife and their little son Yegor. The son is five years old. The family is staying with friends in Germany. The friends approach Sergey about the fact that the little son does not make any contact with them and does not even look at them. Sergey explains that his son has always been a bit slower in his development and he is loved by his wife and him the way he is. The friends recommend that Sergey be examined by a paediatrician friend who works at a social paediatric centre. Since Sergey and his wife do not speak German, the family friend offers translation assistance. Reluctantly, Sergey and his wife follow the suggestion to go to the doctor with their son. The doctor has asked an occupational therapist and a speech therapist to come to the examination. The examining paediatrician, after consulting with the therapists, confronts Yegor's parents with the statement that their son suffers from an autism spectrum disorder and is in urgent need of treatment. The parents do not understand the doctor and the translation of the friends. They ask many questions and want to know again and again why the child must be treated, since their son is doing well and they are now safe.

The following questions are intended to encourage a more thorough exploration of the narratives:

1. Reflect on the roles played by the various participants in the situation. What intentions guide their actions and procedures?

2. How can the behaviour of Bara'a, David or Sergey be explained from a culturally responsive perspective?

3. What do you need to know as an interprofessional team to create a safe space for this individual or family?

4. Which aspects of the interprofessional team members' cultural and professional backgrounds, shaped by their own socialisation and the healthcare system in their country of training, might be perceived or interpreted differently by patients with refugee experience due to differing healthcare experiences and expectations in their country of origin? For example, some healthcare systems emphasise patient autonomy and shared decision-making, which may be unfamiliar to individuals from countries where healthcare professionals make decisions on behalf of patients. In some countries, mental health is highly stigmatised or not recognised as a medical issue, whereas in the local context, seeking psychological support is encouraged.

5. How can you enter into this relationship with cultural humility?

6. How would you as an interprofessional team help and support a patient who suffers from fear associated with forced

migration? What is your role as a professional in the team in this situation?

7. What could person-centred care mean in the situation of Bara'a's and Sergey's family and in David's situation?

8. Please develop a step-by-step plan for an interprofessional approach to build a relationship that is culturally safe, trauma-informed, and anti-oppressive.

9. From your respective professional perspectives, consider which tasks of this plan you could competently complete as a team member and share your thoughts on them.

Conclusion

In conclusion, the health of individuals with refugee experience is a complex issue intricately influenced by cultural dynamics, diversity, and health equity principles. This chapter has delved into these dimensions and tried to offer a comprehensive exploration of key concepts and practical applications within the context of refugee health. Initially, we examined a constructivist understanding of culture, shifting the emphasis from merely understanding cultural nuances to recognizing diversity as a pivotal component of health equity in pluralistic societies that value the diversity of their populations, including the diversity of persons with refugee experience. The role of occupational therapists in fostering social inclusion was highlighted, demonstrating the practical implications of this approach. Importantly, cross-cultural healthcare, as discussed in this chapter, extends beyond the healthcare sector, necessitating a reliable intersectoral approach.

Furthermore, we considered how the unique cultural backgrounds of both patients and health professionals affect their perceptions and interpretations of illness and pain, underscoring the need for a nuanced appreciation of the influence of culture in healthcare interactions. As a consequence, health professionals need to be able to critically reflect on their own cultural influences and biases, as these significantly impact patient interaction. In this context, cultural humility emerges a valuable concept for fostering such critical reflection and professional development. The chapter culminated in a synthesis of international case stories and studies in interprofessional practice, underscoring the collective efforts necessary for culturally responsive care. Overall, this chapter outlined the prerequisites for culturally responsive practice, advocating it as an essential step towards achieving a more inclusive and equitable healthcare environment for persons with refugee experience.

Recommended further reading

The following two reviews show the demands for (and gaps in) culturally responsive healthcare from provider and patient perspective:

Grandpierre, Viviane, et al. 2018. 'Barriers and Facilitators to Cultural Competence in Rehabilitation Services: A Scoping Review', *BMC Health Service Research, 18*, https://doi.org/10.1186/s12913-017-2811-1

Minnican, Carla and Gjyn O'Toole. 2020. 'Exploring the Incidence of Culturally Responsive Communication in Australian Healthcare: The First Rapid Review on this Concept', *BMC Health Services Research, 20*, https://doi.org/10.1186/s12913-019-4859-6

References

Abubakar, Ibrahim, et al. 2022. 'Confronting the Consequences of Racism, Xenophobia, and Discrimination on Health and Health-care Systems', *Lancet, 400.10368*: 2137–2146, https://doi.org/10.1016/S0140-6736(22)01989-4

BAfF e.V., and Leonie Teigler (eds.). 2022. *Mächtige Narrative—was wir uns nicht erzählen: Über den Zusammenhang von Gewalt, Stress und Trauma im Kontext Flucht* [*Powerful narratives—what we don't tell ourselves: On the connection between violence, stress and trauma in the context of flight*] (Berlin: BAfF e. V.).

Ball, Jessica, and Marlene Lewis. 2011. '"An Altogether Different Approach": Roles of Speech-Language Pathologists in Supporting Indigenous Children's Language Development', *Canadian Journal of Speech-Language Pathology and Audiology, 35.2*: 144–158.

Barker, Chris, and Emma A. Jane. 2016. *Cultural Studies: Theory and Practice*, 5th edn (London: Sage).

Battle, Dolores E. 2000. 'Becoming a Culturally Competent Clinician', *Special Interest Division 1: Language, Learning and Education, 7.3*: 20–23, https://doi.org/10.1044/lle7.3.20

Boutain, Doris M. 2005. 'Social Justice as a Framework for Professional Nursing', *Journal of Nursing Education*, 44.9, 404–408, https://doi.org/10.3928/01484834-20050901-04

Cahn, Peter S. 2020. 'How Interprofessional Collaborative Practice Can Help Dismantle Systemic Racism', *Journal of Interprofessional Care*, 34.4: 431–434, https://doi.org/10.1080/13561820.2020.1790224

Callister, Lynn C. 2003. 'Cultural Influences on Pain Perceptions and Behaviors', *Home Health Care Management & Practice*, 15.3: 207–211, https://doi.org/10.1177/1084822302250687

Campesino, Maureen. 2008. 'Beyond Transculturalism: Critiques of Cultural Education in Nursing', *Journal of Nursing Education*, 47.7: 298–304, https://doi.org/10.3928/01484834-20080701-02

Campinha-Bacote, Josepha. 1999. 'A Model and Instrument for Addressing Cultural Competence in Health Care', *Journal of Nursing Education*, 38.5: 203–7, https://doi.org/10.3928/0148-4834-19990501-06

Collins, Patricia H., and Sirma Bilge. 2020. *Intersectionality*. 2nd edn (Cambridge: Polity Press).

Crenshaw, Kimberle. 1989. 'Demarginalizing the Intersection of Race and Sex: A Black Feminist Critique of Antidiscrimination Doctrine, Feminist Theory and Antiracist Politics', *University of Chicago Legal Forum*, Vol. 1989, Article 8, https://chicagounbound.uchicago.edu/uclf/vol1989/iss1/8

Garwood, Candice L., et al. 2022. 'A Multimodal Interprofessional Education Program Including Case-based Problem solving Focused on Pain Management Increases Student's Knowledge and Interprofessional Skills', *Journal of Interprofessional Care*, 36.6: 864–872, https://doi.org/10.1080/13561820.2022.2038102

Gordon, Susan P. 2005. 'Making Meaning of Whiteness: A Pedagogical Approach for Multicultural Education', *Journal of Physical Therapy Education* 19.1: 21–27.

Gordon, Debra B., Judy Watt-Watson, and Beth B. Hogans. 2018. 'Interprofessional Pain Education–with, from, and about Competent, Collaborative Practice Teams to Transform Pain Care', *PAIN Reports*, 3.3: 663, https://doi.org/10.1097/PR9.0000000000000663

Gray, Marion, and Kathryn McPherson. 2005. 'Cultural Safety and Professional Practice in Occupational Therapy: A New Zealand Perspective', *Australian Occupational Therapy Journal*, 52.1: 34–42, https://doi.org/10.1111/j.1440-1630.2004.00433.x

Grossberg, Lawrence. 1997. *Bringing It All Back Home: Essays on Cultural Studies* (Durham, NC: Duke University Press), https://doi.org/10.1215/9780822396178

Hädicke, Maximiliane, and Claudia Wiesemann. 2021. 'Was kann das Konzept der Diskriminierung für die Medizinethik leisten?: Eine Analyse' [What Can the Concept of Discrimination Do for Medical Ethics?: An Analysis], *Ethik in der Medizin* 33: 369–386, https://doi.org/10.1007/s00481-021-00631-4

Helms, Jeb et al. 2023. 'Interprofessional Active Learning for Chronic Pain: Transforming Student Learning from Recall to Application', *Journal of Medical Education and Curricular Development,* 10, https://doi.org/10.1177/23821205231221950

Kluge, Ulrike, et al. 2020. 'Rassismus und psychische Gesundheit' [Racism and Mental Health], *Nervenarzt,* 91: 1017–1024, https://doi.org/10.1007/s00115-020-00990-1

Lerch, Leonore. 2019. 'Psychotherapie im Kontext von Differenz (Macht) Ungleichheit und globaler Verantwortung' [Psychotherapy in the Context of Difference (Power) Inequality and Global Responsibility], *Psychotherapie Forum,* 23: 51–58, https://doi.org/10.1007/s00729-019-0117-y

McGregor, Cass, and Jackie Walume. 2021. 'We Need to Develop Our Approach to Socially Constructed Concepts Including Socioeconomic Factors, Power, Ethnicity and Racism in Pain Care and Research', *Pain and Rehabilitation – The Journal of Physiotherapy Pain Association,* 51: 1–4, https://www.ingentaconnect.com/content/ppa/pr/2021/00002021/00000051/art00001

Mecheril, Paul. 2008. '"Diversity": Differenzordnungen und Modi ihrer Verknüpfung' [Orders of Difference and Modes of Linking them], *Heimatkunde,* https://heimatkunde.boell.de/de/2008/07/01/diversity-differenzordnungen-und-modi-ihrer-verknuepfung

Minnican, Carla, and Gjyn O'Toole. 2020. 'Exploring the Incidence of Culturally Responsive Communication in Australian Healthcare: The First Rapid Review on this Concept', *BMC Health Services Research,* 20: 1–14, https://doi.org/10.1186/s12913-019-4859-6

Miyagawa, Lea Ann. 2020. 'Practicing Cultural Humility when Serving Immigrant and Refugee Communities', *Ethnomed,* https://ethnomed.org/resource/practicing-cultural-humility-when-serving-immigrant-and-refugee-communities/

Morris, David B. 1993. *The Culture of Pain* (Berkeley: University of California Press).

Mortensen, Annette. 2010. 'Cultural Safety: Does the Theory Work in Practice for Culturally and Linguistically Diverse Groups?', *Nursing Praxis in New Zealand,* 26.3: 6–16.

Narayan, Mary C. 2010. 'Culture's Effects on Pain Assessment and Management: Cultural Patterns Influence Nurses' and Their Patients' Responses to Pain', *American Journal of Nursing* 110.4: 38–47, https://doi.org/10.1097/01.NAJ.0000370157.33223.6d

Pillay, Thivian K., Hendrik A. van Zyl, and David R. Blackbeard. 2015. 'The Influence of Culture on Chronic Pain: A Collective Review of Local and International Literature', *Journal of Psychiatry*, 18.2, https://doi.org/10.4172/2378-5756..1000234

Pincus, Fred L., and Bryan R. Ellis. 2021. *Understanding Diversity: An Introduction*, 3rd edn (Boulder, Co.: Lynne Rienner Publ.).

Peltier, Sharla. 2011. 'Providing Culturally Sensitive and Linguistically Appropriate Services: An Insider Construct', *Canadian Journal of Speech-Language Pathology and Audiology*, 35.2: 126–134.

Restall, Gayle J., and Mary Y. Egan. 2021. 'Collaborative Relationship-Focused Occupational Therapy: Evolving Lexicon and Practice', *Canadian Journal of Occupational Therapy*, 88.3: 220–230, https://doi.org/10.1177/00084174211022889

Rohleder, Paul. 2014 'Othering' in *Encyclopedia of Critical Psychology*, ed. by Thomas Teo (New York, NY: Springer, 2014), pp. 1306–1308.

Sharma, Saurab, Pathak Anupa, and Mark P. Jensen. 2016. 'Words That Describe Chronic Musculoskeletal Pain: Implications for Assessing Pain Quality across Cultures', *Journal of Pain Research*, 9: 1057–1066, https://doi.org/10.2147/JPR.S119212

Scherr, Albert. 2008. 'Diskriminierung: eine eigenständige Kategorie für die soziologische Analyse der (Re-)Produktion sozialer Ungleichheiten in der Einwanderungsgesellschaft? [Discrimination: an independent category for the sociological analysis of the (re)production of social inequalities in the immigration society?]', in *Die Natur der Gesellschaft: Verhandlungen des 33. Kongresses der Deutschen Gesellschaft für Soziologie in Kassel 2006* [The Nature of Society: Proceedings of the 33rd Congress of the German Sociological Association in Kassel 2006], ed. by Karl-Siegbert Rehberg (Frankfurt am Main: Campus Verl.), pp. 2007–2017, https://nbn-resolving.org/urn:nbn:de:0168-ssoar-152236

Talero, Pamela, Stephen B. Kern, and Debra A. Tupé. 2015. 'Culturally Responsive Care in Occupational Therapy: An Entry-level Educational Model Embedded in Service-learning', *Scandinavian Journal of Occupational Therapy*, 22.2: 95–102, https://doi.org/10.3109/11038128.2014.997287

Tervalon, Melanie, and Jann Murray-García. 1998. 'Cultural Humility versus Cultural Competence: A Critical Distinction in Defining Physician Training Outcomes in Multicultural Education', *Journal of Health Care for the Poor and Underserved*, 9.2: 117–125, https://doi.org/10.1353/hpu.2010.0233

Williams, David R., et al. 2019. 'Understanding How Discrimination Can Affect Health', *Health Services Research*, 54.S2: 1374–1388, https://doi.org/10.1111/1475-6773.13222

Williams, Raymond. 1983. *Keywords: A Vocabulary of Culture and Society*, rev. ed. (London: Fontana Paperbacks).

Winker, Gabriele, and Nina Degele. 2010. *Intersektionalität: Zur Analyse sozialer Ungleichheiten* [Intersectionality: On the Analysis of Social Inequalities]. 2nd, unaltered edn (Bielefeld: transcript, 2010).

Wittgenstein, Ludwig. 2003. *Philosophische Untersuchungen* [Philosophical Investigations]. 11th edn (Frankfurt am Main: Suhrkamp).

Yeboah, Amma. 2017. 'Rassismus und psychische Gesundheit in Deutschland [Racism and Mental Health in Germany]', in *Rassismuskritik und Widerstandsformen* [Critique of Racism and Forms of Resistance], ed. by Fereidooni, Karim, and Meral El (Wiesbaden: Springer VS), pp. 143–161, https://doi.org/10.1007/978-3-658-14721-1_9

11. Cross-Cultural Communication in Refugee Health

Sandra Schiller and Andreas Wolfs

In the increasingly diverse landscape of modern healthcare, effective communication is paramount. Persons with refugee experience often face unique health needs that necessitate skilled and complex interventions. At the same time, they share the cross-cultural communication needs that are typically characteristic of migrant health. Looking at communication in refugee health, this chapter reflects the paradoxical situation in which persons with refugee experience in the healthcare system are at once comparable to other patients and uniquely distinct. The first section looks at the role of communication in fostering a more equitable health system based on the concepts of inclusive communication and inclusive multilingualism. Counselling from a systems theory perspective is introduced as an analytical framework to be utilized in the context of refugee health, and practical approaches to enhance cross-cultural communication are presented. This chapter emphasizes the importance of creating structures and services that are sensitive and responsive to cultural and linguistic diversity, explores cross-cultural communication strategies at the interpersonal level, and provides information on working with interpreters and cultural mediators. The final section of the chapter highlights the significance of interprofessional collaboration in cross-cultural communication within the context of refugee health.

 https://doi.org/10.11647/OBP.0479.11

The Relevance of Effective Communication in a Diverse Health System

How can health professionals deal with communication barriers in a resource-oriented and productive way? This chapter looks at a process that concerns not just individual health professionals and persons with refugee experience, but also policymakers and organizations responsible for setting up structures and services in the health system, including refugee organisations.

Communication is the process of exchanging information, ideas, thoughts, and feelings between individuals or groups through various mediums and channels, generating meanings within and across contexts and cultures. It is a fundamental aspect of human interaction and vital to achieve understanding and convey meaning in personal relationships, organizations, and society as a whole. Communication can take various forms (including verbal, nonverbal, written, and visual). Healthcare professionals must get to know their patients by understanding their cultural and linguistic backgrounds to ensure that they provide appropriate care. Effective communication is an essential basis for fostering good interpersonal relationships and significantly enhances the efficacy of service delivery in healthcare, thereby leading to better results and improved goal attainment.

A resource-oriented approach to addressing language barriers in healthcare recognizes the value of multilingualism and linguistic diversity. Instead of framing language barriers as a negative aspect of care, a resource-oriented approach emphasizes the importance of language access as a resource for improving the quality of care and promoting positive health outcomes. One way to express this approach is to focus on language access as a valuable resource for enhancing communication and building trust between healthcare providers and patients. Another way is to focus on the benefits of language access for promoting patient autonomy and empowerment. In today's culturally and linguistically diverse society, two essential guiding principles can provide the foundation of culturally responsive communication in healthcare:

1. The concept of inclusive communication represents a process in which different strategies are applied to allow people with communication vulnerabilities to feel acknowledged and respected in the communication and to become actively involved in society. Consequently, inclusive communication is adapted to the individual communication strengths and needs of the persons seeking information and requires accessible, individualized resources together with appropriate communication partners that have the necessary skills, knowledge, experience, and attitude (Money et al. 2016).

2. The concept of inclusive multilingualism values the interactive strategies or communicative modes applied by participants in multilingual interactions who use different means to achieve mutual understanding (Backus et al. 2013). This recognizes the importance of linguistic diversity and acknowledges that all communication partners contribute to efficient communication. In the context of refugee health this could mean affirming and valuing the patients' cultural backgrounds, prior experiences and linguistic resources as a contribution to patient agency.

Currently, however, healthcare systems—much like other societal systems and structures—in Europe, including those in countries with significant immigration, are not consistently aligned with these principles. Interpretation services, for instance, are not regarded as an integral part of healthcare provision but often must be organized and financed in a cumbersome manner by patients or healthcare institutions themselves (Robertshaw et al., 2017; Kwan et al. 2023).

The guiding principles of inclusive communication and inclusive multilingualism should be applied to the field of refugee health because communication plays a crucial role in the context of refugee health as it promotes understanding, addresses the specific needs and challenges faced by persons with refugee experience and facilitates delivery of appropriate health services (Patel et al. 2021). Cultural and linguistic barriers reinforce the power asymmetry between service providers and service users, resulting in poorer adherence to treatment plans or a patient's reluctance to engage in rehabilitation. On the contrary, if patients are given the opportunity to adequately express their symptoms and treatment wishes, unnecessary examinations can be prevented, which are often carried out because clear communication could not be established (especially with regard to symptom and complaint descriptions). At the same time, it is possible to be more responsive to the patients' treatment wishes (Peters et al. 2014). A literature review by Kwan et al. (2023) shows that "patients receiving 'language discordant care' are more prone to adverse events and potentially life-threatening conditions at different stages of hospital care including delay in treatment diagnosis at admission, poor communication for surgical procedure and at discharge which inevitably lead to hospital readmissions and an increase in healthcare costs".

A qualitative study by Pandey and colleagues (2021) examined the effects of English language proficiency on healthcare access, utilisation, and outcomes among immigrants. On page six, the study includes a figure illustrating the adverse impact of insufficient language proficiency on healthcare provision for immigrants, such as reduced access to care, suboptimal quality of care, and patient dissatisfaction.

1. Do you know these factors from your own work?
2. Do additional factors need to be taken into account in the area of refugee health?
3. Which strategies could help to address:

- the ability of persons with refugee experience to access health information and services?
- the ability of persons with refugee experience to develop a therapeutic alliance with healthcare providers?
- challenges associated with engaging language interpreters?
- existing gaps in healthcare provision and improve health outcomes?

In the subsequent sections of this chapter, key approaches are presented that can contribute to enhancing the communication skills of health and social care professionals in a way that fosters inclusive communication and reflects the appreciative stance of inclusive multilingualism. As an essential foundation for this, the next section describes the counselling process in the context of refugee health from a systemic-constructivist perspective. This is rooted in the fundamental belief that persons with refugee experiences are first and foremost individuals, like all other people, and that the design of any interaction and communication situation in health and social care must primarily reflect that each person is unique and that refugee experience is only one, albeit a highly relevant, factor.

Counselling in the Context of Refugee Health

Counselling is always a highly individual process. People who provide counselling as part of their professional role, such as therapists or social workers, encounter a variety of distinct situations with unique individuals for whom they must find goal-oriented solutions.

The fact that there are different perspectives on counselling underscores this individuality. One such perspective is offered by systems theory, which, generally speaking, assumes that all parts of a system are in contact with each other and work towards a common goal (Forrester 1972: 9). Systems theory aids in abstracting the specifics of a counselling situation while simultaneously allowing for flexible consideration of the characteristics of the client and the counsellor. Hence, systems theory provides an analytical framework for retrospectively analysing counselling scenarios and prospectively preparing for future counselling sessions.

The following overview aims to show how the systems theory approach provides a structured understanding of counselling situations involving people with refugee experience. First, the basic principles of counselling processes are presented (see Figure 11.1 below): the structural coupling of the participants in the counselling process, viability, connectivity, and the experience of difference regarding counselling content. Then, the concepts of perturbation tolerance and contingency are introduced as analytical tools to explore possible resistance and obstacles.

A systemic perspective rarely produces entirely new or unknown insights. Rather, it helps to recognize known but possibly misunderstood mechanisms and patterns of action and communication. This is important because only patterns that are consciously perceived can be reflected upon. Reflection, in turn, forms the basis for learning. Ultimately, a systemic perspective offers professionals the opportunity to further develop their counselling skills.

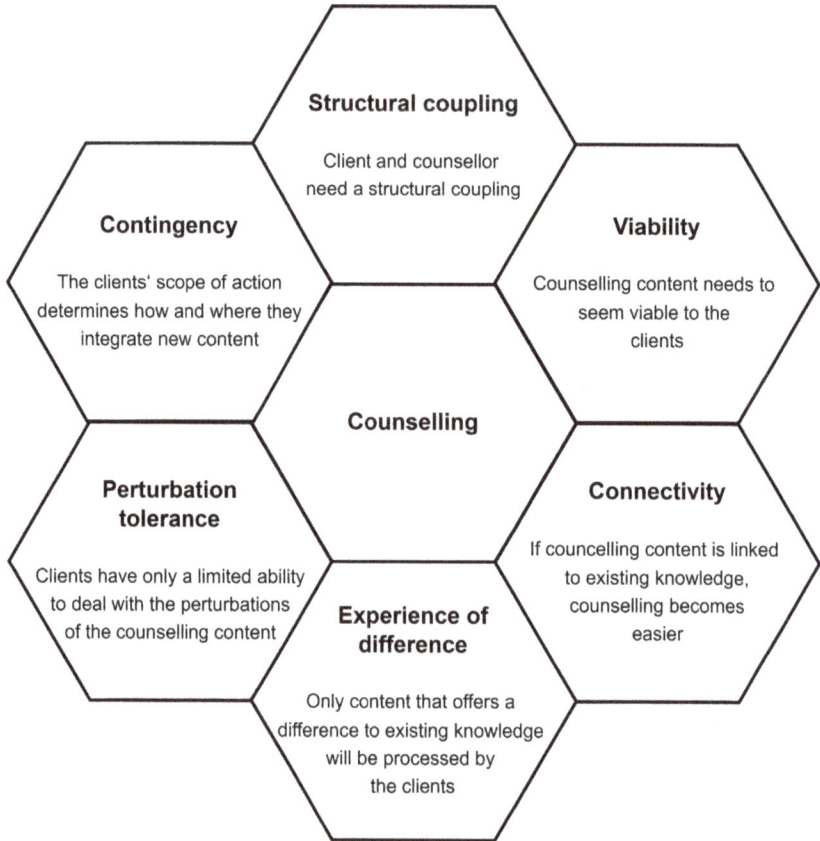

Fig. 11.1 Basic principles of counselling. ©Andreas Wolfs, CC BY.

Basic Aspects of Counselling

Seeking and receiving advice is omnipresent in people's lives. Whether it is for shopping, choosing a holiday destination, or in healthcare or social work, counsel is offered or sought in many different ways. It is not only an explicit service, such as a coaching session with a trained professional or learning guidance in an educational context; often, it is also an implicit part of health or social services or when dealing with the authorities.

In these instances, the professionals providing the counselling may be experts in their specific fields but may have little or no ability to provide person-oriented advice. Individuals with refugee experience may seek counselling in any of these situations. Being a refugee or asylum seeker might be the reason for the counselling situation, e.g., when people seek assistance with administrative matters. However, an individual may also seek advice for reasons unrelated to their refugee status.

Counselling situations vary considerably not only in terms of content but also in person-oriented approaches. Therefore, the counsellor needs explicit skills to address the individuality of each counselling situation. This includes the ability to determine the appropriate amount of technical content to provide and the level of support needed to enable clients to develop self-learning skills.

In general, in any counselling situation, those who seek counselling and those who provide counselling are of particular importance. In addition, the specific context of the counselling situation needs to be taken into account.

The differences among those seeking counselling, i.e., the clients, are apparent. Each individual has a unique biography, which also encompasses their own counselling biography, including personal experiences with situations in which they have initiated or attended counselling. Additionally, the client's biographical knowledge includes insights into the subject of the counselling, as well as their own interests and inclinations. The same is true for those who provide counselling, i.e., the counsellors. They also have experience and knowledge, such as an understanding of which approaches have proven beneficial or obstructive in various situations for different clients.

Counsellors must continually reflect on whether they are being approached in their formal, professional capacity or whether they are dealing with a more informal request. In both cases, they should clearly identify their respective role and clarify it with the client. However, it should be borne in mind that individuals seeking counselling in a professional context will often assume that the counsellor is acting in a professional capacity, even in informal settings, despite the counsellor making it clear that they are speaking outside their professional remit or expressing their personal opinion. For the benefit of those seeking advice, professionals should err on the side of caution and refrain from making statements outside their professional scope in such situations.

With respect to the specific context of the counselling situation, the various media that can be employed will be briefly addressed. For example, it is important to distinguish whether the information in the counselling session is presented orally or in writing. If written information is used, it is essential to ascertain whether the available documents are tailored individually for the client or whether a general information brochure is used. In the case of verbal counselling, for example, distinctions must be made between face-to-face meetings, telephone calls, or video calls. Additionally, the necessity for interpreting services for language mediation is a relevant consideration. Each of these setups brings its own relevant aspect to the counselling process. For example, if a general information brochure is used, it is important to assess whether their content adds value for the specific client in the given counselling context, or whether it might actually be more of a hindrance. Counselling based on the maxim 'more is better' is only beneficial in the rarest of cases. In the scenario of consultations conducted via video calls, the skills and technical equipment of all participants need to be taken into account. Depending on the tools and telephone network used, the quality of communication may be unreliable. Each of these factors can lead to significant disruptions, particularly at the onset of the consultation, when the counsellor and client are becoming acquainted with each other.

This brief overview of the relevant aspects of explicit and implicit counselling, whether by professionals or laypersons, the biographical backgrounds of counsellor and client, and the different media used, illustrates the complex nature of counselling. The perspectives on and descriptions of counselling situations are as varied as counselling itself. A systemic perspective is adopted here to analyse counselling scenarios in general, and specifically with persons with refugee experience. The systemic approach allows for the identification of underlying patterns, while at the same time allowing for a detailed examination of specific situations. This analytical framework facilitates both retrospective analysis of past counselling scenarios and prospective preparation for future sessions.

In the following, we will frequently refer to the client, i.e., the person seeking counselling, and the counsellor, i.e., the person providing it, in order to succinctly identify the two main roles in a counselling session: the one seeking an answer and the one assisting in finding that answer. In the following sections, we will explain why counsellors should be cautious about 'giving advice', and instead see themselves as companions on the client's journey of seeking advice.

The Structural Coupling of Those Involved Forms the Foundation of Counselling or the Counselling System

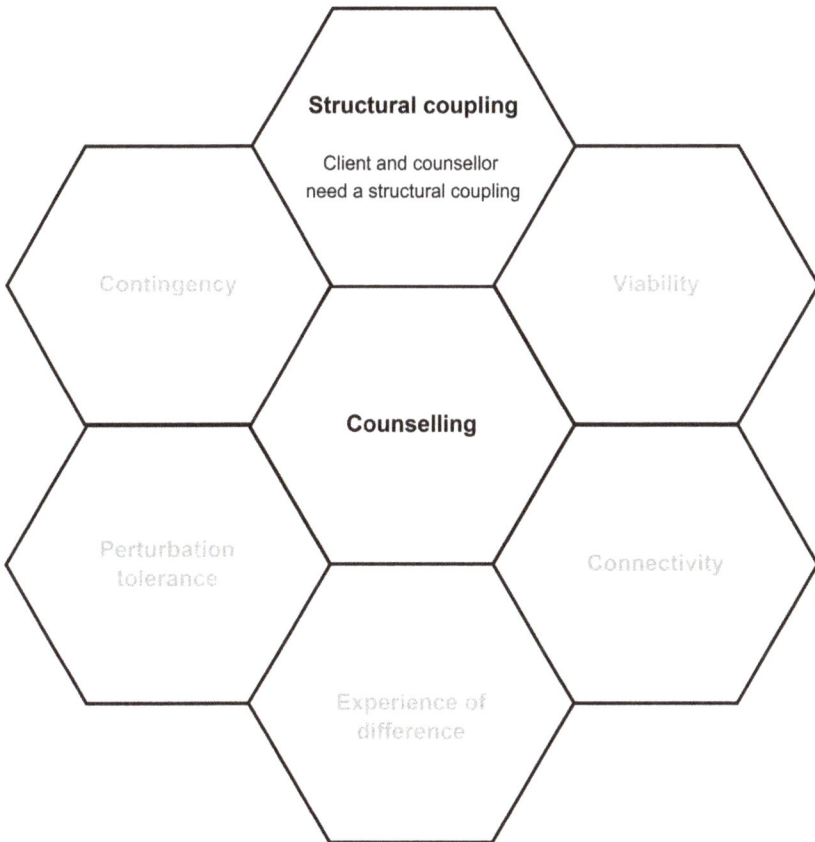

Fig. 11.2 Structural coupling. ©Andreas Wolfs, CC BY.

In a systemic approach, individuals are regarded as self-contained systems that are initially closed to all external influences, including interactions with other people. This approach is based on self-reference, which is characteristic of all closed systems (Luhmann 1985: 403). In humans, statements such as "I'm fine the way I am" or "Why should I learn anything new? I'm fine the way I am" exemplify this concept. Similarly, people seeking advice may express sentiments such as "What can this person tell me that I don't already know?" or "What qualifies this person to be an expert in my situation (or in my life)?". Individuals initiating a counselling situation or seeking answers often adopt these or similar attitudes. Conversely, counsellors can use this self-reference to adopt perspectives such as "The way I counsel is the right way to counsel" or "Why won't the client understand what I'm explaining?". When such positions dominate the counsellor's actions, they clearly get in the way of focusing on the client's needs.

Another consequence of the closed nature of such systems in relation to external influences is that they can only be observed from the outside. Luhmann (1985: 405) describes this phenomenon as a "black box", explaining that this lack of transparency is often compensated for by assuming that the processes and decision-making patterns in other systems are comparable to one's own. Applied to counselling situations, this means that counsellors perceive the actions or words of the clients without recognizing the actual intentions behind them. The counsellor will automatically seek explanations for what has been said that are consistent with their own perspective. To counteract this automatic tendency—especially when understanding the reasons behind the statements is crucial—the counsellor should rely less on their own biased perceptions and instead inquire directly from the client. However, even explanatory words are open to interpretation, so the counsellor can only judge whether the explanations seem coherent. A clear assessment of the inner decision-making patterns is therefore not possible.

From a systems theory perspective, this isolation from external influences can be broken through structural coupling with another system (another person) (Maturana & Varela 1984: 85). The basis of such a coupling is primarily the common interests and common goals of those involved (Siebert 2009: 95).

Basic common goals in counselling may include the desire to solve a problem, clarify a situation, or obtain an answer to a question. Conversely, unsolicited or unintentional counselling initiated by the counsellor is likely to lack these basic elements. It is possible that the other person, not yet in the role of the client, may develop an interest in the proposed topic through the counsellor's initiative, but this requires at least some common interests. Without common interests and goals, it is highly likely that the systems will remain metaphorically side-by-side without structurally binding. In such cases, the counsellor's content may, metaphorically speaking, 'bounce off' the (non-)client and miss its target, while the counsellor might assume that the information has been received. Common interests may relate to the content of the counselling or to aspects independent of it, provided they are comparable for the people involved. The interests of the counsellor and the client must be aligned. This phenomenon explains why individuals with questions about their health situation or healthcare often trust the advice of someone they know more than that of medical specialists or therapists who, despite their professional competence, are initially unknown to them. This trust can only develop once a sustainable structural coupling, based on common goals and interests, has been established. It is important to note that longer-established structural couplings are likely to be more intense and resilient. In conflict situations or when faced with contradictory information, this may mean that clients are more likely to trust those with whom they have long-standing structural couplings, regardless of their professional qualifications.

From a critical perspective, counsellors should also consider the influence of the power imbalance inherent in the counselling situation, particularly when persons with refugee experience are confronted with the authorities' assessments of their circumstances, communication difficulties, psychological stress such as the effects of trauma, and the limited communicability of personal experiences.

The existence of a common language is highly relevant to the establishment of structural coupling. Without a common set of signs, it is far more difficult to find common goals or interests. One way to mitigate this is to involve interpreters. The interpreter must be structurally coupled with all parties in the counselling system. In practice, there is often an acquaintance gap; either the client or the counsellor already knows the interpreter. Both lack of acquaintance and well-established connections can have a negative impact on the transfer of information. If the structural coupling is weak, the interpreter may not be trusted; if the structural coupling is strong, the interpreter may be reluctant to convey the real content and instead present what they personally believe to be valid. Regardless, bias remains inevitable, for example due to time lags between non-verbal and verbal aspects of communication or potential mistranslations due to misinterpretation of the content of the consultation.

Furthermore, persons with refugee experience often encounter rejection regarding healthcare in the host country (Patel et al. 2021; Nowak & Hornberg 2023). Barriers to access, language barriers, discrimination, and the perceived discrepancy between the healthcare they are accustomed to and that which they experience in the host country hinder the establishment of trust (Nowak & Hornberg, 2023). Power asymmetries can arise from diverse linguistic contexts—where one person speaks the official language and is perceived as an authority figure, while the other is a patient who does not speak the language— which can complicate communication and trust within the process (Dressler 2009).

Cultural aspects can result in situations, actions, and messages being perceived and interpreted differently. Cultural influences can shape the extent to which interactions are contextualised, affecting the emphasis placed on verbal and non-verbal elements of a message, as well as situational information, such as the relationship between participants in the interaction (Altorfer & Käsermann 2021). To identify and address misunderstandings arising from these differences, an initial awareness is required. On the other hand, there is also a risk of culturalization, i.e., overemphasizing cultural factors. This may lead to misunderstandings being consistently attributed to culture, thereby overlooking the actual causes (Frederickson 2015). Another structural cause of language barriers is prejudice. Prejudices influence perceptions of individuals and create biases that can affect, for example, the extent of empathy shown by professionals towards people, the level of attentiveness provided to them, or assessments of their competence based on the language they speak. This can also impact the general willingness to engage in interaction (Altorfer & Käsermann 2021). Without awareness of these factors, disruptions such as misunderstandings may occur and remain unrecognized or unresolved. This needs to be taken into account as a factor negatively affecting structural coupling in refugee health.

In general, if there are common goals and interests, possibly supported by additional commonalities such as a common language, structural coupling can be successfully initiated, laying the foundation for counselling. In this case, the participants form a new system or counselling system that is distinct from the environment. It is crucial that both the counsellor and the client remain unchanged and independent within this new system; they are only connected through the structural coupling that has been formed (Becker & Reinhardt-Becker 2001: 65).

Once structural coupling has been initiated and counselling progresses, circumstances may arise that alter the interests or goals of the client—whether over several sessions or within a single appointment. Changes in interests and goals should not necessarily be viewed negatively, as counselling often involves change, which can lead to shifts in goals and interests. This aspect is particularly relevant when counselling individuals with refugee experience; sessions that begin in the context of displacement may take very different directions as they progress. If counsellors lose the structural coupling with their client because they fail to acknowledge these changes, or if the structural coupling weakens, the impact on both future outcomes and those already achieved can be detrimental.

Despite these challenges, changes can either weaken or, in extreme cases, break the initially strong structural coupling, ending the counselling system. Counsellors must therefore continuously monitor the current coupling during the counselling process and recognize or inquire about changes in the client's goals and interests.

Making Counselling Content 'Palatable' for the Client: Viability, Connectivity and Experience of Difference

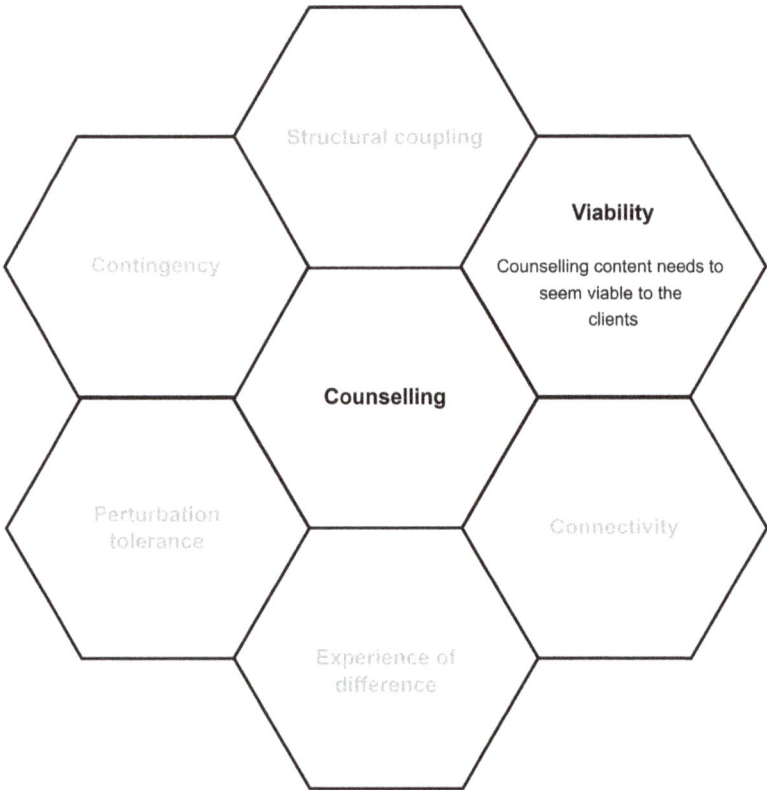

Fig. 11.3 Viability. ©Andreas Wolfs, CC BY.

Establishing a sustainable structural coupling based on common interests and goals is the basis for, but not a guarantee of, successful counselling. Another element to consider is the viability of the counselling content. In systems theory, viability is defined as content that appears relevant, meaningful, or feasible to the client (Glasersfeld 2012: 30). This can be quite challenging for the counsellor. This is especially the case when the counsellor has not only the necessary skills for person-centred counselling but also professional skills in the respective counselling context. It is easy to explain what is relevant and important from the perspective of a knowledgeable person. However, this content may be of little or no relevance to the client. Information that is not relevant for the client is ignored and, to use another metaphor, bounces off the outer shell of the client's closed systems.

It should also be borne in mind that cultural differences, limited health literacy in relation to the organisation of the healthcare system in the host country, and specificities of the legal situation, among others, pose particular challenges in achieving or formulating viable counselling content. Additionally, it is crucial whether or not the counsellor is aware of the client's experience of displacement. While such awareness may enable the counsellor to take this factor into account, there is also a risk of relying on stereotypes, which can be counterproductive.

The counsellor should filter out aspects that are likely to be relevant. It may be helpful to ask questions first, for example, about the reason for seeking the advice and the exact interest in knowledge, before answering questions quickly. In addition to a clarifying viability, the client's goals can also be specified, and if the counsellor agrees with the goals, the structural coupling can be further strengthened.

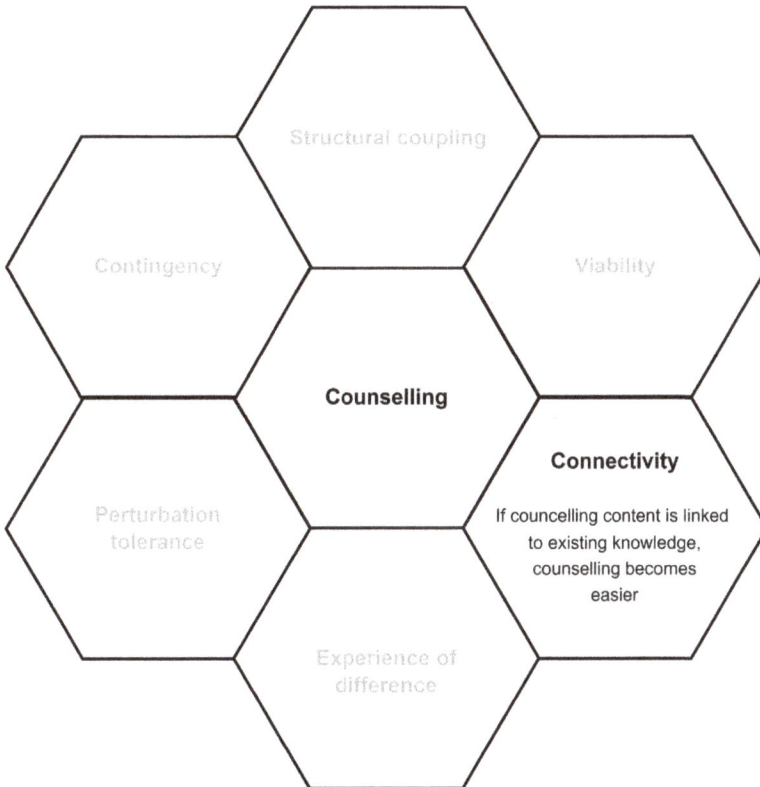

Fig. 11.4 Connectivity. ©Andreas Wolfs, CC BY.

Questioning and the associated experience of prior knowledge and other biographical aspects also promote another relevant aspect: connectivity. Counselling content is connectable if it can be linked to what is already known. This can refer to aspects of the content context of the respective counselling, e.g., in the case of educational guidance, if they are linked to existing information about the desired further education. But it can also refer to aspects that are independent of the content of the counselling. In the example above, counselling content on educational measures could be presented in the context of a hobby or private interest of the client.

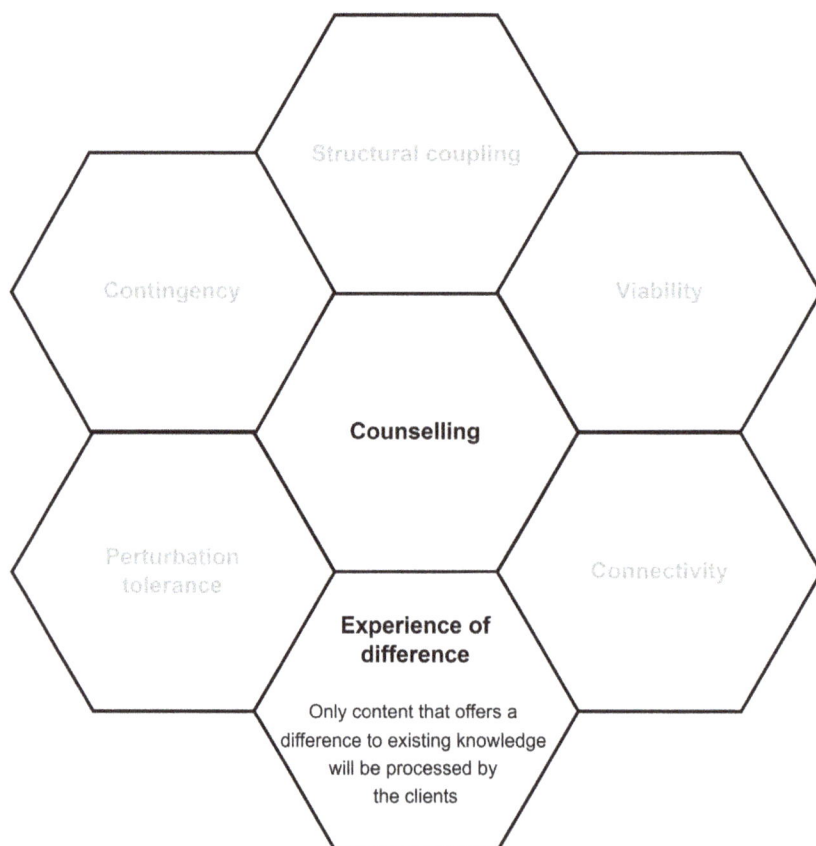

Fig. 11.5 Experience of difference. ©Andreas Wolfs, CC BY.

If counselling content is connectable, it is more likely to be integrated into the client's knowledge network (Arnold 2007: 69). However, connectivity can also result in content from counselling sessions being connected to content other than that intended by the counsellor. It is up to the counsellor to check as best as possible whether the information given has actually been 'received'. This can be done, for example, by asking follow-up questions or by reviewing the action steps resulting from the counselling. However, there is no definitive certainty. The client alone decides whether and where counselling content is linked to existing knowledge.

One aspect that determines whether counselling content is connected, is the answer to the question "Do I already know this?". If the information is already known to the client, i.e., if it does not represent sufficiently an experience of difference from the client's own knowledge, it will also bounce off the outer shell—to stay with the metaphor. What is labelled as "I already know!" is also decided exclusively by the client. In the case of counselling systems that extend over several sessions, the challenge in relation to the experience of difference is for the counsellor to make sure of the client's current status at the beginning of each session. This is not only useful to ensure the appropriate difference in the counselling content, but also helps to review the objective and thus the viable counselling content.

During counselling, counsellors walk a tightrope between content that is compatible, i.e., as close as possible to the client's existing knowledge, and a lack of experience of difference on the part of the client, i.e., when the content is 'too close' or in line with what the client already knows. At the same time, it is always important to look back at the goals that have been set, i.e., to ascertain whether the current path can lead to the agreed goal. This is the only way to ensure the relevance, i.e., the viability, of the current counselling content.

One conclusion to be drawn from the tension described above is that counsellors should give as little advice as possible, but instead support clients in finding the information they need themselves or deriving it from the known and the unknown. When clients are actively involved in achieving the goal and help shape the process and content, it can be assumed that aspects that lack viability or connectivity will often be directly excluded. Information that offers clients too little experience of difference is also unlikely to be included. This type of accompanying advice requires a high degree of flexibility from the counsellor and, if possible, a willingness to accompany people along paths to solutions that the counsellors themselves would not have chosen on the basis of their own experience. Ultimately, it's about finding content that is connectable and offers an experience of difference. A practical tip could be 'listen and ask questions'. On the other hand, this does not mean that the counsellor should sit back and 'let the client do everything', which would most likely also have a negative impact on the structural coupling. The responsibility for the process and the design counselling remains with the counsellor.

The viability, connectivity, and experience of difference of individual counselling topics are anchored and rooted in the individual biographies of the people involved. People who have experienced forced displacement have often experienced significant breaks and drastic events in their lives. It is less important to compare the severity of these events with those experienced by people without refugee experience. Rather, the different nature of these events is of great importance from the perspective of the counsellor. It is important to regularly question and reflect on situations, counselling content, but also on the objectives and connectivity of the content. This can be done individually, for example by using guiding questions, as well as in a group setting with other counsellors who design counselling situations with clients who have experienced forced displacement. Due to the highly individual nature of each counselling situation, it is also possible to involve the clients themselves. This can take place both during and after a counselling session. For example, it is possible to ask a single question at the end of a counselling session, such as "How did you find the counselling?", or to use a standardized feedback form, preferably written in the client's native language. At this point, it is important to note that (former) clients will only comply with the request for substantive feedback if they recognize the viability, i.e., the relevance of the feedback, and the participants are still connected by means of a structural link. Ultimately, in all forms of reflection, counsellors can only test content, procedures, and questioning techniques, evaluate the results retrospectively and, on this basis, develop ideas for possible future use prospectively. There is no certainty as to which intervention will lead to which result.

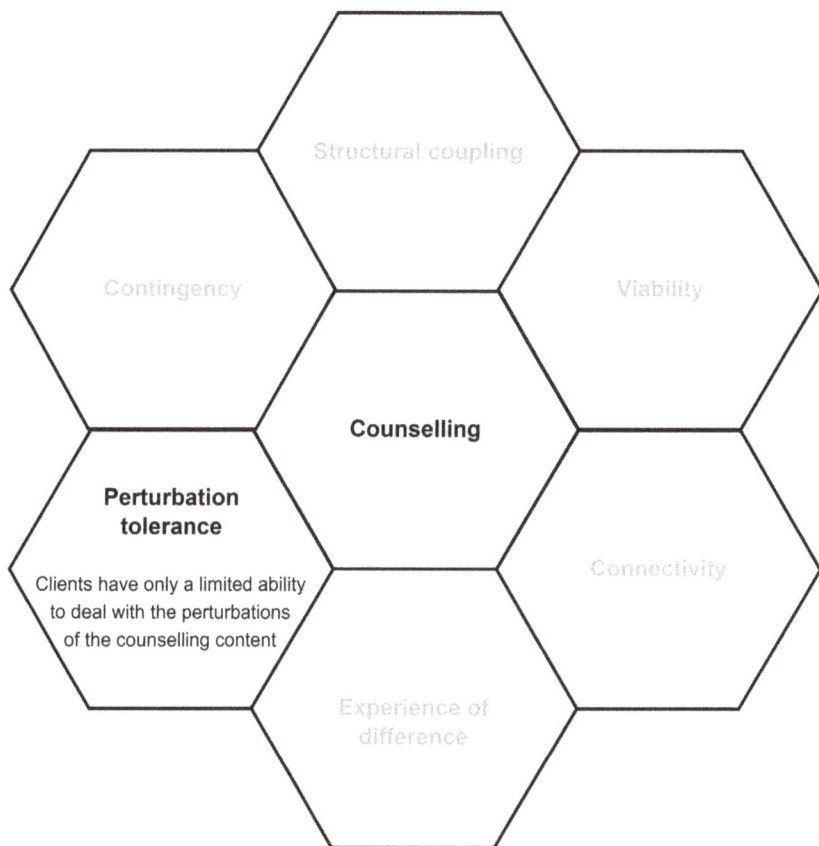

Fig. 11.6 Perturbation tolerance. ©Andreas Wolfs, CC BY.

New Information as a Disturbance of the Known: Perturbation Tolerance of the Clients

Section 2 on structural coupling has already described how external stimuli to closed systems are initially perceived as disturbances— systemically: perturbations—and, metaphorically speaking, bounce off the outer shell of the system. Information, such as that perceived during counselling sessions, is also a stimulus and initially has a perturbing effect. However, as Section 3 has shown, counselling content can be integrated into the client's knowledge network, provided that it is viable for them, designed to be connectable, and offers an experience of difference. The basic prerequisite for this is the structural coupling of all relevant participants.

The diverse perturbations that individuals with refugee experience have endured in their lives can, on the one hand, contribute to a significantly reduced tolerance for perturbation. On the other hand, such experiences may also strengthen their ability to cope with external disturbances. Perturbation tolerance can also vary considerably between individuals with similar experiences of forced displacement, even within families. As the disruptive effect of individual counselling content can also vary, a high degree of flexibility and empathy is required on the part of the counsellor.

Even if the perturbing effect can be minimized in individual cases through high-quality structural coupling as well as viable and connectable content, the counselling content still remains disruptive to the client's system. In addition to the counselling content itself, all other stimuli in daily life also have a perturbing effect. This means that counselling can also lead to double perturbation.

Firstly, the individual counselling content perturbs the client's system. If the new content is connected and changes behaviour, further perturbations may arise due to reactions from the client's environment. Unfortunately, it is not possible to make a general statement as to whether an early indication in the context of counselling, in the sense of 'Be prepared for the fact that your environment might react if you change your behaviour', has a mitigating effect on the expected perturbations. On the one hand, clients are prepared for reactions that are new and perturbing for them; on the other hand, this may lead to the new elements not being integrated at all or being integrated differently into their behavioural patterns, which may lead to different feedback or reactions from the environment.

The reference to the family illustrates another aspect of perturbation tolerance, which has already been described in connection with structural coupling: people from the client's environment, such as family members, may also be relevant to the counselling process although they are not directly involved in it. This is partly due to the structural coupling that the client has with these people. In addition, their perturbation tolerance may directly or indirectly influence the client's potential for change. For example, clients may be ready for the changes initiated by the counselling, partly due to a high tolerance of perturbation, while their (family) environment may react negatively, possibly due to a low tolerance of perturbation. For instance, the client may want to undergo a specialist (preventive) medical examination as a result of the counselling they have received, but refrain from doing so because of negative reactions from their personal (family) environment. The more strongly the connection between the client and their environment is anchored in the client's biography, the more likely it is that the client will take into account the needs of others and postpone their own changes. Through such connections, people from the client's wider environment, who may be unknown to the counsellor, can also be highly relevant to the design of the counselling, highlighting the importance of attentive inquiry and questioning of the context.

In the case of counselling sessions that involve several individual meetings, counsellors should be prepared for such situations and should also question possible patterns of client response that may result from these causes.

In conclusion, it should be noted that the level of perturbation of each individual piece of information, i.e., each stimulus, is just as variable as the amount of perturbations a person can 'tolerate' before their own perturbation tolerance is exceeded and they tend to reject new content across the board, regardless of connectivity or viability. In addition, perturbation is highly dependent on topic and situation. Finally, counsellors must always bear in mind that the counselling situations are only a part of the perturbations to which clients are exposed on a daily basis.

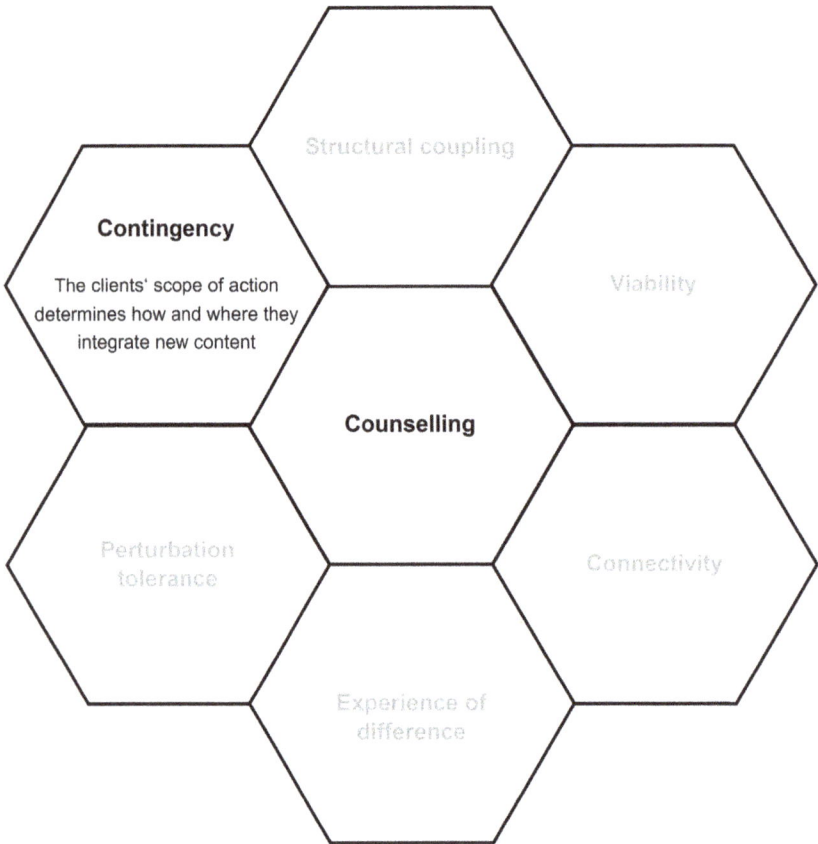

Fig. 11.7 Contingency. ©Andreas Wolfs, CC BY.

A Person's Scope of Action Determines the Integration of the New: The Contingency of the Clients Seeking Advice

In the context of connectivity, one aspect has already been mentioned in a previous section and will be discussed in more detail in this section: clients connect new content to their own knowledge network in a way that seems reasonable or viable from their point of view. These alternative courses of action are also called contingencies (Willke 2006: 249). In other words, one's own contingency determines whether, how, and where new content is integrated into one's own knowledge network and, moreover, what effect this information has and whether, and if so, how it changes one's own actions. The contingencies of the participants in a counselling system differ, and actions or reactions may seem surprising or irritating to the other participants, even though they seem perfectly logical and consistent to the person involved.

The client's scope of action is also important in counselling persons with refugee experience. Contingency, as a result of one's own biography, is characterized by the experience of flight as a drastic life event as well as by one's previous life and events before the displacement. These biographical aspects are supplemented by the experiences that have been incorporated into one's own biography since the flight. People with similar experiences of forced displacement may have very different contingencies due to their previous lives. For counsellors, this can be a reason to ask about the circumstances of their clients' lives before they fled. It is always important to bear in mind that it is very likely that the reasons for fleeing and the traumatic events associated with it are also hidden here. The particular scope of action of clients with refugee experience, which can result from the possible influences of this tripartite biography, can be perplexing or confusing for their counsellors. The same is true of possible changes in the scope of action. Counsellors need a high degree of flexibility in dealing with their clients' contingencies and also need to be mindful of the goals and potential solutions that have been set.

In a counselling system, this effect is particularly noticeable when clients, due to their contingency, connect information in unexpected ways, resulting in seemingly illogical actions. From a systemic point of view, however, these actions are not wrong but rather logical, at least for the actors, i.e., the clients. Counsellors need to adapt to this unpredictability of reactions and evaluate them individually.

One evaluation criterion is whether the client's reaction counteracts the agreed goal or represents a potential solution. This requires a high degree of flexibility, as it is not about the path the counsellors themselves would take, but about a path that the clients consider relevant for them. Depending on the outcome of this assessment, a (corrective) response may be necessary or a change in the counsellor's own solution may be required.

Another assessment criterion is the client's perturbation tolerance, as described in the previous section. If, in the counsellor's opinion, this tolerance is exhausted, the counsellor's own reaction should be assessed with particular sensitivity to possible disturbance of the structural coupling.

Given the above arguments, it seems logical that the ability to assess the contingency of the clients as accurately as possible is particularly relevant for counsellors. On the one hand, it helps if the counsellor has experience of counselling on comparable issues or people in comparable contexts. On the other hand, the duration of the counselling is important. If it takes place over several sessions, experience from previous sessions can be transferred to the current session. However, counsellors should always be prepared for the unexpected. Contingencies may change over the course of a series of counselling sessions, or even within a single session. Ultimately, there should even be changes within the contingency, as the implicit goal of counselling is often to change the client's scope of action, i.e., the contingency.

Each counselling situation and each client must be considered individually. No matter how much experience the counsellor has, the client's contingency remains a black box.

What Is the Benefit of a Systemic-Constructivist Approach to Counselling in Refugee Health

Overall, counsellors should be seen more as facilitators in the counselling process. Once the goal has been set and the establishment of structural coupling has begun, it is beneficial for the clients themselves to discover the viable aspects and identify the appropriate content. This approach helps to mitigate the risk of a lack of exposure to experience of difference, as the clients can directly reject non-viable information and move on to more appropriate content. Counsellors should act as companions in this process, respecting the autonomy of the clients and supporting them on their individual paths to the agreed goal, possibly providing guidance or helping to structure complex contexts.

This more reserved role can be particularly difficult for counsellors, especially if they believe, perhaps from years of experience, that the path chosen by the client may not lead to the desired goal. It requires a great deal of flexibility and courage to suggest possible paths and then to accept if the client chooses a different one.

As a consequence, asking questions is more important than 'giving advice'. It is never about asking 'why?' with an implicit demand for justification, but about understanding the client's current situation and biography. This understanding is one of the keys to person-centred counselling: on the one hand, the biographical context provides the basis for the client's scope of action and starting points for new information. On the other hand, the current situation provides clues to other relevant people who should also be involved in the counselling process through structural couplings.

When asking questions, the aspect of observation, already mentioned in connection with structural coupling, must be considered. Closed systems can only be observed from the outside. Applied to the counselling system, this means that counsellors can never be sure that clients' responses are not primarily tailored to what they believe is appropriate for the situation. When counsellors are on an official, regulatory mission, clients, especially those with refugee experience, may draw on patterns of interaction with officials in their home countries. This can lead to disruptions in structural coupling or in the connectivity of counselling content.

The quality of the counselling can be assessed by counsellors on the basis of correctness, for example in terms of regulatory or scientific evidence. However, this is of much less importance in systemic counselling. The quality assessment is more likely to be done by the clients. Criteria here could include aspects such as suitability for everyday life and a focus on participation. These are far more subjective than technical, content-related criteria. For example, a counsellor may have 'done everything right', but the counselling was not found helpful by the client. In evaluating their own performance, counsellors should rely on the clients' feedback and accept their 'judgment'. This requires the ability, energy, and willingness to continuously question, reflect on, and adapt one's own counselling skills. In essence, it is not just about content or professional skills, but also about person orientation. Person orientation involves creating and maintaining resilient counselling systems through sustainable structural linkages and developing skills to accompany clients in their search for solutions, for example through topic structuring and follow-up questioning techniques.

A systemic-constructivist approach promotes and necessitates the individual design of counselling sessions and can explain a variety of counselling situations. Establishing a structural coupling and identifying relevant, viable counselling content that provides clients with experiences of difference is the basis for successful counselling. By also considering the client's individual, situational perturbation tolerance and contingency, the main obstacles in counselling sessions can be anticipated and analysed, if not completely eliminated. All these aspects are particularly relevant in counselling sessions with people who have experienced forced displacement.

Building on this conceptual foundation, which preserves the individuality of patients with refugee experience and aims to make refugee health more person-oriented and participatory, the subsequent sections of this chapter present strategies that facilitate effective and respectful cross-cultural communication in patient care across language barriers.

Strategies for Effective Cross-cultural Communication in Refugee Health

Setting Up Culturally Responsive Structures and Services

If patient care is to take into account the cultural backgrounds of patients from the perspective of self-determination and equity, appropriate structural conditions must be created. Without suitable structures and space to implement measures, even culturally responsive staff cannot act effectively. Uniform, universally applicable structures must be created at all organisational levels in which culturally responsive patient care is standard (Peters et al. 2014). Measures should include improving workforce diversity, conducting structural analysis, and ensuring competence in planning, policy formulation, and practice (Spitzer et al. 2019). The scoping review by Grandpierre et al. (2018) found that patients and caregivers expressed an appreciation for services that incorporated cultural awareness into practice protocols. This involved services that used culturally appropriate materials and tailored care to meet their needs. Another recommendation was extending the appointment times for patients who do not speak the service language.

An international review conducted by Krystallidou and colleagues (2024) examines the barriers faced by migrants and refugees in accessing mental health services, and highlights the convergence and interconnectedness of communication needs, barriers, and strategies experienced by patients, carers, and professionals alike. A combination of systemic, interpersonal, and intrapersonal factors contribute to a fragmented landscape of language support options, which ultimately affects the quality of communication and, in turn, the uptake and quality of service provision and mental healthcare among migrants and refugees. The review advocates for enhanced cultural and structural competence within the education of health and social care professionals, as well as greater linguistic diversity within the healthcare workforce to better reflect the varied experiences of migrants and refugees. Both patients/clients and professionals appear to strongly prefer communication in the same language, ideally with a shared cultural background as well. Where this is not possible, both groups generally prefer high-quality professional interpreters and translators, which are, however, often lacking or unavailable in mental health settings. Policy makers are encouraged to adopt a systems thinking approach to understanding the complex interactions that influence access to mental health services. In the context of increased global migration and forced displacement, coupled with the high prevalence of mental health disorders among migrants and refugees, the authors assert that language skills should not be viewed merely "as part of individual lifestyle factors, but as an underlying factor permeating all social determinants of health" (Krystallidou et al. 2024).

The Health Evidence Network (HEN), an information service for public health decision-makers in the WHO European Region, has published a report on strategies that have been implemented and evaluated in European countries to address communication barriers for refugees and migrants in healthcare settings (McGarry et al. 2018). This report includes the following policy recommendations (McGarry et al. 2018: ix):

The main policy and practice considerations based on the findings of this review in the WHO European Region are to:

- encourage collaboration between statutory healthcare organisations, non-statutory organisations such as NGOs with an interest in migrant health, and academic institutions to develop and implement strategies to address communication barriers for refugees and migrants in healthcare settings;

- establish intersectoral dialogues on cultural mediation and interpretation among academic, policy, healthcare, and professional organisations and NGOs concerned with refugee and migrant health to:

- clarify the terminology used to describe the role(s) of mediating and interpreting, and

- develop and implement consistent systems across countries for training, accreditation and professionalisation;

- provide training for healthcare staff in working effectively with cultural mediators and interpreters in cross-cultural consultations with refugees and migrants;

- ensure the use of professionals who have been trained and accredited for mediating and interpreting roles in healthcare settings;

- establish incident reporting systems in healthcare settings where strategies to address communication barriers are being implemented to provide a system level mechanism for reporting, monitoring, and responding to problems and barriers to implementation;

- involve migrants in developing and implementing strategies to address communication barriers; and

- develop a national policy that emphasizes the importance of formal strategies to effectively address communication barriers experienced by refugees and migrants in healthcare settings.

These recommendations underscore that effective cross-cultural communication in healthcare can only be guaranteed if the necessary measures and strategies are implemented at the macro, meso, and micro levels. However, the HEN report also shows that knowledge of a wide range of successful interventions at these three levels already exists. These interventions have been tested and evaluated in practice, and can be utilized by others to minimize the negative effects of communication barriers experienced by persons with refugee experience.

Cross-cultural Communication Strategies at the Interpersonal Level

Effective and Respectful Communication in Patient Care across Language Barriers

Effective communication forms the foundation for culturally responsive care, establishing mutual understanding and fostering patient engagement. Collaborative strategies are instrumental in promoting patient engagement and building partnerships. Key strategies involve comprehending the patient's overall situation, tailoring practices to suit the individual's circumstances and ensuring the patient's comprehension of therapeutic procedures. Patients recommend that practitioners be aware of language barriers and speak slowly to ensure comprehension (Grandpierre et al. 2018). In cases where language barriers persist, alternative forms of communication, such as nonverbal cues, gestures, or drawing, may be necessary to gather information.

In addition, according to the review by Grandpierre et al. (2018), patients and caregivers emphasize the significance of their relationships with healthcare practitioners and the need for collaborative partnerships within those relationships. They value practitioners who share information about their lives, including social, cultural, and historical aspects. Patients and caregivers also express the importance of having a consistent therapist to facilitate long-term relationships. It is often beneficial when the practitioner shares a similar cultural background or gender, as they may be perceived as more familiar with cultural taboos. However, it is worth noting that some patients also express concerns about maintaining confidentiality within their communities when such facilitators are present (Grandpierre et al. 2018).

In situations where refugees and staff are under pressure, maintaining a friendly, patient, and attentive demeanour may prove challenging. Various factors, such as anger, insecurity, fatigue, and pre-existing prejudices, can impede refugees' ability to express themselves, while also hindering staff members' active listening and respectful actions. Additionally, the power imbalance between refugees and staff can limit open communication, create unrealistic expectations, and heighten tensions (UNHCR n.d.).

When communication problems remain unresolved at the institutional level, it can lead to frustration, which negatively impacts subsequent patient encounters. Barriers that hinder healthcare professionals from fulfilling their professional roles increase the likelihood of patients experiencing discrimination and mistreatment (Lewicki 2021).

Self-reflection exercise:

The UNHCR published a document with tips and strategies for effective and respectful communication in forced . Please have a look at this document, which is available at: https://www.refworld.org/docid/573d5cef4.html

Read the key considerations at the beginning of an intervention and the key considerations during an intervention.

Think of the way interactions with patients or service users are typically organized in your workplace:

1. Which of the UNHCR's recommendations do you already observe?

2. Where would micro- or meso-level changes be needed to enable you to implement the suggested actions?

3. Where would you need support from other professionals, volunteers, etc., to enable you to follow the strategies recommended by the UNHCR?

Utilizing Translation Tools or Services

There are numerous digital resources, such as translation software and apps, that can provide quick and convenient translations for simple conversations. Generative artificial intelligence (AI), such as Chat GPT, can also be asked to translate into other languages. However, it is important to recognize the limitations of these tools and seek professional translation or interpretation services for more nuanced or critical discussions.

Experiment with your own phone: try Google Translator, DeepL, ChatGPT or other translation apps by typing in sentences, or using voice input. Try to use simple language in your native language. Try translating into another language that you speak and check the translation for errors. The further the language you try is from English, the more errors will occur.

Utilizing Non-verbal Communication

While language is a primary means of communication, nonverbal cues, such as facial expressions, gestures, and body language, can also convey meaning and facilitate understanding. Utilizing these cues, particularly when combined with limited shared language, can help to bridge gaps in communication.

You can watch the following animated video explaining the concept of positive body language: https://www.youtube.com/watch?v=6vT6sqjBFrs&ab_channel=KristenOber

Please note, however, that this video does not include a cross-cultural perspective.

Using Visual Aids

In addition to verbal communication, visual aids such as pictures, diagrams, pictionaries, and other written materials can help convey meaning and facilitate understanding. These tools can be particularly useful in situations where language barriers are severe or when working with individuals who may have limited literacy skills.

You can find specific software for pictograms used in your country. This is an example from Germany. Have a look at the video on the site to get an impression of how to use pictograms: https://www.metacom-symbole.de/metacom_en.html

Another internationally used set of picture communication symbols can be found via Board Maker: https://goboardmaker.com/pages/picture-communication-symbols

You can also use booklets with pictograms. Here is an example of a translation aid for Ukrainians: https://piktuu.com/de/piktuu-health-care-digital/ in German, English and Ukrainian. You can order the booklet or use the online version for free.

Investing in Language Learning

Learn a few words of the language as an icebreaker and to facilitate deeper connections with individuals from different linguistic backgrounds. Learning a new language can also broaden your cultural understanding.

Working with Interpreters and Cultural Mediators

A worldwide strategy to overcome linguistic barriers is the provision of professional services by interpreters or cultural mediators. These individuals are trained to accurately convey the meaning and intent of spoken or written language, ensuring that there are no misunderstandings or miscommunications. A review by Kwan et al. (2023) shows that the use of professional interpreters reduced interpretation errors that have potential clinical consequences and could improve understanding of discharge diagnoses; in contrast, the use of ad hoc interpreters, or going without the use of an interpreter altogether when the patient needed one, increased interpretation errors. In other words, in situations where language barriers are particularly pronounced or the stakes are high, enlisting the services of a professional interpreter or cultural mediator is strongly advised.

Whereas interpreters are typically only responsible for verbally translating spoken information from one language to another, cultural mediators facilitate mutual understanding by also providing advice on cultural understandings of healthcare issues. According to McGarry et al. (2018) cultural mediation has three main components: language interpretation, a responsibility to mediate cultural differences or facilitate intercultural communication, and knowledge about a specific healthcare topic or health service.

ASHA, the American Speech-Hearing Association, has created a reminder that the interprofessional team should include a variety of experts to enable successful cross-cultural communication. Find out more here: https://www.thatsunheardof.org/learn-now/whos-on-your-cultural-iq-team/

Sometimes patients will refuse the use of an interpreter. Several factors could account for this, and it may be beneficial to allocate time to discuss and explain the role of the interpreter. In this way, health professionals can make clear why an interpreter is necessary to ensure effective communication. This approach can reduce the pressure on the patient by shifting the responsibility for decision-making to the service provider.

Despite all the evaluations that show the positive effect of trained interpreters on preventing mistreatment, improving patient adherence to treatment, and reducing healthcare costs, in many countries access to interpretation services is still limited for health professionals. As a consequence, these professionals are regularly obliged to enlist the help of lay interpreters, i.e., staff or family members. This has a massive impact on the quality of the service and thus on the quality of the content of the information. For example, Grandpierre et al. (2018) found that services that failed to provide an interpreter and assumed that the patient would bring someone who could translate were seen as creating a barrier that could negatively affect attendance.

Many communities have organizations that specialize in working with refugees and may have staff or volunteers who are proficient in the languages spoken by refugees. Connecting with these organizations can provide a valuable resource for facilitating communication and supporting refugees as they navigate in the health system.

Using family members for interpretation services is generally considered to be highly problematic. Family members are emotionally biased and only pass on the content of conversations in an adapted form. Children in particular are exposed to content that is not suitable for them. In addition, unwanted role shifts in the family may occur.

Recommended Further Information on How to Work with Interpreters

ASHA, the American Speech-Hearing Association, has published information on steps to take before collaborating with an interpreter to ensure a successful collaboration: https://www.thatsunheardof.org/learn-now/collaborating-with-an-interpreter/

American Speech-Language-Hearing Association (n.d.), *Collaborating with Interpreters, Transliterators, and Translators* (*Practice Portal*). Available at: www.asha.org/Practice-Portal/Professional-Issues/Collaborating-With-Interpreters/

Blackstone, Sarah W., David R. Beukelman, and Kathryn M. Yorkston. 2015. *Patient Provider Communication: Roles for Speech-language Pathologists and Other Health Care Professionals* (San Diego, CA: Plural Publishing)

Clarke, Sarah. 'How to Use Interpreters Effectively to Create a Healing Environment: A Guide for Refugee Service Providers' (10 min.): https://www.youtube.com/watch?v=flB3DLEOsmg

Langdon, Henriette W., and Terry I. Saenz. 2016. *Working with Interpreters and Translators: A Guide for Speech-Language Pathologists and Audiologists* (San Diego, CA: Plural Publishing)

Migrant & Refugee Women's Health Partnership. 2019. *Guide for Clinicians Working with Interpreters in Healthcare Settings.* Available at: https://culturaldiversityhealth.org.au/wp-content/uploads/2019/10/Guide-for-clinicians-working-with-interpreters-in-healthcare-settings-Jan2019.pdf

Migrant & Refugee Women's Health Partnership. 2019. *Culturally Responsive Practice: Working with People from Migrant and Refugee Backgrounds. Competency Standards Framework for Clinicians.* Available at: https://culturaldiversityhealth.org.au/wp-content/uploads/2019/02/Culturally-responsive-clinical-practice-Working-with-people-from-migrant-and-refugee-backgrounds-Jan2019.pdf

UN High Commissioner for Refugees (UNHCR). 2009. *Self-Study Module 3: Interpreting in a Refugee Context.* Available at: https://www.refworld.org/docid/49b6314d2.html

Self-reflection exercise:

1. What is the situation like in your own workplace? Do you know how to contact available interpretation services or cultural mediators in your workplace or municipality?

2. Can you give examples of situations when you used an interpreter (or would have liked to use one)? Whose services did you employ (or could you employ)?

Enhancing Cross-cultural Communication through Interprofessional and Intersectoral Collaboration

When different health and non-health services work together and coordinate their efforts, it helps improve how service providers communicate and coordinate with each other to meet the needs of persons with refugee experience. The health sector plays a crucial role in collaborating with other organizations that deal with migration, social issues, welfare, education, and development. This collaboration is essential for promoting the health of refugees and migrants. Refugees often have complex healthcare needs, which means it's important to have a team of professionals from different fields working together. This kind of team helps organize and coordinate healthcare services to address the diverse needs of individuals requiring complex care (Iqbal et al. 2022).

As the European review by McGarry et al. (2018) highlighted, strategies were often put into action by teaming up people from different areas, like healthcare providers, community organizations, and academic institutions. These worked together to come up with plans that could be implemented in one place or spread across a whole region. Evaluation of these strategies showed in most cases that refugees and migrants gained better knowledge about health, improved their health habits, and got easier access to healthcare services. This shows how crucial it is for different sectors to collaborate and for regional and local authorities to create and carry out official plans that tackle communication issues faced by refugees and migrants in healthcare settings throughout the area.

According to Iqbal et al. (2022), there are nevertheless only very few interventions that focus on training or encouraging interprofessional teams in delivering healthcare services. This is in stark contrast to the fact that by working together, these different professions can ensure that patients receive comprehensive, culturally-responsive care and help to identify and address systemic barriers to care, such as inadequate interpreter services or lack of access to culturally sensitive health information. Healthcare professionals, such as physicians, nurses, allied health professionals, psychologists, and psychiatrists can collaborate with interpreters; social workers and community health workers can, for example, ensure that:

- service users understand their diagnosis, treatment options, and care plan;
- service users and their families receive education and support;
- service users receive appropriate care and treatment;
- service users receive support to navigate the healthcare system and connect with community resources and services;
- service users can advocate for their rights and work to reduce barriers to care;
- service users who may be experiencing trauma, anxiety, or depression receive mental health services;
- service users have access to health promotion and illness prevention.

Self-reflection exercises:

What can you learn from others? In this short video, physiotherapist Philip Rynning Coker shares his ideas and experiences: https://www.youtube.com/watch?v=cinUwtgQHfo

- What is your own perspective regarding the value of interprofessional teamwork to overcome communication barriers when working with persons with refugee experience?

A practical example illustrating interprofessional and intersectoral cooperation with a focus on communication is provided in a video produced by the Philadelphia Refugee Mental Health Collaborative (PRMHC). Voices of Care: Promoting Wellness in Refugee Health – Communication: https://www.youtube.com/watch?v=sJ5nqghC6l0

In the video, the following scenarios are shown:

- introduction to the patient
- navigating language barriers
- communicating the referral process
1. What recommendations are provided in the video? Are they relevant to your own work?

2. How does the video demonstrate the value of interprofessional cooperation in cross-cultural communication with persons with refugee experience?

3. Are there any similar cross-cultural health networks in your own area? Health professionals who have not yet worked with such networks are encouraged to research which health facilities, community services, and refugee organizations they could establish interprofessional or intersectoral collaborations with to enhance their capacity for cross-cultural communication.

In addition to direct interpersonal communication, the creation of culturally and linguistically appropriate education or information material can also be useful to increase the health literacy of persons with refugee experience and contribute to community empowerment processes. The following case story by Lokken and colleagues (2023) provides an example of how interprofessional health service delivery for persons with refugee experience can be improved with the help of educational videos. The videos produced in the project can be accessed here: https://www.youtube.com/channel/UC35cwxMBKJiR0CYELAWkbUw?view_as=subscriber

This exemplary case story can be used to engage with the topic in the following way:

1. Identify the issue at hand and the cultural and linguistic barriers that presented themselves.

2. Recognize the different professions involved in the initiative and assess the importance of interprofessional collaboration in addressing cultural and linguistic barriers.

3. Evaluate the significance of support from volunteers and community members.

4. Outline the steps taken by the team to address the issue.

5. Assess the outcome and determine what is needed to make it sustainable.

6. Research and identify similar collaborative projects in refugee health within your own area.

Exercise: Interprofessional Collaboration to Prepare Information Material

Working in small interprofessional teams, participants will be asked to create posters that address different aspects of cross-cultural communication in refugee health. These posters should encapsulate the perspectives of the different professions represented in each team, using strong visual elements (such as pictograms) and minimal text. The posters will then be presented during the plenary session, where participants will explain their design choices.

Key topics for consideration include:

1. Strategies for building trust and facilitating effective communication in the practice of health professionals, and the critical of robust interprofessional teamwork in achieving this.

2. Approaches to enhancing interprofessional collaboration to improve access to healthcare services for individuals with refugee backgrounds, thereby ensuring improved health outcomes.

Conclusion

To date, cross-cultural communication in refugee health has predominantly been addressed in a rather unsystematic manner. By initiating a reflection on the creation of participatory, person-centred communication environments that effectively address language barriers and challenges in cross-cultural understanding, we aimed to provide a comprehensive framework that goes beyond mere language barriers. Recognizing the potential burden placed on health and social care practitioners due to insufficient institutional and structural support, we focused on the concepts of inclusive communication and inclusive multilingualism as foundational to overcoming these challenges, as these align with the feedback provided by migrants and persons with refugee experience in existing research on enhancing cross-cultural communication in migrant and refugee health contexts. To expand on these ideas, the principles of counselling from a systemic-constructivist perspective were adapted for the context of refugee health. This perspective provides a structural framework for locating refugee experience as a relevant part of a person's biography in the context of the person's entire history. It can also support interdisciplinary communication and reflection between various health and social care professionals by providing uniform dimensions. With this in mind, specific strategies for effective and respectful intercultural communication in patient care across language barriers were presented at the micro level of individual healthcare professionals and at the meso level of healthcare institutions, such as utilizing translation tools or services, working with interpreters or cultural mediators and enhancing cross-cultural communication in refugee health through interprofessional and intersectoral collaboration.

References

Altorfer, Andreas, Käsermann, Marie-Louise (2021). 'Die Bedeutung des Nonverbalen in der Kommunikation,' [The Importance of the Non-verbal in Communication] in *Transkulturelle und transkategoriale Kompetenz: Lehrbuch zum Umfang mit Vielfalt, Verschiedenheit und Diversity für Pflege-, Gesundheits- und Sozialberufe* [Transcultural and transcategorical competence: Textbook on the scope of diversity for nursing, health and social professions], ed. by Dagmar Domenig. 3rd, completely revised and expanded edition (Bern: Hogrefe).

Arnold, Rolf. 2007. *Ich lerne, also bin ich, Eine systemisch-konstruktivistische Didaktik* [I Learn, Therefore I Am: A Systemic-constructivist Didactics] (Heidelberg: Carl Auer, 2007).

Backus, Ad, et al. 2013. 'Inclusive Multilingualism: Concept, Modes and Implications', *European Journal of Applied Linguistics,* 1.2: 179–215, https://doi.org/10.1515/eujal-2013-0010

Becker, Frank, and Elke Reinhardt-Becker. 2001. *Systemtheorie: Eine Einführung für die Geschichts- und Kulturwissenschaften* [Systems Theory: An Introduction for History and Cultural Studies] (Frankfurt am Main, New York: Campus).

Dressler, Dominique. 2009. *Interkulturelle Kommunikation in der stationären Rehabilitation nach Unfällen* [Intercultural Communication in Inpatient Rehabilitation after Accidents] (Göttingen: Cullivier).

Forrester, Jay. W. 1972. *Grundsätze einer Systemtheorie: Principles of Systems* (Wiesbaden: Gabler).

Frederickson, George M. 2015. *Racism: A Short History* (Princeton: Princeton University Press) (Princeton Classics).

Glasersfeld, Ernst von. 2012. 'Konstruktion der Wirklichkeit und des Begriffs der Objektivität [Construction of Reality and the Concept of Objectivity]', in *Einführung in den Konstruktivismus* [Introduction to Constructivism], ed. by Heinz von Foerster (München: Piper).

Grandpierre, Viviane, et al. 2018. 'Barriers and Facilitators to Cultural Competence in Rehabilitation Services: A Scoping Review', *BMC Health Services Research*, 18.23, https://doi.org/10.1186/s12913-017-2811-1

Iqbal, Maha P., et al. 2022. 'Improving Primary Health Care Quality for Refugees and Asylum Seekers: A Systematic Review of Interventional Approaches', *Health Expectations*, 25.5: 2065–2094, https://doi.org/10.1111/hex.13365

Kwan, Michelle, et al. 2023. 'Professional Interpreter Services and the Impact on Hospital Care Outcomes: An Integrative Review of Literature', *International Journal of Environmental Research and Public Health*, 20.6: 5165, https://doi.org/10.3390/ijerph20065165

Krystallidou, Demi, et al. 2024. 'Communication in Refugee and Migrant Mental Healthcare: A Systematic Rapid Review on the Needs, Barriers and Strategies of Seekers and Providers of Mental Health Services', *Health Policy*, 139, https://doi.org/10.1016/j.healthpol.2023.104949

Lewicki, Aleksandra. 2021. 'Gesundheit' [Health], in *Diskriminierungsrisiken und Handlungspotenziale im Umgang mit kultureller, sozioökonomischer und religiöser Diversität: Ein Gutachten mit Empfehlungen für die Praxis* [Discrimination risks and potential for action in dealing with cultural, socio-economic and religious diversity: An expert report with recommendations for practice], ed. by Merx Andreas, et al. (Essen: Stiftung Mercator GmbH), pp. 68–87.

Lokken, James, et al. 2023. 'How Rohingya Language Educational Videos Help Improve Refugee Interprofessional Health Service Delivery in Milwaukee', *AMA Journal of Ethics*, 25.5: E365–374, https://doi.org/10.1001/amajethics.2023.365

Luhmann, Niklas. 1985. 'Die Autopoiesis des Bewußtseins' [The Autopoiesis of Consciousness], *Soziale Welt*, 36: 403.

Maturana, Humberto R., and Francisco J. Varela. 1984. *Der Baum der Erkenntnis: Die biologischen Wurzeln des menschlichen Erkennens* [The Tree of Knowledge: The Biological Roots of Human Cognition] (München: Goldmann).

McGarry, Orla, et al. 2018. *What Strategies to Address Communication Barriers for Refugees and Migrants in Health Care Settings Have Been Implemented and Evaluated across the WHO European Region? Health Evidence Network (HEN) synthesis report 62* (Copenhagen: WHO Regional Office for Europe), https://www.ncbi.nlm.nih.gov/books/NBK534365/

Money, Della, et al. 2016. *Inclusive Communication and the Role of Speech and Language Therapy, Royal College of Speech and Language Therapists Position*

Paper (RCSLT: London), https://www.rcslt.org/wp-content/uploads/media/docs/20162209_InclusiveComms_final.pdf

Nowak, Anna Christina, Hornberg Claudia. 2023. 'Erfahrungen von Menschen mit Fluchtgeschichte bei der Inanspruchnahme der Gesundheitsversorgung in Deutschland: Erkenntnisse einer qualitativen Studie' [Experiences of Persons with Refugee Experience in Accessing Healthcare in Germany: Findings of a Qualitative Study], *Bundesgesundheitsblatt*, 66: 1117–1125, https://doi.org/10.1007/s00103-022-03614-y

Pandey, Mamata, et al. 2021. 'Impacts of English Language Proficiency on Healthcare Access, Use, and Outcomes among Immigrants: A Qualitative Study', *BMC Health Services Research*, 21.741, https://doi.org/10.1186/s12913-021-06750-4

Patel, Pinika, Bernays, Sarah, et al. 2021. 'Communication Experiences in Primary Healthcare with Refugees and Asylum Seekers: A Literature Review and Narrative Synthesis', *International Journal of Environmental Research and Public Health* 18, 1469, https://doi.org/10.3390/ijerph18041469

Peters, Tim, et al. 2014.'Grundsätze zum Umgang mit Interkulturalität in Einrichtungen des Gesundheitswesens [Principles for Dealing with Interculturality in Health Care Institutions]', *Ethik in der Medizin*, 26: 65–75, https://doi.org/10.1007/s00481-013-0289-x

Siebert, Horst. 2009. *Selbstgesteuertes Lernen und Lernberatung: Konstruktivistische Perspektiven* [Self-directed Learning and Learning Guidance: Constructivist Perspectives] (Augsburg: Zentrum für interdisziplinäres erfahrungsorientiertes Lernen).

Robertshaw, Luke, Dhesi, Surindar, et al. 2017. 'Challenges and Facilitators for Health Professionals Providing Primary Healthcare for Refugees and Asylum Seekers in High-income Countries: A Systematic Review and Thematic Synthesis of Qualitative Research', *BMJ Open*, https://www.doi.org/10.1136/bmjopen-2017-015981

Spitzer, Denise L., et al. 2019. 'Towards Inclusive Migrant Healthcare', *BMJ*, 366: 14256, https://doi.org/10.1136/bmj.l4256

Willke, Helmut. 2006. *Systemtheorie I: Grundlagen: Eine Einführung in die Grundprobleme der Theorie sozialer Systeme* [Systems Theory I: Basics: An Introduction to the Basic Problems of Social Systems Theory] (Stuttgart: Lucius & Lucius).

UN High Commissioner for Refugees (UNHCR). 2016. *Community-Based Protection in Action: Effective & Respectful Communication in Forced Displacement* (Switzerland: UNHCR), https://www.refworld.org/docid/573d5cef4.html

12. Advanced Clinical Reasoning

Kathrin Weiß, Amira, Kerstin Berr, Ousman Drammeh and Franziska Grünberg-Lemli

Introduction to Advanced Clinical Reasoning

Advanced clinical reasoning is the process by which healthcare professionals from different disciplines collaborate to understand and address the complex needs of patients. When working with persons with refugee experience, this process becomes particularly important as they may have unique healthcare needs and face challenges such as language barriers and cultural differences. Their potentially complex healthcare needs may require the expertise and input of multiple professionals. Interprofessional advanced clinical reasoning involves the ability to think critically and creatively and to consider the potential long-term impact of different treatment options. The healthcare needs of persons with refugee experience may be more complex and may necessitate longer-term solutions.

When you, as a healthcare professional, first speak with your patient, depending on your work setting, you often know only the diagnosis from the doctor's referral. The following chapter will guide you on how to take more aspects into consideration. You will learn to describe the current components of your patient's health using the International Classification of Functioning, Disability and Health (ICF). Finally, you will take into account narratives of the past and different forms of clinical reasoning. The authentic voices of those who have experienced displacement will stimulate your reflection and enhance your understanding of their extraordinary life situations.

    https://doi.org/10.11647/OBP.0479.12

As essential background information for professionals working with people who have experienced forced migration, it is helpful to first learn about the health risks that are prevalent in the different countries of origin of people who have experienced forced migration. Read the report by Navarese et al. (2022) on the impact of war on a country's ability to provide health services to its citizens. For people working in the health system who have not experienced war and forced displacement, it is often impossible to imagine the serious consequences of a lack of medical services and medication. It is therefore important to bear in mind the major medical and psychological consequences for the individual.

Using the ICF in Advanced Clinical Reasoning in Refugee Health

The life situation of people with refugee experience is complex and characterized by various factors that influence their lives. Knowledge and understanding of these factors are difficult for healthcare workers to develop, because in most cases the circumstances are completely unknown and therefore more difficult to understand. Good interviewing, careful listening, and special empathy skills are necessary to develop a sustainable client-therapist relationship in this context. Special attention must be paid to the context, which in most cases will be very new and perhaps unfamiliar for clients with refugee experiences.

Interprofessionality is essential in this process, as different disciplinary perspectives contribute to a deeper understanding of the client's situation and allow the client more diverse ways of working together with their professionals. The chance of successful collaboration is increased by interprofessionality. Therapists who have developed competencies in the areas of role understanding, communication, teamwork, and ethics in interprofessional collaboration can use these in the collaboration with clients and the team for the development of individually appropriate and sustainable care for people with refugee experiences. As explained by Adamopoulou et al. (2022: 74), "Therapeutic teams work interprofessionally in this field to be able to address the multiple needs of refugees' health through multiple coordinate professional competences".

One key aspect of interprofessional advanced clinical reasoning is the ability to consider the patient's overall context and life circumstances, rather than simply focusing on their immediate healthcare needs. This includes taking into account factors such as social, cultural, and economic issues that may have an impact on the patient's health and well-being.

As a healthcare professional you will probably be used to working with the International Classification of Functioning, Disability, and Health (ICF) (WHO 2001). The ICF describes the components of health to identify the constituents of health. You can use this model to understand the complex health situation beside the specific medical problem of people with refugee experience. Additionally, the ICF provides a common language for describing health and health-related states that facilitates interprofessional communication.

This approach is, for example, underpinned by the research project 'Using the International Classification of Functioning, Disability and Health (ICF) to describe the functioning of traumatized refugees':

> The aim of this project was to use the International Classification of Functioning, Disability and Health (ICF) to develop an interdisciplinary instrument consisting of a Core Set, a number of codes selected from ICF, to describe the overall health condition of traumatized refugees. We intended to test 1) whether this tool could prove suitable for an overall description of the functional abilities of traumatized refugees before, during and after the intervention, and 2) whether the Core Set could be used to trace a significant change in the functional abilities of the traumatized refugees by comparing measurements before and after the intervention (Jørgensen et al. 2010: 57).

The results of the project suggest that the examination of the ICF can be particularly useful in working with people with a refugee background in order to capture the whole person and enable a comparison of the situation before and after rehabilitation.

> By focusing on five very important components of functioning, Body Functions, Body Anatomy, Activity and Participation, Environmental Factors and Personal Factors, ICF offers an overall view of the human aspects of functioning. Considering the very complex situation of traumatized refugees, this perspective seems crucial since traumatization

of refugees impacts the mental, physical, and social functioning. This advocates for an interdisciplinary approach emphasizing rehabilitation, which includes treatment, as a part of the effort. ICF seems to be an appropriate instrument to describe the overall health condition of a patient or client and to document and monitor rehabilitation. ICF focuses on functioning rather than symptoms and diagnosis. It takes into account impairment as well as resources of the person, which creates a good basis for an assessment of all aspects of the person's health conditions.

We successfully developed a Comprehensive Core Set with 106 codes describing common and important aspects of traumatized refugees' health conditions. The result might have been a little different if the procedure had been carried out by international experts selected by certain criteria, but probably not in any decisive way (Jørgensen et al. 2010: 57).

Have a look at the interaction between the components of ICF:

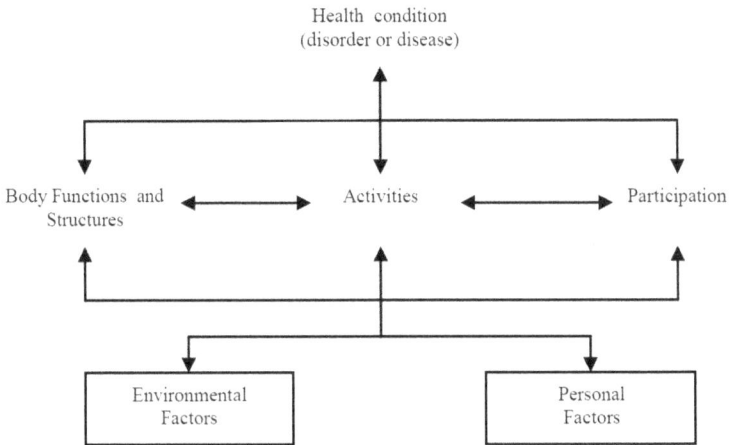

Fig. 12.1 World Health Organization 2001. International classification of functioning, disability and health: ICF. World Health Organization. https://apps.who.int/iris/handle/10665/42407

Regarding the specific needs of people with refugee experience, healthcare professionals will focus also on the contextual factors such as environmental and personal factors to gain a better understanding of the current health problem. They play an important role in establishing a diagnosis and providing treatment. The ICF provides a list of contextual factors, which help you to consider and classify contextual factors.

The following videos offer an in-depth exploration of the International Classification of Functioning, Disability and Health (ICF). The first video provides a detailed overview of the interplay among the individual components of the ICF:

https://www.youtube.com/watch?v=Vj7cF63egGU

The following video will deepen your understanding of the ICF by explaining the contextual factors of the ICF and providing you with an example of how to use them:

https://www.youtube.com/watch?v=j0495iwCX0&ab_channel=PranayJindal

Examining these tables of the ICF contextual factors will assist health professionals in identifying additional potentially relevant aspects for the individuals with whom they work. The ICF classification facilitates the systematic assessment of these determinants of health.

	Environmental Factors
e1:	Products and technology e.g., food, drugs, assistive devices, assets
e2:	Natural environment and human-made changes to environment e.g., land forms, demographic change, plants, animals, climate, sounds, air quality
e3:	Support and relationships e.g., family, friends, people in positions of authority, care providers, strangers
e4:	Attitudes e.g., individual attitudes of family, friends, people in positions of authority, care providers; societal attitudes, social norms, practices and ideologies
e5:	Services, systems, and policies Concerning e.g., housing, utilizes, communication, transportation, civil protection, law, association, media, social security, social support, health, education, labour and employment, politics

Table 12.1 Environmental factors.

	Personal Factors
i1:	General characteristics such as age and gender e.g., calendrical age, biological sex
i2:	Physical factors e.g., physical characteristics
i3:	Mental factors e.g., personality factors, cognitive factors, amnestic factors
i4:	Attitudes, skills, and habits e.g., attitudes, competencies (language competence, self-competence), habits (communication or sleeping habits)
i5:	Living situation e.g., employment status, housing situation

Table 12.2 Personal factors.

The tables 12.1 and 12.2 are based on ICF Praxisleitfaden 4 (2016). Bundesarbeitsgemeinschaft für Rehabilitation (BAR) e.V.: https://www. bar-frankfurt.de/service/publikationen/produktdetails/produkt/1-04-025-icf-praxisleitfaden-4-berufliche-rehabilitation-120.html

The ICF serves as a tool for assessing the current components of health but does not encompass the individual's history. Consequently, it is essential to be attentive to personal narratives. To gain a comprehensive understanding of the health issues at hand, it is important to consider the individual's past as well as the historical aspects of their environment. Adopting an open conversational attitude that encourages client narratives is crucial for understanding the person's preferences and expectations. These narratives are very important for aligning therapeutic interventions meaningfully with the individual's needs.

In addition to the effective utilization of the ICF, incorporating other assessments can be advantageous. Good interprofessional cooperation enables the coordinated use of profession-specific assessments. Given their unique focus on the respective subject areas of different health professions, these assessments can yield valuable insights that benefit the interprofessionally coordinated therapeutic process. Moreover, interprofessional coordination of assessments helps to prevent duplication of assessment procedures and avoids inefficiencies and unnecessary burdens for the client. It also fosters mutual knowledge within the interprofessional team, facilitating the development of an effective team reasoning process for therapeutic decision-making.

It may be useful to explore the topic further by writing down a specific case and analysing it based on the ICF. Use advanced clinical reasoning to promote a better understanding of the whole person. Use the ICF to get an idea of the different aspects and components of health. Add aspects of the patient's past if relevant.

For healthcare professionals working with persons with refugee experience, advanced clinical reasoning may necessitate consideration of the impact of factors such as trauma, displacement, and limited access to resources and their impact on the patient's health. It may also require understanding the unique cultural and linguistic needs of these individuals, including the use of interpreters or other language support services as needed.

In order to broaden understanding of the life situation of people with refugee experience and to enable more in-depth professional reasoning, two personal experience reports are detailed in the following sections of this chapter. The original voices of people with a refugee background are important sources of information in understanding their life situations. These personal experience reports will provide the reader with the opportunity to mentally scrutinize and apply the framework and content discussed in the preceding sections of this chapter.

What Language Means to Me: A Personal Story

The following text was written by Amira* (*name changed), a 45-year-old freelance journalist and children's book author from Damascus, Syria, and a single mother of three children. In 2015, she fled Syria via the Balkans with her youngest daughter and her elder son and came to Germany. It was only four years later that Amira managed to bring her middle son—shortly before his 18th birthday—to Germany via a family reunification procedure. For the first few years, Amira lived with her children in various refugee shelters in southern Germany. Since 2019, Amira has been living in her own flat with her daughter and middle son. Today, her sons live in shared flats in the same city.

Her co-author is Kerstin Berr, MSc, in Occupational Therapy, employed at Bosch Health Campus GmbH, Stuttgart. In 2016, I (Kerstin) met Amira and her family through my volunteer work in refugee aid and we became friends. Today we live in close proximity to each other and meet every week. While we only communicated in English in the beginning, we have exclusively been speaking German with each other since 2018. The text is based on our conversations. We recorded our conversation and I wrote it down and summarized it. Together we discussed the text. It is only a small part of Amira's story, but an attempt to give her feelings a voice.

I love writing! As a child I used to write and read the texts to my mother. If my mother thought it was good, it was good enough for me. If she didn't like something about my writing, then I wasn't happy either. I always tried to write. I often sat in my room for hours and created stories.

But it was a long way until I found my way to writing as a career. After my school education, I started a family early and spent the next years of my life taking care of my family and raising the children. During this time, there was little room for writing. But whenever I found the opportunity to take time out, I read and put my story into words.

When the children started school, I finally got the chance to work for an agency that produced children's books. They published books for children from 1 to 12 years old. My job was to check the texts first. During this time, a colleague of mine found out that I write texts myself and asked me if I could show her some of my texts. She read my texts and was enthusiastic. I told her that I only write for myself, without a bigger plan. She asked me if we could show the texts to our boss. And so, I started writing for the publishing house.

I worked a lot during that time—copywriting, graphic design and I wrote my own stories on the side. But then the unrest in the country began and finally the war broke out. That's when I started working as a clandestine journalist. I travelled to places that were affected by the war and reported on the situation on the ground. I talked to many people and documented the crimes. It was very stressful work, but I wanted to help and give people a voice through my reports. The texts were then taken abroad. It was very dangerous work. After two years it became too dangerous and I was afraid for my children. My mother finally told me to leave the country.

Then the publishing house I worked for also left the country. In my office there was a drawer with all my written work. There were many notebooks that I had filled by hand. I only wanted these texts. It was my story—the story of my life so far. But I was told they were all destroyed. I didn't care so much about the children's books, but much more about my private texts. I didn't have a copy; it was all handwritten. But I didn't get anything back.

Then came the escape.

I fled with my youngest daughter and my older son. Actually, we wanted to go to the Netherlands, but with a group of refugees we finally ended up in Germany.

At first, I thought I could manage everything, learn the language quickly, and catch up with my son within a few weeks. I thought I only needed one year and then I could work as a writer again—or so I had heard. You only need one year to learn the language and then you move on. But I experienced one trauma after another in Germany. The first camp was very bad. We shared a room with many other people, the food was very bad, we had little money, and no idea what to do.

I had no orientation and didn't know what to do to change this state of waiting. It was very hard for me—always waiting. I was in the country for seven months without access to a language course. I tried to learn the language through YouTube videos. I learned a few simple phrases, like "My name is ...; I have children...". I kept asking for a language course, but I was told that I couldn't take part in any language courses without papers. When we moved to the next accommodation, my daughter got a place at school. Every day I had to take her to school and pick her up. It was only in the third accommodation after a year in Germany that I was able to start my first language course.

Before that, I could only communicate in English, and in the camps, there were sometimes projects run by volunteers. When I heard about them, I went and learned a bit. That's why I was able to join the first official language course at A2 level. At first, I was very good, but then I don't know exactly what happened. Maybe it was because I was very unhappy at the camp or because of my stressful situation? I had imagined everything so differently. Everything was incredibly difficult—learning the language, finding work, worrying about my children and the many foreign people around me.

And when I sought medical help, I had to understand everything that was said, but I didn't. That made me very angry and sad. But I swallowed my anger—all day long. All the difficulties in everyday life: with the social welfare office, the job centre, the situation of my children, and I still had no residence status and no papers.

I didn't ask for help and instead tried to sort everything out in English, but my head was often too full. Too full to understand everything and I just felt sad. And I really tried to learn, but I don't know why what I learned didn't stay in my head. I've had the problem for a long time that I forget a lot. But I thought I could do it: I can learn German, I can work, I can start a new life. But I have lost that feeling.

I don't know. I tried to talk to a doctor, but it didn't help me. They don't have time to listen and help me and that makes me even sadder. I was recommended therapy at a counselling centre.

I wanted to try everything to make it better and I started a trauma therapy. There they tried to explain my situation to me. There is no certainty, but maybe I have a trauma and because of this trauma this blockage in the brain happens. My head wants to protect me and that's why I can't remember. I don't know.

One year after therapy I still have the feeling I am very deep down and I need a lot of time to come up again. And for that I need a lot of energy, a lot of strength and time. I hate it when I need help. I hate the feeling and, so far, I need a lot of help—with translations of letters from the authorities, with financial questions, just for everything, and I hate this feeling. And I hate it when I have to ask my children for help. And it makes me sad and angry when my children say to me that I need to do more. I feel bad and stupid when I have to ask for help. My head is empty.

I have told a lot—talked a lot, a lot, because I want to help myself. And the therapists have said that this is good. It's good if I can talk about the past and they noticed that I have a lot of information about mental health problems. I said, "Yes, I am interested in this". And they said this is the first important step. I understood that right away and talked diligently. But I want to understand! Why do I have such a problem? I asked my mother, friends, and the therapists. But they only said, maybe it's a big problem—maybe you saw a murder, for example, or it comes from my war experiences...—but maybe it's a very small problem, but very important for me and it broke something? And I answered "Excuse me, many people in Syria have experienced disasters, but they go on, they have a life and they are happy. They also have beautiful memories. Like my mother, she didn't have a wonderful life, but she has everything in her head and if you ask her something she has answers. Why not me? Am I stupid?" But they said that's not true. But then what? Why can't I write anymore, for example? That's a big problem. I don't want to write for other people, but for myself—I feel myself when I write.

But what should I do? What can I do? It's like my teacher said: language is the key here in Germany. If you don't know the language, you don't have the key. For example, when I get a letter and I don't understand anything. I have to translate everything and still I don't understand it properly. I have done very stupid things because I didn't understand. I never said I didn't understand and I usually try to manage on my own. My problem is, I have read and translated a word a thousand times and then I have forgotten it again. Why does this happen? It makes me very sad—where is my voice, where has my language gone?—I miss writing.

In order to develop a deeper understanding of Amira's situation, it can be helpful to engage with the following questions on your own or in conversation with another person who has also read Amira's story:

1. When in your life have you ever felt that you could no longer pursue an activity, hobby, or occupation, or others prevented you from pursuing it?

- What feelings did this trigger in you?
- What did you do about it?
- Who or what helped you in this situation?

2. Discuss these questions related to the situation Amira describes in her story:

- What prevents Amira from pursuing her activities and occupations?
- What feelings does she describe?
- What could Amira do about the situation?
- Who or what could be a help in the situation?

3. Share Amira's situation in relation to your specific professional focus (subject area). What concrete benefits can interprofessional cooperation bring for Amira?

4. Read the following article on occupational disruption:

Helen C. Hart. 2023. 'Imagined futures: Occupation as a means of repair following biographical disruption in the lives of refugees', *Journal of Occupational Science*, 30:1, 24-36, https://doi.org/10.1080/14427591.20 22.2038249

- Summarize the key messages of the text.

- What further possibilities for supporting Amira arise from the text?

- Develop a series of statements about the connection between the consequences of trauma and language learning or other important activities.

The content of the following interview with Ousman should also contribute to a better understanding of the life situation of people with refugee experience and enable more in-depth professional reasoning.

The Meaning of Illness and Education: A Personal Story

The following summarized text describes the current life situation of Ousman D. He comes from the Gambia and is now 23 years old. The interview with Ousman took place in October 2023. A lengthy escape, an initial stay in Italy and his arrival in Germany as an unaccompanied minor refugee preceded the interview. Ousman arrived in Germany in 2017. He completed his schooling here up to year 10. Ousman now speaks very good German and trained as an occupational therapist from 2019–2023. He has been working as an occupational therapist in Germany since 2023.

The interview and the text were developed by Kathrin Weiß, MSc in Occupational Therapy, employed at the University of Applied Sciences and Arts Hildesheim/Holzminden/Göttingen (HAWK) und at Schule für Ergotherapie, Bildungsakademie GENO, Bremen. In 2018, she met Ousman D. during the application process for professional training at the school for occupational therapy. Since then, they have remained in casual contact.

The interview provides insight into the experiences and important aspects of the life of a person with refugee experience and is intended to emphasize some aspects of advanced clinical reasoning within the context of interprofessional collaboration.

The unique situation of individuals who have fled with a serious illness or significant health restrictions, often in pursuit of better health outcomes abroad, should be particularly emphasized. The challenges of this huge transition—which involves not only leaving one's continent and home country, but also acclimatizing to a new ethnic group, social system, and language—demand tremendous adaptive efforts. Ousman's aspiration to become an occupational therapist emerged from this transformation, which he accomplished with enormous commitment and perseverance. His learning situation in a class of prospective occupational therapists was characterized by his profound thirst for knowledge, open-mindedness, self-confidence, and commitment. Inclusion in a cooperative learning group, alongside a reliable educational supervisor and empathetic teachers supported Ousman in his ambition to become an occupational therapist.

Ousman offers the following insights into his everyday life, daily routine, and leisure activities.

Insights into everyday life:

I am currently still on holiday and have not yet commenced my new job, which I will begin next month. I mainly spend my days at home, where I engage in sport to clear my mind. Additionally, I work at my part-time job three times a week. I also like to watch TV to relax and recharge before starting work.

Daily routine:

When reflecting on my daily routine, I must admit that I do not currently enjoy waking up early. I often spend my evenings watching TV until late at night, which results in me falling asleep around half past two and waking up around eleven in the morning. This habit is not just a result of being on holiday, but has also manifested itself during other phases of my life. However, once I start working, I will need to adjust my rhythm.

Leisure activities:

In my free time, I am passionate about sport. I regularly go to the gym and play football, occasionally serving as a coach for youth teams. One of my favourite things to do at home is cooking; I enjoy trying new dishes as well as connecting with my culture through traditional food.

In the context of clinical reasoning, it is essential for healthcare professionals who aim to treat individuals with refugee experience to understand these preferences and their importance in a person's life. It is equally important to discuss their significance with the client, including within the interprofessional team. This can only be achieved by creating spaces for conversations in a relaxed and trusting atmosphere, allowing stories to be shared. These narratives not only help in understanding the person and discovering their cultural needs but also in considering their preferences in therapeutic planning and medical care (narrative reasoning) (Mattingly 1991: 1000). Knowledge of relevant and important activities, such as cooking and football, can provide important clues for therapy planning and intensive dialogue (Hart 2023: 29).

Ousman also provides insight into how he manages his illness and assesses the services provided by the medical system. His narrative illustrates the reality of his life, his coping mechanisms for illness, and the burden of stress.

Health:

When asked about my health, I disclose that I have lived with a serious illness all my life. However, thanks to the medical care in Germany, I have the disease well under control. Despite occasional impairments due to changes in climate and the associated discomfort, I never give up. With perseverance and a willingness to face challenges, I manage to lead a largely normal life. Although hospitalization is sometimes necessary, I strive to live in harmony with my illness and build a kind of relationship with it that enables me to remain healthy and strong despite everything.

Medical care:

I have been living with a particular illness since childhood, and it will probably accompany me for the rest of my life. Nevertheless, thanks to the medical care available here in Germany, it is possible to alleviate the symptoms and manage the disease better than would ever have been possible in my home country. Taking medication regularly and having regular check-ups with doctors approximately every six weeks are essential for keeping the illness under control. Checking my blood and liver values is particularly important, as it allows me to ensure that everything is going well. Compared to my home country, where medical appointments were infrequent and usually not attended for financial reasons, this represents a significant improvement.

It reassures me to know that, in the event of illness, quick and straightforward assistance is available without the need for immediate financial resources—a stark contrast to my experiences in my home country. This healthcare system has a stabilizing influence on my life and ensures that I feel free from unnecessary stress despite my illness.

To underscore the importance of communication in the healthcare system, I would like to stress the importance of encouraging staff who work directly with people who have experienced displacement to familiarize themselves with their culture and traditions. This can help to create a deeper connection and a better understanding of each person's unique needs. One of my own experiences highlights the importance of this aspect: a friend of mine from Guinea would never agree to have his blood drawn for fear that it could be sold. Such misunderstandings and fears can only be overcome through effective communication and an understanding of cultural differences.

During my time in the hospital, I frequently noticed that communication problems exist not only between patients and medical staff but also within the medical team itself. It is therefore essential that everyone involved, from doctors to therapists, communicates regularly and works together to ensure holistic care. My experience shows that when such team agreements take place, patient care can be significantly improved.

Furthermore, the healthcare system should be open to persons with a migrant background, both in patient care and in employment opportunities within the system. This could pave the way for a more inclusive and diverse healthcare environment that benefits everyone. I have often discussed with friends who, out of insecurity, take on physically demanding jobs rather than explore opportunities in the healthcare sector. Such an opening could encourage many to broaden their professional horizons.

Finally, research is another critical area that needs to be improved in order to sustainably strengthen and expand the healthcare system. Self-help groups in particular offer a valuable resource for individuals facing similar challenges.

They provide not only knowledge and support, but also a sense of community and understanding that is difficult to find outside of the clinical setting.

To summarize, I would say that effective communication, cross-cultural understanding, teamwork, and ongoing research are the pillars on which a robust and inclusive healthcare system should rest. It is my hope that by promoting these aspects, everyone, regardless of their background or experience, will be able to access quality healthcare and feel at home within the German healthcare system.

While I have no immediate family in Germany, I am surrounded by friends from my home country who also feel well cared for here. Most of them have not experienced any major problems with the healthcare system, apart from one friend who tragically died because his illness was recognized too late—a fate he might also have suffered in our home country. These experiences illustrate that, overall, the German healthcare system provides reliable support for individuals like me who have come to this country for various reasons.

Although my friend's issue was recognized, it was unfortunately too late to do much about it. A few months later, my friend passed away, which is a tragic reminder of the importance of timely medical intervention. That said, I have observed that many of my acquaintances have fewer health problems, apart from the stress caused by the system itself. In fact, I myself sometimes feel the pressures and stresses of the system. Nevertheless, I strive to come to terms with it and live with it; adaptation is a part of life here in Germany.

Navigating a foreign healthcare system can be a significant challenge for ill people who have experienced displacement. Making themselves understood, explaining their needs, building trust in unfamiliar procedures, but also being surprised about the 'free' access to medication and therapies can be overwhelming and stressful. From the perspective of clinical reasoning, the aim for healthcare professionals is to enquire about a person's life and illness conditions and strive to understand them (conditional reasoning) (Crabtree 2012: 122). "It involves imagination on the part of the therapist to see the client across time, in the past, present and future and refers to the way a therapist engages the client in a shared vision of his or her future" (Fleming 1991). Given the backdrop of completely different socialization, achieving this understanding requires a high level of reflection and empathy. As Sodemann (2022: 17) notes, "It is hard to understand the extreme stress of having experienced severe trauma and at the same time having to live alone with this trauma in a country where you neither speak nor understand the language". Interprofessional dialogue about the conditions of a person's life and illness can lead to a more comprehensive understanding. Contributions from colleagues in the healthcare system who have personally experienced displacement and understand life in a foreign country are particularly valuable. Building interprofessional teams with a high degree of diversity is a crucial task for the future.

Ousman D.'s educational path highlights aspects of his personality characterized by strength, determination, and self-confidence despite facing significant resistance, misunderstandings, and illness. From the perspective of clinical reasoning, it is evident that these personal values can be revealed through trusting interactions (interactive reasoning) (Crabtree 2010: 119). Discussing the client's personality within the interprofessional team and with the client themselves enhances the likelihood of providing individualized and maximally supportive therapy and consultation.

Professional career:

Regarding my professional career, I am about to embark on my new role as an occupational therapist. After arriving in Germany, I faced numerous challenges to discover and pursue this career path. Training to become an occupational therapist was demanding, but also very fulfilling. I successfully graduated and received numerous job offers. I have chosen a position that is close to my heart and am excited to start in November.

School education:

My early education in the Gambia and later in Senegal was complicated due to my health problems. However, these challenges did not deter me. I was not fortunate enough to have access to adequate education or medical care in my home country, which motivated me to change my life and come to Germany.

Key moment:

A key moment in my journey was discovering the profession of occupational therapy at a job fair. This encounter influenced my career direction and motivated me to pursue this path. My search for an internship eventually led me to a private practice that was willing to provide me with an opportunity to familiarize myself with the profession and gain practical experience.

The healthcare system in Germany has opened up new perspectives for me, not only in terms of my own healthcare, but also in terms of my professional development. It has demonstrated to me the value of access to quality healthcare and the importance of contributing as part of this system.

The insight into Amira's and Ousman's life has been profoundly impressive and enlightening for me (Kathrin) as a teacher, therapist, and researcher. These insights are incredibly valuable. They inspire me to facilitate narratives, practice deep and repeated listening, trust in the power of the confidence and hope of people with displacement experiences, and support them in their aspirations.

The value of interprofessional exchange in advanced clinical reasoning and the sharing of responsibility within the healthcare system enables a new perspective on clients. As Adamapoulou et al. (2022: 74) suggest,

> to be able to address the multiple needs of refugees' health through multiple coordinate professional competencies [...] [c]ollaboration enables health professionals to achieve better health outcomes as it allows them to exercise their expertise in their specific area of practice while communicating their different perspectives with other professionals working with the same service user (Zwarenstein et al. 2009).

This creates a more adaptive and stable starting point for clients in the healthcare system on their path to better health.

Further reading:

The textbook *What You Don't Know Will Hurt the Patient: Cross-cultural Clinical Medicine and Communication with Ethnic Minority Patients* by Danish author Morten Sodemann is, as he himself writes, "not a substitute for medical or surgical textbooks. The book deals with everything that we don't know about patients from a different background compared to patients we are familiar with. As the Danish poet, Piet Hein put it: 'Knowing what you do not know—is, however, a kind of omniscience'. This book is intended to highlight the known unknowns about migrant health and hopefully through that insight to awaken a professional curiosity among health professionals in their encounter with refugees, migrants and ethnic minority patients. It is about everything that we forget, overlook, ignore, misinterpret, minimize, or simply give up on. And then there are the small things that are rare, strange, and which we are not used to". The book is a compendium of experience, knowledge, and empathy.

Morten Sodemann is a Danish physician and professor renowned for his work in global health and migration. He is a specialist in infectious diseases and has extensive experience in migrant health, including social determinants of health and improving access to health services for marginalized groups. He works at the University of Southern Denmark and heads the migrant clinic programme at Odense University Hospital.

The book is available as a free download (www.ouh.dk/textbook).

Conclusion

This chapter highlights the importance of advanced clinical reasoning, which involves critical and creative thinking, especially when working with individuals from refugee backgrounds who face unique challenges like language barriers and cultural differences. The chapter emphasizes using the International Classification of Functioning, Disability and Health (ICF) to provide a comprehensive assessment of patients' health beyond immediate medical conditions. The ICF framework facilitates interprofessional communication and allows healthcare professionals to consider contextual factors like social, cultural, and economic issues impacting the patient's wellbeing.

The chapter includes narratives and case studies, such as Amira's struggle to rebuild her life in Germany and Ousman's journey to becoming an occupational therapist, showcasing how personal stories can enrich clinical reasoning. By understanding personal and cultural contexts, healthcare professionals can offer more empathetic and effective care. The chapter also advocates for interprofessional collaboration, emphasizing that diverse disciplinary perspectives enhance the understanding and treatment of complex health needs, fostering better patient outcomes. The narratives from the refugees underscore the need for health professionals to engage with the patient's past and personal circumstances, promoting a holistic approach to patient care.

References

Adamopoulou, Eileni, Sarah Scheer, and Margarita Mondaca. 2022. 'Creating Brave Spaces in Higher Education: A Short Interprofessional Education Exchange to Support Refugees' Psychosocial Needs', *International Journal of Higher Education*, 11.6: 73–85, https://doi.org/10.5430/ijhe.v11n6p73

Crabtree, Michael. 2010. ,Images of Reasoning: A Literature Review', *Australian Occupational Therapy Journal*, 45.4: 113–123, https://doi.org/10.1111/j.1440-1630.1998.tb00792.x

Fleming, Mary H. 1991. 'The Therapist with the Three-Track Mind', *The American Journal of Occupational Therapy*, 45.11: 1007–1014.

Hart, Helen C. 2023. 'Imagined futures: Occupation as a means of repair following biographical disruption in the lives of refugees', *Journal of Occupational Science*, 30.1: 24–36, https://doi.org/10.1080/14427591.2022.2038249

Jørgensen, Ulla, et al. 2010. 'Using the International Classification of Functioning, Disability and Health (ICF) to Describe the Functioning of Traumatised Refugees', *Torture*, 20.2: 57–75.

Mattingly, Cheryl. 1991. 'The Narrative Nature of Clinical Reasoning', *The American Journal of Occupational Therapy*, 45.11: 998–1005, https://doi.org/10.5014/ajot.45.11.998

Navarese, Eliano P., et al. 2022 'The Spoils of War and the Long-Term Spoiling of Health Conditions of Entire Nations', *Atherosclerosis*, 352: 76–79, https://doi.org/10.1016/j.atherosclerosis.2022.05.012

Sodemann, Morten. 2022. *What You Don't Know Will Hurt the Patient: Cross-cultural Clinical Medicine and Communication with Ethnic Minority Patients* (Odense: Odense University Hospital), https://ouh.dk/media/5evcuqm4/morten-sodemann-2022-what-you-don-t-know-will-hurt-the-patient-final_09-03-2022-red-05-04-2022.pdf

Zwarenstein, Merrick, Joanna Goldman, and Scott Reeves. 2009. 'Interprofessional Collaboration: Effects of Practice-Based Interventions on Professional Practice and Healthcare Outcomes', *Cochrane Database of Systematic Reviews*, 3.CD000072, https://doi.org/10.1002/14651858.CD000072.pub2

13. Advocacy and Empowerment in the Context of Refugee Health

Sandra Schiller with Kass Kasadi

Advocacy and empowerment are closely related concepts. Advocacy refers to efforts to support the rights and needs of a particular group or individual, while empowerment involves the process by which individuals or groups acquire the knowledge, skills, and resources necessary to take control of their own lives and advocate for their own needs. The first section of this chapter looks at 'health advocacy'. It emphasizes that a human-rights framework in refugee health requires health and social care professionals to engage in actions that advance the rights of individuals and groups towards social justice objectives. Following this, the next section introduces the concept of empowerment as it is commonly applied in health and social care, highlighting both political-activist and psychosocial perspectives. In order to illustrate the relevance of advocacy and empowerment in practice, the last section of the chapter provides a case example of a current project in which the fight against female genital mutilation (FGM) is closely linked to the empowerment of African women living in the federal state of Lower Saxony in Germany.

Health Advocacy

Following the definition of medical advocacy suggested by Earnest et al. (2010: 63), the concept of health advocacy can be seen as "action by a [healthcare professional] to promote those social, economic, educational and political changes that ameliorate the suffering and threats to human health and wellbeing that he or she identifies through his or her professional work and expertise." This requires health professionals to have good knowledge of the rights that individuals are entitled to and why these rights need to be inviolable rights for everyone, regardless of their legal status. Based on this knowledge, professionals also need to be willing to take action to assist persons with refugee experience in achieving these rights.

Article 25 of the Universal Declaration of Human Rights (United Nations 1948: 76) addresses health as a fundamental human right: "Everyone has the right to a standard of living adequate for the health and well-being of himself and of his family, including food, clothing, housing and medical care and necessary social services, and the right to security in the event of unemployment, sickness, disability, widowhood, old age or other lack of livelihood in circumstances beyond his control." Similarly, the Constitution of the World Health Organization (2020/1948: 1) recognizes health as a fundamental human right, stating: "The enjoyment of the highest attainable standard of health is one of the fundamental rights of every human being without distinction of race, religion, political belief, economic or social condition."

However, for persons who have experienced forced displacement, health is not a given in many European countries. Current national and international studies show that people who have experienced forced displacement are not only exposed to specific health risks before and during their flight but also to influences from the living conditions in the country of arrival (WHO 2022). Accommodation in a collective accommodation centre, an insecure residence status or an uncertain legal situation, limited access to healthcare, experiences of racist protests including attacks and right-wing populist agitation, discrimination, and a lack of social participation have a negative impact on the health of those affected in many European countries (Nowak & Hornberg 2023; Stevens et al. 2024). Furthermore, refugees and asylum seekers "face legal restrictions with regard to their access to healthcare in many countries of the European Union" although this practice violates their right to health (Bozorgmehr et al. 2017). Against this background, promoting the health and well-being of persons with refugee experience is an ethical challenge that calls on health professionals to advocate for social justice and equity.

The *Advocacy Toolkit for Diaspora Organizations* (Danish Refugee Council 2023: 4) defines advocacy

> as a process of supporting and enabling people to express their views and concerns, access information and services, defend and promote their rights and responsibilities, and explore their choices and options in life. Advocacy, in that sense, can be understood as an organised effort to influence social or policy change, whereby action can be directed towards both political decision-makers or society as a whole.

In refugee health, advocacy typically includes efforts to lobby for persons with refugee experience to have access to quality health services and to ensure that healthcare services are culturally and linguistically appropriate, taking into account the specific living situation of persons with refugee experience.

Advocacy in refugee health cannot be pursued without the strong involvement of persons with refugee experience themselves to avoid the risk that their real interests will be ignored. Legitimacy and accountability are crucial concepts that need to be considered before taking up advocacy work (Danish Refugee Council 2023). Networks and organizations by and for persons with refugee experience have published guidelines and other works offering valuable information on how to prevent the exclusion or tokenization of persons with refugee experience in (health) advocacy (Global Refugee-Led Network 2019).

In this context, it should be noted that although research in the area of refugee health has significantly increased over the last two decades, substantial gaps in the current knowledge base have been criticized. These gaps are considered to stem from a lack of meaningful participation of individuals with refugee experience in this research (James et al. 2021; Kronick et al. 2021; MacFarlane et al. 2024). As MacFarlane et al. (2024) emphasize, explicit, critical attention must be given to the voices that are heard, the voices that are left out, and the voices of those who are ignored because they do not even have a seat at the table.

To narrow this gap, participatory health research—a research paradigm originating from the Global South—has been promoted as a methodology to follow a human rights advocacy perspective in order to strengthen knowledge translation and promote social justice (Kronick et al. 2021; MacFarlane et al. 2024). However, the intensification of the above-mentioned restrictive refugee policies, as reflected in the asylum compromise adopted by the European Union (EU) member states in 2023, renders a transformative, evidence-based, and rational design of European healthcare systems a distant prospect (Bozorgmehr & Gottlieb 2023).

Self-reflection exercise:

1. Which refugee associations, networks, or self-help group exist in your local context?

2. How can you support them in acting as advocates for refugee health?

A human rights framework challenges the historical division between systemic change efforts and individual casework in health and social care, advocating for the integration of actions that advance social justice and the rights of individuals and groups in all practices. All health and social care professionals working with persons with refugee experience have a responsibility to advocate for the improvement of the conditions in which care is provided, and advocacy is often written into their ethical code and scope of practice (Gallagher & Little 2017; Stoddart et al. 2020).

However, many health professionals who have not been trained in refugee health are uncertain about what this entails in practice and whether they possess the necessary skills to advocate for the health and well-being of persons with refugee experience. For example, Claire O'Reilly, a physiotherapist working in refugee health, describes the initial feeling of self-doubt: "Probably one of the first challenges was that idea that I didn't necessarily interpret advocacy as part of my role. So, I think there's that element of do I have time to take this on? But it was also much more, do I have the skills? Am I the best person to be doing advocacy?" O'Reilly has experience from various conflict zones and is particularly interested in how humanitarian health responses can be sustainable. In an interview created within the EU-funded project PREP (Physiotherapy and Refugee Education Project) she discusses advocacy strategies: https://soundcloud.com/maria-alme/emer-mcgowan-advocacy-intervie w?si=4d3a7dfd322f4bab807871fed425cfc5

A transcript of the interview can be found here: https://hvl. instructure.com/courses/19115/pages/Transcript%20of%20 discussion%20McGowand%20and%20O%27Reilly?titleize=0

Health advocacy "dictates that practitioners do not shy away from conflict where this is necessary to promote a human rights and agenda" (McAuliffe 2022: 67). Health and social care professionals working in countries where refugees and asylum seekers are not granted access to regular healthcare, or who work in specific settings such as immigration detention centres, are regularly confronted with conflicts between their obligation to act in the best interests of their patients and the demands placed on them in "a system that expects clinicians to deliver diminished standards of care and violate patients' rights to health" (Stoddart et al. 2022). The competing demands of "dual loyalty" towards the patients and the employer (Solomon 2005) make advocacy an important professional role to lessen experiences of moral distress.

An Australian study by Stoddart and colleagues from 2020 documents the personal views and experiences of Australian medical and health professionals advocating for the health of refugee and asylum-seeker populations in mandatory immigration detention. The study provides insights into how advocacy is related to contemporary medical ethics and understandings of core professional roles. It examines which factors have an influence on healthcare professionals' motivation to engage and persevere with advocacy, and what role health advocates can play "in systems that diminish patients' health rights." The participants of this study saw advocacy as both a personal and professional duty in the face of the challenges offered to their obligations as professionals. They identified three key motivations for engaging in advocacy: proximity, readiness, and personal ethics. Proximity involved their awareness and closeness to injustices faced by detained asylum seekers, often stemming from personal or professional experiences. Readiness depended on their ability to advocate given their personal circumstances, such as holding citizenship or permanent resident status. Personal ethics aligned with their core professional responsibilities, leading to two types of advocates: accidental advocates and "jigsaw advocates", the latter seeing advocacy as "a final piece of a personal puzzle" in their pursuit of social justice and humanitarian efforts.

Self-reflection exercise:

1. How well can you relate to the experiences of health professionals described in this section?

2. What are you passionate about? Which aspects of the healthcare system you work in need to be changed in relation to refugee health? Make a plan for an advocacy strategy for working towards this.

3. How do your personal and professional ethics support you in a role as health advocate?

4. Which rewards and challenges are associated with the role of being a health advocate for persons with refugee experience?

Advocacy is one strategy to raise levels of familiarity with an issue and promote health and access to quality healthcare and public health services at the individual and community levels. When trying to gain political commitment, policy support, social acceptance and systems support for a particular public health goal or programme, a combination of individual and social actions may be used to try to affect change (European Centre for Disease Prevention and Control 2009).

Effective advocacy typically requires a combination of strategies that address both the broader policy context and the needs of individuals. Systems and policy advocacy involve advocating for changes in legislation, regulations, policies, and practices to allow increased funding for refugee healthcare, access to interpreters and other language or cultural support services, and training for healthcare providers on cultural humility and refugee health (MacDonald & Stymiest 2023). This advocacy strategy includes providing information about the healthcare needs of persons with refugee experience and the challenges they face to policymakers and the public to help build support for policies and practices that address these needs. For advocacy to be effective, there is a need to clearly document and define the problem, target a specific audience/group that can affect change, propose a solution, and use evidence and data as a basis for proposed action (MacDonald & Stymiest 2023).

Another type of advocacy is case advocacy, which focuses on providing direct support to individuals and families with refugee experience as they navigate the healthcare system (MacDonald & Stymiest 2023).

Ultimately, advocacy in refugee health needs to be founded on building partnerships and coalitions by working with community organizations, advocacy groups, and other stakeholders as a way to help amplify the voices of persons with refugee experience and increase the impact of individual advocacy efforts.

It is no coincidence that advocacy is one of the three main strategies promoted by the Ottawa Charter for Health Promotion (WHO 1986) as it plays a crucial role in formulating policy programmes or planning for the future, taking into account the social determinants for health that impact health equity. From this perspective, advocacy becomes necessary whenever a group of people or a socio-political goal, such as health, is not considered to be sufficiently articulate and assertive (Lehmann et al. 2020). Approaches to cross-sectoral cooperation can be found at all national and international levels (e.g., federal, state, and local) (Lehmann et al. 2020). An interprofessional and intersectoral approach in health and social care is the basis for effectively designing and planning health promotion programmes for people with refugee experience. Health and social care professionals need to address fundamental issues such as the appropriateness and feasibility of integrating health promotion programmes for refugees into mainstream health promotion structures, the specific needs arising from diverse backgrounds, living conditions, and environments, and how to plan and implement socio-culturally sensitive health promotion in a way that considers the diversity within the refugee population (Kooperationsverbund Gesundheitliche Chancengleichheit 2021).

Community health, or primary healthcare, is promoted by the WHO (2023) as the most promising way to achieve universal health coverage, despite recent setbacks. Primary healthcare is seen as:

> the most inclusive, equitable, cost-effective and efficient approach to enhance people's physical and mental health, as well as social well-being. It enables universal, integrated access to health services as close as possible to people's everyday environments. It also helps deliver the full range of quality services and products that people need for health and well-being, thereby improving coverage and financial protection (WHO 2023).

This point is illustrated by the case example of Carol, an occupational therapist working in the Pathway Homeless team in the UK, who describes how she fulfilled her role as an advocate by assisting a person with refugee experience to find suitable housing. This case story was created in the EU-funded project PREP (Physiotherapy and Refugee Education Project): https://hvl.instructure.com/courses/19115/pages/case-study-advocacy-for-people-from-a-refugee-background

Self-reflection exercise:

1. How can you collaborate with community health centres or other facilities aiming to increase access to essential primary and preventative care services, particularly for people who experience restricted access to health services?

2. How can you utilize their expertise and support them as part of your professional role? Where do you see the potential of interprofessional collaboration?

Advocacy in refugee health will only be successful if it is not primarily seen as a task for particularly committed 'lone fighters,' but as a collective responsibility supported or initiated by employers in the outpatient, inpatient, or rehabilitation sector, and in the context of intersectoral health promotion, community-oriented work, educational institutions, professional associations, and (inter)professional networks. McAuliffe (2022: 71–72) highlights the critical role played by interprofessional cooperation in such a collective approach:

> Collective action and collaborative partnerships between people of different professional disciplines provide excellent opportunities for strong advocacy and activism through the pooling of intellectual and skills resources. There are many examples across different workplaces of people coming together to work on projects, community action initiatives, research studies and therapeutic interventions with the explicit aim of joining with others and connecting knowledge and know-how. Part of interprofessional education is learning how to find out about what others can offer, and how others position themselves in terms of their value base, ontology and epistemology.

Most importantly, the experiences and expertise of health and social care professionals who have personal experiences of forced displacement are vital as advocates. They can build bridges to local, national, and international refugee communities, organizations, and networks, ensuring that health advocacy efforts have the legitimacy and the necessary skills to act in the interests of the health and wellbeing of people experiencing displacement.

To further illustrate the importance of advocates who have first-hand experience of the unique healthcare issues with which specific refugee and migrant communities are faced, the last section of this chapter demonstrates how advocacy can be practically applied through community-based initiatives by introducing a real-world example. In recent years, a network dedicated to health and inclusion within African communities living in Germany has increasingly made the fight against female genital mutilation/cutting (FGM/C) the central focus of its work. This case example demonstrates how advocacy is not solely the responsibility of individual health and social care professionals but involves collective community action to ensure equitable healthcare access.

Empowerment in the Context of Refugee Health

Empowerment has become a fashionable concept in various disciplines and can be understood in many different ways (Herriger 2020; Mohseni 2020). In social work or health promotion, empowerment typically signifies a shift from a deficit-oriented, hierarchical, and devaluing view of patients or clients to one that focuses on their resources and strengths. According to Herriger (2022: own translation),

> empowerment describes encouraging processes of self-empowerment in which people in situations of helplessness and powerlessness begin to become aware of their abilities and strengths, actively shape the reality of their lives and learn to use their resources to lead a self-determined life. Empowerment—in a nutshell—aims at (re)establishing self-determination over the circumstances of one's own life.

From an empowerment perspective, people who have experienced displacement are not seen as 'passive victims', but as competent actors who successfully managed their displacement thanks to their significant abilities and resources, their inner strength, and their networks.

Self-reflection exercise:

1. What understanding(s) of empowerment is common in your own profession?

2. What (inter)professional empowerment approaches are applied in your field of work?

3. How well does this apply to refugee health?

Empowerment is originally a strategy used by disadvantaged social groups to defend themselves against unequal opportunities for participation and an unfair distribution of resources resulting from existing social and political power structures. This strategy was developed primarily in the women's and civil rights movements of the 1960s and 1970s and in the self-help movement of the 1970s in the USA. Empowerment stands for the ability to find one's own voice individually and collectively through joint political action, to use one's own resources, and thus to develop agency (Herriger 2020). The empowerment of people with refugee experience is therefore not about the (self-)empowerment of individuals, but about complex, interconnected, individual, collective, and structural power-building processes at the micro, meso and macro levels, the aim of which is to achieve greater democratic participation and political decision-making power. The activist and political engagement of self-organized groups of people with refugee experience—from local initiatives to international movements—play a vital role in bringing public attention to their struggles against exclusion and racism, and their fight for a life free from inhumanity. As a result,

> empowerment benefits not only one group or community, but all citizens. A real perspective for persons with refugee experience also means a new perspective for the respective host country. For us, empowerment means that decisions are made with us, not for us. We want to have a say in all matters that affect us and we want to have a say in the future of the country in which we live. But the basis for this is a level playing field and equal civil rights (Amoah et al. 2023: 15).

Empowerment also plays an important role in health promotion, "the process of enabling people to increase control over, and to improve, their health" (WHO 1986). Empowerment in the health sector often refers to supporting the development of health literacy by making relevant health information accessible in appropriate ways, for example by working with language and cultural mediators. Good interprofessional and intersectoral networking is important here, including, for example, cooperation with self-help organizations that support migrants and people with refugee experiences. Empowerment in healthcare typically involves support of community-based healthcare initiatives. In refugee health, by supporting the development of initiatives that are led and controlled by persons with refugee experience themselves, healthcare professionals can contribute to empowerment processes that will allow persons with refugee experience to take an active role in their own healthcare and the healthcare of their communities. This is demonstrated, for example, in the interactive, community-based training programme for cross-cultural trauma-informed care described by Im and Swan (2022). Another area is supporting people with refugee experience in accessing services in the healthcare system. Finally, empowerment refers to the implementation of structures and practices in the healthcare system that fundamentally benefit people with refugee experiences. Here, there are many overlaps with advocacy.

Empowerment refers to a process of collective self-empowerment in which individuals and groups acquire the knowledge, skills, and resources they need to take control of their own lives and advocate for their own needs. As a professional support service, empowerment is inevitably based on a tension between self-determination and heteronomy, autonomy, and dependency (Lindmeier & Meyer 2020). It is therefore important to be clear about what health and social care professionals can and cannot do in relation to their patients' or clients' empowerment processes. Empowerment approaches in the tradition of social movements understand empowerment "as a healing, empowering experience between people with equal rights" (Flory et al. 2020). Health and social care professionals without refugee experience can use their privileged position in society and act in solidarity. This, however, cannot replace empowerment by or with other people who have had similar experiences. Health and social care professionals with refugee experience can both engage in empowerment processes themselves and support others to do so. Their experiences and knowledge are a valuable source for developing the field of refugee health in the future.

Empowerment requires not only "a tireless emancipative, radical and courageous practice by those who protect and defend their human dignity and empower others to do the same. It also requires: listening, openness to learning, allies, power-sharing [...], stepping back from decision-making processes and positions, as well as resources, resources, resources" (Haschemi et al. 2023: 406; own translation). There can be no concrete instructions for the empowerment process, as its goals and elements depend on the specific experiences of the people with refugee experience and their personal coping skills, needs, and demands (Flory et al. 2020). The characteristics of the psychosocial attitude of empowerment, which can form the basis for interprofessional collaboration, include a fundamental trust in the ability to shape one's own life, a strength- and resource-oriented view, motivational interviewing to enable more self-determination, identifying strengths and resources together, and creating opportunities to experience self-efficacy, recognizing the patients or clients as experts in their own cause, and negotiating and sharing responsibilities as partners (Projekt Kompass F 2018).

Health and social care professionals can support and promote the (individual) development process of empowerment by contributing to the establishment of networks and the creation of spaces where people with refugee experience can create empowerment in exchange with others (Benbrahim 2017). Empowerment processes can only emerge from the needs, interests, and life situations of refugees, and specific content and methods are suitable for initiating these processes with regard to structural disadvantages (Projekt Kompass F 2018). Key elements include creating protected spaces, such as peer-to-peer environments that bring together people with common experiences of discrimination, such as Muslim women refugees or LGBTTIQ* refugees. Additionally, low-threshold activities for refugee groups, such as meeting cafés and creative activities, can strengthen exchange and self-help potential, promote cohesion, and contribute to normalizing everyday life. Providing access to knowledge through workshops and seminars by refugee self-organizations can offer information on legal rights and opportunities for political participation. Establishing, using, and expanding networks by promoting interest- and target-group-specific contacts and cooperation with self-organizations, self-help groups, political groups, NGOs, and regional working groups is also crucial. Finally, linguistic empowerment involves making marginalized voices and perspectives visible, for example, in local decision-making processes and public relations work. Such an approach calls for sound interprofessional and intersectoral collaboration, which is also reflected by the World Health Organization's (2023) Global Research Agenda on Health, Migration and Displacement.

When empowerment is applied in professional help contexts in the health and social sector, there is a risk of individualizing unequal power relations by focusing on individual patients or clients and their resources. This is why health and social care professionals need to be able to recognize and critique unequal structural and social power relations, and to advocate for structural change that may also challenge their own privileges. Health and social care professionals, who have structural power and institutional access, are called upon to engage in power sharing (in the sense of power distribution and power access, Rosenstreich 2006) when working with people with refugee experience. A fundamental prerequisite for power sharing is to get to know and take seriously the perspectives, problem definitions, positions, and interests of people with refugee experience. This may require a willingness to change one's own actions and attitudes. It is also important to avoid a paternalistic attitude and not to speak for people with refugee experience, but to support them in pursuing their own interests (Rosenstreich 2006).

Empowerment in the context of forced migration has particularly been criticized with regard to the following points: Firstly, empowerment becomes a diversionary tactic when the same problems are named over and over again while their causes are only sought in people with refugee experience themselves, and a self-critical public discussion of "inadequate and outdated structures, legal situations or blatant violations of humanity" in the host country is avoided (Amoah et al. 2023: 14; own translation). Secondly, the establishment of parallel and inexpensive alternative structures in the form of voluntary support groups or peer offers of psychosocial support carries the risk that such services do not come close to the professional care to which persons with refugee experience are entitled (Flory et al. 2020). Thirdly, there should be no illusion that the empowerment approach can lead to cooperation on an equal footing with people with refugee experience, whose life situations are largely determined by their residence status, who experience a wide range of discrimination and who are dependent on support, but often face long waiting lists (Flory et al. 2020). Taking this criticism into consideration, the aim in European countries should be to enable the empowerment of persons with refugee experience within the structures of an established healthcare system that is sensitive to the needs of diverse groups in society and that promotes strong intersectoral collaboration as a crucial means to enhance the health and well-being of persons with refugee experience.

Self-reflection exercise:

1. What can you contribute to power sharing and empowerment in refugee health?

2. How can the empowerment of persons with refugee experience be supported within the context of your country's health and social care system?

Empowerment in refugee health necessitates collaborative, context-sensitive and nuanced approaches. The following section underscores how empowerment is operationalized within African communities through peer-to-peer health promotion and active engagement against practices like female genital mutilation/cutting (FGM/C). This case highlights the intersection between empowerment and advocacy, illustrating that empowerment efforts are most effective when they are community-driven and culturally resonant. By directly involving community members in health initiatives and advocacy projects, the case study exemplifies how participatory approaches can promote health equity and provide individuals with the tools necessary for self-advocacy and self-determination.

The Need for Networking to Promote the Health of African Migrants and Refugees

In order to illustrate the concepts explored in the previous two sections, Kass Kasadi, the founder of baobab—zusammensein e.V., an association focused on advocacy and the empowerment of women and families from the African community, provides a practical case example describing the association's work. Among other things, he works as a project manager for the project Elikia.

The association baobab—zusammensein ('zusammensein' means 'being together'), founded in 2013, emerged from the heterogeneous African communities in the German federal states of Lower Saxony and Bremen. In the course of its existence, it has increasingly developed from a project in the field of disease prevention to a network for health and participation. Baobab—zusammensein e.V. offers a low-threshold counselling service for basic questions on the topics of childrearing, integration, health, education, work, and assistance with everyday issues, e.g., housing and living. Many women and families from the African community are looking for support, counselling, and advice, particularly with regard to female genital mutilation/cutting (FGM/C), as there is currently no appropriate contact point for the community.

Due to the strong desire and commitment of the community members to become involved in the areas of health and integration, the need for exchange, training programmes, participation, and support has increased. This is provided by means of:

1. participatory, emancipatory and eye-level (peer-to-peer) health promotion by and for Africans in the federal state of Lower Saxony;

2. establishing and anchoring self-help groups in the African community;

3. the fight against female genital mutilation/cutting (FGM/C) by combining community-based awareness-raising, direct support for affected individuals, intersectoral networking, and preventive protection work, all within a framework of empowerment and cultural sensitivity;

4. HIV/AIDS/hepatitis prevention through multilingual education, culturally sensitive outreach, peer mediation, support in health system navigation, and cooperation with professional agencies, all tailored to the specific needs of migrant and refugee communities in Hannover;

5. support during medical treatment and therapy to increase patient adherence to advice and treatment in the German healthcare system;

6. promoting the participation of communities in the development and organisation of services and approaches that promote health, integration, and transculturality;

7. training and further education programmes for professionals working in the health and integration sector on African lifestyles and societies;

8. promoting empowerment and combating stigmatisation;

9. supporting the continuation of health promotion in African communities;

10. social services/social mediators.

Currently, the association is run from three offices: the main office in Hanover, and a small one in Walsrode and Osnabrück, respectively; and has five full-time employees. Most importantly, the network is supported by a large number of volunteers, the majority of whom are women, representing the diverse African communities in Lower Saxony.

These volunteers are of such a great importance because they are part of their communities, hence they are heard—and they hear what issues are being discussed; they know what the main problems are, because these are their problems as well. These volunteers are trusted, so they can put forth and discuss solutions. In other words, the problems discussed in baobab—zusammensein are problems of daily life, not problems drawn from theoretical discussions.

The following languages are spoken in the network: Kabwe, Ewe, Kotokoli, Twi, Medumbe (Bamileke), Lingala, Lari, Kikongo, Kizombo, Swahili, Tshiluba, Tetela, Peul, Yoruba, Ibo, Wolof, Djoula, Bete, Kreol, Mandingue, Arabic, Tigrini, Somali, Kinyarwanda, Kirundi, Shona, Ndebele, Twi, Bambara, Abron, Haoussa, Baoulé, German, French, English, Portuguese, and Spanish.

With the project 'Elikia', which was launched in the spring of 2024, baobab—zusammensein aims to take up the fight against FGM/C in Lower Saxony in order to offer those affected a contact point so that they can come to terms with the suffering inflicted on them. Elikia also aims to carry out low-threshold prevention and awareness-raising work in the communities. In this context, 'contact point' must also be understood as a place that can change. Not only is a fixed counselling centre offered where people can go, but the staff of baobab—zusammensein go to the people, i.e., they move around in the communities. This outreach work is time-consuming and labour-intensive, but it also serves to build trust, which is the basis for any collaboration. It is only from this position of trust that effective cooperation can take place with those affected, those at risk, and husbands or fathers.

Baobab—zusammensein has already implemented two projects focusing on FGM/C, both of which, however, have regional or spatial limitations. With funding from the state capital of Hanover, the 'Mouharaba' project has been implemented for Africans living in Hanover since 2019. At state level, the project 'Ntafe' was launched in 2021, which aims to help overcome FGM/C through awareness-raising at the Lower Saxony state reception centre for asylum seekers.

The project 'Elikia' has three target groups: African women; African men; and finally a group made up of educators, primary school teachers, professionals in projects and institutions, and medical doctors.

The first target group is African women and in particular mothers. This is about educational work. Education and discussion about this rite are necessary, because the reasons for its practice lie in tradition. Circumcision is part of cultural identity and is deeply rooted in it. Female genital mutilation is a tradition that primarily underpins the strong role of men. Since, depending on the type of circumcision, the woman has little or no sexual desire afterwards, and often experiences severe pain during sex, FGM/C is also intended to 'protect' her from being unfaithful.

However, women and mothers are often responsible for forcing their daughters to undergo this cruel practice. Girls are often circumcised at a very young age so that they cannot defend themselves or refuse the practice, and so that the circumcisions are protected from state persecution—as female genital mutilation is now banned in many countries.

In modern Africa, however, there are already many awareness campaigns by various groups, organisations, and governments. But people who have emigrated find it harder to give up their customs. They are more likely to cling to the traditions and associated values of their home country.

The second target group is African men. A lot of educational work and persuasion is needed here. Many men from countries with a tradition of FGM/C who live here bring their traditional way of thinking with them to Europe. They do not want an uncircumcised woman because they have been brought up with the idea that if a woman is not circumcised, she is not pure. If she is not circumcised, she is considered a whore. Most immigrants from Africa are convinced that an uncircumcised woman cannot lead a good life. No one wants to marry her; her community shuns her. This is ingrained in them. These attitudes need to be addressed and clarified.

Both African men and African women need to be made aware of the social and legal values that also determine their lives in Germany.

The third target group (educators, primary school teachers, professionals in projects and institutions and medical doctors) are to be reached through events and workshops. The initial aim here is to raise awareness of the problem of FGM/C: how can I tell if a girl is about to be circumcised, what happens during the procedure, why do mothers (especially), but also fathers, do this to their daughters?

The project is implemented through two main strands: counselling/ support and awareness-raising/prevention, with the latter targeting communities and professionals in authorities and institutions. The primary aim is to prevent FGM/C among African women living in Germany—in particular, among young girls between the ages of 3 and 12, as this is the age group in which most of the victims of this practice are found.

Another key objective is to raise awareness of the issue. This includes the third group of educators, primary school teachers, professionals in projects and institutions, and medical doctors. Further training programmes and campaigns are implemented to educate this target group on this sensitive topic and to ensure their commitment to fight against this ritual.

In order to successfully combat this serious violation of girls' and women's rights, the education of African women and men should be carried out by an African network that has proven access to the communities, enjoys their trust, and has a proven track record in disease prevention and health promotion. There is a need for an intensive, personal outreach approach by African women to African women for the purpose of education and prevention in the various communities: this is indispensable.

The project started with a needs assessment of the target group, from which specific educational activities were then derived. The process accompanying the needs assessment phase included the following steps:

1. Promoting the acceptance of the project among the communities.

2. Involving as many volunteers as possible.

3. Promoting the project and cooperation with day-care centres, schools, medical doctors, independent churches, mosques, counselling centres, youth welfare offices, and health authorities, etc.

4. Training sessions for the full-time and volunteer staff of the project by various specialists.

5. Training sessions for professionals on transcultural competence in dealing with those affected or at risk.

Indicators of goal achievement:

1. Ability to act independently.

2. Contact and cooperation with the further help systems of state institutions and welfare organisations (KSD/Johanniter/ AWO/Caritas/Diakonie, Red Cross, etc.).

3. Involvement as multipliers within the communities—people who have sought counselling become counsellors themselves.

4. Those affected take responsibility for themselves and others; they become health mediators.

The multipliers should carry out low-threshold education and prevention work in their respective place of residence/district (this is known as 'the baobab principle') and receive ongoing training and further education.

In principle, there are two strands to the implementation phase: the first is the organisation and implementation of both the further training programmes for African communities, and the further training programmes as well as the continuous provision of information for the schools, kindergartens, advice centres etc., and the medical sector. Contacts with the medical sector are also intended to serve the subsequent medical care of the women concerned. The second strand aims to strengthen the existing African networks. Future participants and multipliers will be recruited from these contacts to the African communities.

Contact:

baobab—zusammensein e.V.
Georgswall 3
30159 Hannover, Germany
+49-511 – 47 26 26 77
info@baobab-zs.de
www.baobab-zs.de

For more information on the project 'Elikia': www.elikia.baobab-zs.de

Conclusion

This chapter highlighted the intricate relationship between advocacy, empowerment, and the health of persons with refugee experience, demonstrating how these elements are essential for promoting health equity in diverse societies. Through the exploration of health advocacy, professionals are encouraged to incorporate a human rights framework into their practices, ensuring that they engage in concrete action towards social justice and equity. This involves understanding the social and political challenges faced by refugee communities and actively working to influence change at systemic and policy levels.

In parallel, the empowerment of persons with refugee experience was described as a vital component of effective health and social care delivery. By shifting the focus to the strengths and resources of individuals, health and social care professionals can facilitate processes that enable persons with refugee experience to advocate for their healthcare needs. Lastly, the case example included in the chapter underscored that meaningful empowerment can only come from collaborative efforts and community-driven initiatives, where individuals with lived experiences lead and shape the interventions that affect them. The work of the association baobab—zusammensein provides a practical illustration of how advocacy and empowerment can be operationalized through community networks. This initiative exemplifies how integrated approaches can effectively address pressing issues such as female genital mutilation/cutting (FGM/C) while promoting broader health improvements and social integration. The empowerment strategies employed by baobab—zusammensein, such as fostering self-help groups and training for community leaders, align with the empowerment approaches discussed in this chapter, demonstrating the transformative potential of enabling migrants and persons with refugee experience to advocate for themselves. Ultimately, this showcases the necessity of an interprofessional and intersectoral approach to refugee health. Without strong connections between health and social care professionals, community organizations, and individuals with lived experiences, inclusive and equitable healthcare environments cannot be created.

Advocacy by healthcare professionals and advocacy by associations by and for persons with refugee experience must therefore go hand in hand. Furthermore, empowerment within the context of refugee health means first and foremost that health and social care professionals acknowledge their role in supporting and facilitating opportunities for persons with refugee experience to influence their own health matters through collective political and societal engagement.

References

Amoah, Stephen, et al. 2023. 'Empowerment als Ablenkungsmanöver [=Empowerment as a Diversionary Tactic]', *Impu!se für Gesundheitsförderung* 120: 14–15, https://www.gesundheit-nds-hb.de/impulse/

Benbrahim, Karima. 2017. 'Empowerment-Räume als Orte der Sichtbarmachung von Rassismus- und Diskriminierungserfahrungen im Kontext von Flucht und Asyl [Empowerment Spaces as Places to Make Experiences of Racism and Discrimination in the Context of Displacement and Asylum Visible]', in *kontext.flucht: Perspektiven für eine rassismuskritische Jugendarbeit mit jungen geflüchteten Menschen* [Perspectives for Youth Work with Young Displaced Persons That Is Critical of Racism], ed. by Koch, Kolja (Düsseldorf: Informations- und Dokumentationszentrum für Antirassismusarbeit in Nordrhein-Westfalen (IDA-NRW)), pp. 23–26, https://www.ida-nrw.de/fileadmin/user_upload/brosch_flyer/IDA-NRW_Reader_kontext.flucht.pdf

Bozorgmehr, Kayvan and Nora Gottlieb. 2023. 'Gesundheitspolitik für Migrant: innen: Politische Entscheidungsmacht zwischen Evidenz, Transformations- und Identitätspolitik [Health Policy for Migrants: Political Decision-making Power between Evidence, Transformation and Identity Politics]', *Impu!se für Gesundheitsförderung,* 120: 3–4, https://www.gesundheit-nds-hb.de/impulse/

Bozorgmehr, Kayvan, Wenner, Judith and Oliver Razum. 2017. 'Restricted Access to Health Care for Asylum-seekers: Applying a Human Rights Lens to the Argument of Resource Constraints', *The European Journal of Public Health,* 27: 592–593, https://doi.org/10.1093/eurpub/ckx086

Danish Refugee Council. 2023. *Advocacy Toolkit for Diaspora Organizations* (Copenhagen: Danish Refugee Council), https://pro.drc.ngo/media/jwrn2plf/advocacy-toolkit-for-diaspora-actors-2.pdf

Global Refugee-Led Network. 2019. 'Meaningful Refugee Participation as Transformative Leadership: Guidelines for Concrete Action', Global Refugee-Led Network, https://www.asylumaccess.org/wp-content/uploads/2019/12/Meaningful-Refugee-Participation-Guidelines_Web.pdf

Earnest, Mark A., Shale L. Wong, and Steven G. Federico. 2010. 'Perspective: Physician Advocacy: What Is It and How Do We Do It?', *Academic Medicine,* 85.1: 63–67, https://doi.org/10.1097/acm.0b013e3181c40d40

European Centre for Disease Prevention and Control. 2009. *Health Advocacy* (Solna: European Centre for Disease Prevention and Control), https://www.ecdc.europa.eu/en/health-communication/health-advocacy

Flory, Lea, et al. 2020. *Trauma, Empowerment und Solidarität: Wie können wir zu einem verantwortungsvollen und ermächtigenden Umgang mit Trauma beitragen?* [Trauma, Empowerment and Solidarity: How Can We Contribute to a Responsible and Empowering Approach to Trauma?] (Berlin: Bundesweite Arbeitsgemeinschaft der Psychosozialen Zentren für Flüchtlinge und Folteropfer – BAfF e. V.).

Gallagher, Siun, and Miles Little. 2017. 'Doctors on Values and Advocacy: A Qualitative and Evaluative Study', *Health Care Analysis,* 25.4: 370–85, https://doi.org/10.1007/s10728-016-0322-6

Haschemi, Golschan Ahmad, Verena Meyer, and Pasquale Virginie Rotter. 2023. '"Slow Slow (Run Run)": Empowerment, Sichtbarkeit und Teilhabe in der Offenen Jugendarbeit ["Slow Slow (Run Run)": Empowerment, Visibility and Participation in Open Youth Work]', in *Empowerment und Powersharing: Ankerpunkte – Positionierungen – Arenen* [Empowerment and Powersharing: Anchor points – Positioning – Arenas], ed. by Chehata, Yasmine, and Birgit Jagusch, 2nd edn (Weinheim: Beltz, 2023), pp. 415–426.

Herriger, Norbert. 2022. 'Empowerment' [online], in *Socialnet Lexikon* (Bonn: socialnet), https://www.socialnet.de/lexikon/411

Herriger, Norbert. 2020. *Empowerment in der Sozialen Arbeit: Eine Einführung* [Empowerment in Social Work: An Introduction], 6th edn (Stuttgart: Kohlhammer).

Im, Hyojin and Laura E.T. Swan. 2022. '"We Learn and Teach Each Other": Interactive Training for Cross-Cultural Trauma-Informed Care in the Refugee Community', *Community Mental Health Journal*, 58: 917–929, https://doi.org/10.1007/s10597-021-00899-2

James, Rosemary, et al. 2021. 'Migration Health Research in the European Region: Sustainable Synergies to Bridge the Research, Policy and Practice Gap', *The Lancet Regional Health—Europe*, 5: 100124, https://doi.org/10.1016/j.lanepe.2021.100124

Kassam, Azaad, Olivia Magwood, and Kevin Pottie. 2020. 'Fostering Refugee and Other Migrant Resilience through Empowerment, Pluralism, and Collaboration in Mental Health', *International Journal of Environmental Research and Public Health*, 17: 9557, https://doi.org/10.3390/ijerph17249557

Kooperationsverbund Gesundheitliche Chancengleichheit. 2021. *Gesundheitsförderung mit Geflüchteten: Lücken schließen – Angebote ergänzen* [Health Promotion with Refugees: Closing Gaps – Supplementing Services] (Berlin: Kooperationsverbund Gesundheitliche Chancengleichheit), https://www.gesundheitliche-chancengleichheit.de/fileadmin/user_upload/pdf/Handreichungen/21-02_Handreichung_Gesundheitsfoerderung_mit_Gefluechteten.pdf

Kronick, Rachel, Eric G. Jarvis, and Laurence J. Kirmayer. 2021. 'Refugee Mental Health and Human Rights: A Challenge for Global Mental Health', *Transcultural Psychiatry*, 58.2: 147–56, https://doi.org/10.1177/13634615211002690

Lehmann, Frank, Carolin Chwaluk, and Alf Trojan. 2020. 'Anwaltschaft: Vertretung und Durchsetzung gesundheitlicher Interessen [Advocacy: Representation and Enforcement of Health Interests]', in *Leitbegriffe der Gesundheitsförderung und Prävention: Glossar zu Konzepten, Strategien und Methoden* [Key Terms in Health Promotion and Prevention: Glossary of Concepts, Strategies and Methods], ed. by Bundeszentrale für gesundheitliche Aufklärung (BZgA) (Köln: Bundeszentrale für gesundheitliche Aufklärung), https://leitbegriffe.bzga.de/alphabetisches-verzeichnis/anwaltschaft-vertretung-und-durchsetzung-gesundheitlicher-interessen/

Lindmeier, Bettina, and Dorothee Meyer. 2020. 'Empowerment, Selbstbestimmung, Teilhabe: Politische Begriffe und ihre Bedeutung für die inklusive politische Bildung' [Empowerment, Self-determination, Participation: Political Terms and their Meaning for Inclusive Civic Education], in *Grundlagen und Praxis inklusiver politischer Bildung*

[Principles and Practice of Inclusive Civic Education], ed. by Meyer, Dorothee, Wolfram Hilpert and Bettina Lindmeier (Bonn: Bundeszentrale für politische Bildung).

McAuliffe, Donna. 2022. *Interprofessional Ethics: Collaboration in the Social, Health and Human Services*, 2nd edn (Cambridge etc.: Cambridge University Press)

MacDonald, Noni and Laura Stymiest. 2023. *Advocacy for Immigrant and Refugee Health Needs* (Ottawa, ON: Canadian Paediatric Society), https://kidsnewtocanada.ca/care/advocacy

MacFarlane, Anne, et al. 2024. 'Normalising Participatory Health Research Approaches in the WHO European Region for Refugee and Migrant Health: A Paradigm Shift', *The Lancet Regional Health—Europe,* 41: 100837, https://doi.org/10.1016/j.lanepe.2024.100837

Mohseni, Maryam. 2020. *Empowerment-Workshops für Menschen mit Rassismuserfahrungen: Theoretische Überlegungen und biographisch-professionelles Wissen aus der Bildungspraxis* [Empowerment Workshops for Persons with Experiences of Racism: Theoretical Considerations and Biographical-Professional Knowledge from Educational Practice] (Wiesbaden: Springer VS, 2020).

Nowak, Anna Christina, and Claudia Hornberg. 2023. 'Erfahrungen von Menschen mit Fluchtgeschichte bei der Inanspruchnahme der Gesundheitsversorgung in Deutschland – Erkenntnisse einer qualitativen Studie', *Bundesgesundheitsbl* 66: 1117–1125, https://doi.org/10.1007/s00103-022-03614-y

Projekt Kompass F. (ed.). 2018. *Diskriminierungsschutz in der Sozialen Arbeit mit geflüchteten Menschen: Prävention und Interventionen* [Protection against Discrimination in Social Work with Persons who Have Fled: Prevention and Interventions] (Köln: Projekt Kompass F/ARIC-NRW e.V.), https://www.kompass-f.de/publikationen/

Rosenstreich, Gabriele. 2006. 'Von Zugehörigkeiten, Zwischenräumen und Macht: Empowerment und Powersharing in interkulturellen und Diversity Workshops' [Belongings, Spaces in between and Power: Empowerment and Power Sharing in Intercultural and Diversity Workshops], in *Spurensicherung: Reflexion von Bildungsarbeit in der Einwanderungsgesellschaft* [Securing Evidence: Reflecting on Educational Work in the Immigration Society], ed. by Elverich, Gabi, Annita Kalpaka and Karin Reeindlmeier (Frankfurt am Main: Iko-Verlag für Interkulturelle Kommunikation), pp. 195–231.

Solomon, Mildred Z. 2005. 'Healthcare Professionals and Dual Loyalty: Technical Proficiency Is Not Enough', *MedGenMed: Medscape General Medicine,* 7:14, https://www.ncbi.nlm.nih.gov/pmc/articles/PMC1681654/

Stevens, Amy J., et al. 2024. 'Discriminatory, Racist and Xenophobic Policies and Practice against Child Refugees, Asylum Seekers and Undocumented

Migrants in European Health Systems', *The Lancet Regional Health—Europe*, 41: 100834, https://doi.org/10.1016/j.lanepe.2023.100834

Stoddart, Rohanna, Paul Simpson, and Bridget Haire. 2020. 'Medical Advocacy in the Face of Australian Immigration Practices: A Study of Medical Professionals Defending the Health Rights of Detained Refugees and Asylum Seekers', *PLoS One*, 15, https://doi.org/10.1371/journal.pone.0237776

United Nations. 1948. *Universal Declaration of Human Rights. General Assembly Resolution, 217 A* (Paris: United Nations), https://www.un.org/en/about-us/universal-declaration-of-human-rights

World Health Organization. 2020. *Constitution of the World Health Organization.* Basic documents: forty-ninth edition (including amendments adopted up to 31 May 2019) (Geneva: World Health Organization), https://www.who.int/about/governance/constitution

World Health Organization. 2023. *Universal Health Coverage (UHC)* (Geneva: World Health Organisation), https://www.who.int/news-room/fact-sheets/detail/universal-health-coverage-(uhc)

World Health Organization. 2022. *World Report on the Health of Refugees and Migrants* (Geneva: World Health Organisation, 2022), https://www.who.int/publications/i/item/9789240054462

World Health Organization. 1986. *Ottawa Charter for Health Promotion: First International Conference on Health Promotion Ottawa, 21 November 1986* (Geneva: World Health Organization/Regional Office for Europe), https://iris.who.int/handle/10665/349652

World Health Organization. 2023. *Global Research Agenda on Health, Migration and Displacement: Strengthening Research and Translating Research Priorities into Policy and Practice* (Geneva: World Health Organization), https://iris.who.int/handle/10665/373659

V. Social and Occupational Determinants of Mental Health for Refugees

---

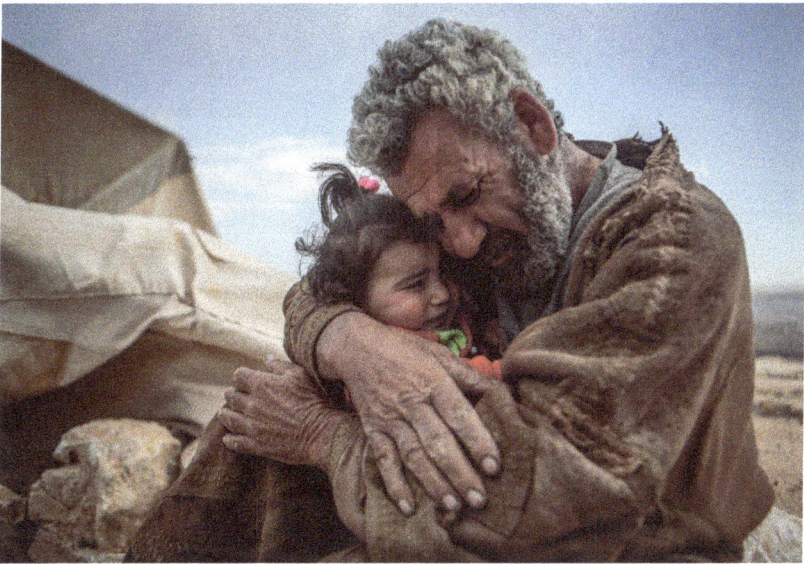

14. Flight and Post-Traumatic Stress: Their Influence on a Person's Identity

Christine Spevak-Grossi

This chapter describes the impact of refugee experiences and post-traumatic stress disorder (PTSD) on a person's identity. In addition, the author aims to show ways in which refugees with PTSD can be supported in their recovery by focusing on their identity. To do this, she uses the Identity Work approach.

Based on Heiner Keupp's socio-psychological theory of identity work and Gary Kielhofner's occupational therapy Model of Human Occupation (MOHO), it is important to pay particular attention to the following targets when working with refugees with PTSD (Spevak, 2022a, 2022b):

- analysing one's occupational roles in life;
- implementing routines;
- strengthening personal causation and occupational performance;
- reflecting on narrative during therapy;
- the role of healthcare professionals as health advocates in the client's environment;
- client-centred goal setting.

To understand the term 'identity' in this context, it is important to assume that it is subject to a constant process of change. This dynamic process

  https://doi.org/10.11647/OBP.0479.14

allows people to constantly adapt to their ever-changing environment (Keupp 2000; O'Brien 2017).

In order to adapt to these environmental changes, people need to be or become able to act. The ability to act is often reduced in people with PTSD. This makes it difficult to adapt to environmental changes. In the case of refugees, this is exacerbated by the fact that they are experiencing severe environmental change (Grinberg & Grinberg, 2010).

In the country of arrival, refugees suffer from occupational deprivation. This means that environmental conditions prevent people from taking action, for example when an asylum seeker is not allowed to work for legal reasons. Environmental conditions, such as economic, social, and political factors prevent refugees from participation in society. This can exacerbate illness. In the sense of occupational justice, it is the task of the health professions to demonstrate that a limited ability to act and the prevention of individually meaningful occupation have a negative impact on a person's identity and thus severe negative consequences for their health (Whiteford, 2011; Wilcock, 2015). This feeds the vicious circle of PTSD: uprooting through flight, loss of identity, and illness. This needs to be broken. One possible approach is identity work, as described in this chapter using occupational therapy interventions.

Mental Health of Refugees

Many refugees suffer from the psychological consequences of flight and their experiences in their home country, as well as from stressors in the host country after migration. This group of people is up to ten times more affected by mental illness than the autochthonous population of Western countries (Fazel et al. 2005; Crumlish & O'Rourke 2010). As a result, diseases such as depression, anxiety disorder, adjustment disorder, and post-traumatic stress disorder (PTSD), among others, often occur (Heeren et al. 2014). The study (Switzerland) by Heeren et al. (2014) found that 41.4% of the refugees and 54% of asylum seekers whose data was analysed exhibited symptoms of PTSD. In addition, the study has shown that mental illness persists even after asylum, i.e., refugee status, has been granted. This suggests a need for ongoing and comprehensive psychosocial support for people with refugee status (Heeren et al. 2014).

Another study from 2015 showed that 64% of the 283 refugees analysed had a psychiatric diagnosis. Among them, PTSD was the most common diagnosis. This suggests that psychiatric and psychological care is extremely important and should begin as soon as possible after refugees arrive in the host country (Richter Lehfeld & Niklewski 2015). The length of the asylum procedure is a key factor in the increasingly poor quality of life of refugees and the rising prevalence of mental disorders, while access to healthcare is inadequate (Gerritsen et al. 2006).

The challenges and expectations placed on refugees are also counterproductive and can even form a further episode in the traumatisation process. They have lost all areas of their psychosocial environment due to the loss of their home, homeland, profession, social network, and in a number of cases family members (Klingberg 2011). In addition, the uncertainty regarding residence status, as well as uncertain prospects for the future, and the confrontation with many new things, are extremely stressful (Stock-Gissendanner et al. 2013: 64).

A study (Netherlands) confirms a higher suicide rate among male asylum seekers than among the autochthonous population. However, suicide attempts are higher among both genders compared to the majority population. The reasons given were the length of the application period, being in the refugee camp, loneliness and no contact with the outside world, losses, no future prospects, and mental illness (Goosen et al. 2011).

Trauma and PTSD and the Importance of the Ability to Act

Fischer and Riedesser defined psychological trauma in 2003 (revised version from 2009) as:

> a vital experience of discrepancy between threatening situational factors and the individual's ability to cope, which is accompanied by feelings of helplessness and defenceless abandonment and thus causes a lasting shattering of self-awareness and understanding of the world (Fischer & Riedesser 2009: 84)

The shattering of the understanding of oneself and the world refers to the loss of self-confidence and self-efficacy as well as the disillusionment of possibly being close to death at many moments in our lives. Everyone needs a certain amount of illusion in order to face reality without fear. For example, when we get into a car, we assume that we will reach our destination safely and without incident. Without this illusion we would be constantly anxious and try to avoid many situations. People need a certain capacity for illusion in order to cope with everyday life. However, if this is lost, people suffer from hyperarousal, withdrawal, hopelessness, and a lack of prospects for the future (Fischer & Riedesser 2009: 90). In a threatening situation, people respond with actions such as fleeing or fighting to save themselves. The situation becomes a trauma because the person experiences that these actions do not protect them from the danger. This destroys their confidence in their own ability to act (Fischer & Riedesser 2009: 98; Bering 2011: 29). It can be concluded that the restoration or expansion of the ability to act is important for the recovery of traumatized people. Spontaneity and creativity, which are necessary to cope with change, new situations, and social contacts, are also reduced (Blaser & Csontos 2014: 135). For health professionals, this means promoting the ability to act, spontaneity, and creativity in their work with clients.

The extent to which the traumatizing experience causes a lasting shock in the sense of the definition depends on the level of threat, and the coping strategies of the person at the time of the event (Fischer & Riedesser 2009: 90). Reddemann distinguishes between three types of events and their degree of impact on mental health. "Personal" traumatisation has the strongest impact on the person's psyche, as the traumatizing experience only affects "me" and is caused by another person. This includes physical or sexual violence, torture, neglect, or witnessing violence. There is also a distinction between this and "a personal" traumatisation, which refers to situations that cannot be influenced by people, such as natural disasters, accidents, or diseases. These can be defined as a stroke of fate. Another threatening situation can be war or flight, which are defined as "collective" traumatic experiences. Feeling that you are not the only one affected, and that you can share what you have experienced, helps you to cope. Of course, these types of events can also occur in combination, which leads to an increased or decreased risk of severe traumatisation (Reddemann 2006). A distinction is also made according to the temporal component, depending on the frequency with which the traumatic event is repeated. In 1979, Leonore Terr distinguished between type I, with a single event, and type II, with multiple repetitions of the event. The more often the situation occurs and the more threatening it is, the greater the impact it has on mental health (Reddemann 2006; Wintersperger 2006).

However, it cannot be ruled out that a person who has experienced a traumatic event will be able to process it through their own resources. It is not possible to predict whether this will be possible without support. The post-exposure stress reaction sets in after the experience. In this phase, people initially avoid thinking about the event. Over time, uncontrolled memories and thoughts of the situation keep coming back, which is known as intrusion. According to the American psychoanalyst Mardi Horowitz, the unfinished action is organized and completed through the recurring alternation of denial and intrusion. Completion is when the person can consciously remember the event and control whether or not they think about it (Fischer & Riedesser 2009: 98). Symptoms of PTSD do not always occur immediately after the traumatizing experience, but only become apparent after weeks or years. Whenever these symptoms occur, if they do not subside within six months of their first appearance, they are referred to as post-traumatic stress disorder (PTSD) (Reddemann & Dehner-Rau 2006: 26).

According to ICD-11 6B40, PTSD is a delayed reaction to a threatening situation. The typical symptoms on a psychological level are flashbacks and intrusions, whereby the traumatizing situation is relived. Further characteristics of the disorder are: a lack of emotion and indifference towards other people as well as apathy and avoidance behaviour towards situations that could be reminiscent of the traumatic experience. Other symptoms include: anxiety, depression, sleep disturbance, increased vigilance, and an overexcited nervous system, as well as suicidal thoughts. The course can last for weeks or months but can also take a chronic course over many years until the personality changes (Dilling et al. 1991).

Social consequences result from the psychological symptoms. Avoidance behaviour, flashbacks, and chronic overexcitement have a serious impact on the social life of those affected and their relatives.

Withdrawal or cancellation of social contacts, mistrust of people with whom one is close, etc., are a heavy burden on relationships (Lindert 2016: 389).

As already mentioned, the probability of PTSD occurring is related to the cause and frequency of traumatisation. In terms of epidemiology, there is a 50% prevalence of PTSD after rape and among victims of war, displacement, and torture; 25% for violent crimes other than rape; and 10% of road accident victims and serious organ diseases such as heart attacks (Flatten et al. 2011).

The next section takes a closer look at action and its function as a therapeutic tool. Occupational therapy focuses on the ability to act and the meaning of action for the individual.

Activity and Occupational Therapy

There is a lot of talk about activity, but what is it? Here are some of the characteristics of action.

Activity is purposeful and conscious, which means that the person sets a goal, which must be realistic in order to be satisfactorily achieved. A debilitating environment prevents people from setting goals. Activities are structured. Each activity follows a plan of action, has a beginning and an end, and has a goal. After completion, the activity is evaluated by the performer and the environment. Activity is influenced by environmental factors and opportunities. Conversely, people shape their environment through their activities. Actions and their meanings change over the course of life, which means that activities change, and so do the roles and possibly the groups in which I participate. However, this requires the ability to adapt actions and respond flexibly to environmental conditions. People are constantly changing through their activities and therefore constantly redefining themselves.

PTSD limits a person's ability to act, which has a major impact on their daily life. The flexibility to adapt to new situations or respond to problems that arise is also reduced by the condition. This requires support to promote action and creativity. Occupational therapy addresses both aspects in its work with clients.

Occupational Therapy and People with PTSD

The aim of occupational therapy when working with people with PTSD is to improve their ability to act in the areas of life that are subjectively important to the client. Occupational therapy is less trauma-focussed and more resource-oriented. The present, the here and now, takes centre stage (Döring et al. 2008).

Occupational therapy uses activities as a therapeutic tool. Activities are individually selected and adapted, and their performance is analysed with the client. In order to be able to perform activities, however, it is also necessary to adapt the environment. Occupational therapy is intensively concerned with human occupation and deals individually with the meaningful occupation of a person (DACHS 2007). Occupational therapy is used at every stage of treatment for people with PTSD. These phases include crisis intervention, stabilisation, trauma processing, reintegration, and rehabilitation (Döring et al. 2008: 5).

The International Classification of Functioning, Disability and Health (ICF), is used interprofessionally. As a result, it supports coherent communication between the health professions. When working with people with PTSD, the following areas should receive particular attention: cognition, communication and interaction skills, social integration, occupational balance, identifying and resuming occupation that is meaningful to the person, the plan of action and problem solving, making decisions, coping strategies and overcoming avoidance behaviour, identifying personal needs, and adapting environmental factors. All in all, working on these areas leads to the improvement of the person's ability to act (Flotho 2009: 369).

Meaningful Activity and Accessibility

The central core of the occupational therapy approach is that meaningful occupation is a basic human need. It is an innate need to express oneself through activity, to be a part of society and thus to fulfil one's role in society (Wilcock 2015: 86-89). Being able to engage in meaningful occupations is a human right (WFOT 2019). What constitutes a meaningful occupation is subjective and is based on socio-cultural and personal factors such as socialisation and abilities. It is therefore important that people are free to choose their activities. However, environmental factors such as economic or socio-cultural aspects can prevent people from performing the activity they experience as meaningful. The possibility of filling time with meaningful occupation is not available to all population groups or classes in a society. In occupational therapy, this is referred to as "occupational injustice" (Whiteford 2011: 304–305; Wilcock 2015: 392; WFOT 2019).

Many refugees experience occupational deprivation in their country of arrival. This refers to reduced or no opportunities to participate in activities that are meaningful to the individual in everyday life. Occupational deprivation has no apparent time limit, and the person concerned has no control over their options for activity. External factors such as social, economic, geographical, historical, or political reasons prevent participation in meaningful activities. Uncertainty regarding residence status, which means uncertain prospects for the future and confrontation with the new environment, is a burden on the recovery from psychotrauma (Herzig et al. 2001; Moser 2021). Occupational deprivation means that refugees are deprived of the opportunity to implement structure, meaning, and coherence in their daily lives through familiar activities (Christiansen & Townsend 2010; Whiteford 2011: 305; Wilcock 2015: 285). If groups of people are unable to perform meaningful occupations, they cannot subsequently fulfil any roles and therefore cannot participate in society (Whiteford 2011).

Being part of society or a group is an important, meaningful factor for every person. Occupational injustice has a negative impact on people's health and can shorten their life expectancy. Ann Wilcock assumes that a person's health is strongly characterized by their opportunities to "do" and consequently by their opportunities to "be", "become", and "belong" (Wilcock 2015: 134–138).

By experiencing participation through independently chosen and initiated activities, people gain an understanding of who they are and who they want to be. This is summarized by the term occupational identity. Based in turn on volition (values, interests, and personal causation), habituation (habits, routines, and roles) and experiences with the resources and limitations of the body, mind, and soul, people create future identity projects and goals (Keupp et al. 2002; Heras de Pablo 2017). These are pursued through meaningful occupations. These identity projects are largely characterized by the opportunities provided by the environment. Identity shaping is a continuous process and accompanies people throughout their lives (Keupp et al. 2002).

Flight and PTSD Influence Identity

People who have experienced displacement frequently suffer from Post-Traumatic Stress Disorder (PTSD) due to drastic environmental changes and extreme demands before, during, and after migration. These can lead to disruption of the identity-building process (Bennett et al. 2012; Stock-Gissendanner et al. 2013). Identity work is a lifelong process that is an important prerequisite for achieving life satisfaction. The context of life is constantly changing and demands continuous adaptation. People are required to adapt their actions, roles, and routines to the demands of their environment (Keupp et al., 2002). In this sense, fleeing to a foreign country requires a great deal of individual identity work. Identity work is particularly important when working with people who have experienced flight and PTSD (Stock-Gissendanner, Calliess, Schmid-Ott, & Behrens, 2013).

In the country of arrival, previously identity-forming occupations, relationships, and behavioural norms are questioned (Sluzki 2016; O'Brien 2017). A process of adaptation and rejection is set in motion. Attempts can be made to replace these identity-forming occupation and behavioural norms with those customary in the country of arrival or to maintain the familiar ones with all one's might. A rejection or idealisation of the society of origin or the society of arrival can be set in motion. Any path to an extreme, over a longer period of time, leads to a destabilisation of identity. If a person reacts by idealizing the society of arrival with a strong adaptation of identity-forming occupation and behavioural norms, the continuous course of the identity process is interrupted. This process needs time and an anchor point through the familiar occupation and behavioural norms of the society of origin. Stagnation or destabilisation of identity can also occur over a longer period of time due to adherence to familiar occupation and behavioural norms (Sluzki 2016; Stock-Gissendanner et al. 2013; O'Brien 2017; Heras de Pablo 2017). At the same time, there is a high demand to adapt one's occupation to the new environment. During the migration process, constant humiliation and ongoing negative events can lead to psychological trauma (Grinberg & Grinberg 2010; Sluzki 2016). Discrimination and negative events put a strain on a person's identity (Stock-Gissendanner et al. 2013). A traumatized basis of the person leads to a further discontinuous course of identity in this adaptation process. The psychological state at the time of arrival and the migration attempt can be responsible for the extent to which this phase manifests itself as traumatic or how the migration proceeds (Grinberg & Grinberg 2010). It would therefore make sense to look at identity as such and in relation to people who have experienced displacement.

Aspects such as environment, identity goal, narrative, personal causation, and roles are essential in the identity process, as is confidence in one's subjective ability to act. This is a prerequisite for the feeling of being able to shape one's own areas of life. Heiner Keupp says about people's ability to act:

> The ability to act represents the most general framework quality of a human and humane existence, in that the availability and mouldability of living conditions forms the antithesis to feelings of being at the mercy of circumstances, of fear and lack of freedom. (Keupp et al. 2002)

A humane existence is made possible through the free and independent organisation of living conditions. The basis for this is the ability to act. Occupational therapy is the profession that aims to (re)enable people to engage in meaningful activities. This in turn is essential for strengthening a person's sense of identity. Aspects of identity work are therefore addressed and described in the following section. We will then look at each of these aspects and how they can be addressed in occupational therapy interventions.

Important Aspects for Identity Work in Occupational Therapy

The following section outlines the aspects that are particularly important for identity work in occupational therapy. The definition of these aspects will therefore be explained in more detail.

Roles: Can be predefined, such as the role of the daughter, or self-chosen. Roles require certain activities. By performing these and participating by doing them, the person can identify with the role. The importance of the individual roles can change and vary (Wook Lee 2017a).

Personal causation: According to the definition of the Occupational Therapy—Model of Human Occupation (MOHO), the term "personal causation" consists of two dimensions called "sense of personal capacity" and "self-efficacy". Sense of personal capacity includes the judgement that a person has of their own physical, mental, social, and intellectual abilities. Self-efficacy defines the conviction of being able to shape and change the environment through these abilities—for example, the confidence to be able to cope with new, unforeseeable situations. The term also includes a person's satisfaction with their own activities. The expectations that a person has of their own ability to act are characterized by experiences and the demands of the environment, and therefore influence their self-image (Wook Lee 2017b).

Narration: Through the narrative, the person expresses themselves and reflects on their life and occupation in the past. From this, they can plan the future. The image a person has of their life and how they choose their activities in the future as a result can be recognized through a person's story about themselves (Keupp et al. 2002).

Environment: Working on and, above all, with the environment is an important aspect of the identity process. In addition to adapting to the physical environment, recognition and belonging must be experienced in the social environment. The term environment also addresses economic, cultural, institutional, and political factors. The environment is constantly changing (O'Brien 2017).

Identity goals: Identity concepts are created in advance. If necessary, these ideas or dreams are communicated to the environment in order to carry out a reality check. This results in concrete identity projects that lead to the identity goal (Keupp et al. 2002).

Capacity to act: The ability to act is the realisation of the person's identity projects. The correct assessment of the ability to act is the basis for matching identity projects with one's own abilities and transforming them into identity projects with their goals. Adequate capacity to act gives the person the confidence to adapt, organise, and cope with everyday life. The ability to act therefore also means being able to comply with norms of behaviour and action established by society or the cultural context, and being part of them. The ability to act enables a self-determined life (Keupp et al. 2002).

> It would appear that building an occupational identity starts with self-knowledge of our capacities and interests from experience and extends to constructing a value-based vision of the future we desire. (Kielhofner 2008: 106)

The following section looks at the practical implementation and opportunities for occupational therapy intervention. The aim is to support clients with PTSD and refugee experience to strengthen their identity. The section is therefore structured according to the aspects of identity work and the Model of Human Occupation (MOHO) (Spevak, 2022a, 2022b).

Roles in Occupational Therapy Intervention

In occupational therapy, those affected deal with their own present, past, and future roles.

Fundamental goals are a necessity for role formation. This means that there must be a certain degree of awareness of one's own ability to act and the effect this has on the environment. In this phase of therapy, the focus is placed on the person's resources and further, familiar activities are thematized and activated again.

Roles can have negative connotations; therefore, caution is advised at the beginning of therapy. Dealing with current roles with negative connotations or the loss of roles should only be addressed at a later point in the therapy. This requires a certain degree of stability on the part of those affected. Later on, it is important to build up new roles or deal with these negative roles.

Future (New) Roles

The occupational therapist supports those affected in finding new roles. These result from the requirements of the environment and the interests of the person concerned. The environment has a significant influence on the opportunities to develop and take on new roles. Examples of these new roles are 'learner' through learning German in language courses or the role of 'worker' in a new, unknown profession, etc.

Current Roles

If necessary, current roles are adapted to the current environment in order to experience more satisfaction.

Past (Old) Roles

The occupational therapist identifies past roles during the interview. These point to activities that were important in the past or in the home country. Being able to perform these activities again conveys a sense of security and strengthens the feeling of identity. Nevertheless, those affected experience a great deal of insecurity when confronting old roles for fear of no longer being able to fulfil them. Dealing with and resuming past roles and the activities that were meaningful at the time is very effective for the recovery of those affected, but requires a high level of sensitivity on the part of the occupational therapist.

By activating past roles, those affected begin to feel anew what they want and what they like (interests). They get to know themselves again through their 'old' activities (personal causation).

Dysfunctional Roles

Dysfunctional roles, in other words roles that lead to activities that cause long-term physical and/or psychological damage, are addressed later in the course of therapy. The aim is to discard these roles and replace them with functional ones. This is an extremely difficult and long process. It requires a great deal of sensitivity on the part of the occupational therapist. In order to discard dysfunctional roles, work is done on the personal causation. Sensitivity and dialogue in a multi-professional team about possible dysfunctional roles is beneficial for the recovery of those affected, but also for the mental hygiene of the therapist.

Routines in Occupational Therapy Intervention

Routines are essential intervention goals when working with people affected by PTSD and complex PTSD (CPTSD). Routines can create or reinforce a sense of safety. In people with PTSD, basic routines have often been broken and need to be rebuilt. This rebuilding process involves observing which routines are already in place and how these can be reinforced. A basic action such as 'eating' is one example. Eating structures everyday life and 'taking care of others' is an important aspect of this activity.

Routines Help in Saving Energy

Psychological energy is often reduced in people who have experienced flight and PTSD or CPTSD. Consequently, it is important to address energy balance and improve energy management when working with the target group. Activities that encourage sleep are identified to establish a consistent sleep routine.

Energy management in occupational therapy further includes the analysis of activities and their energy expenditure. Instructions are given on how to save and mobilize energy. An additional goal consists in finding activities that provide energy and can be performed regularly. The objective is to work on occupational balance.

Rituals in Therapy Sessions

As rituals provide a sense of safety and stability, they constitute an important part of therapy sessions with people from the target group. The sequence is always the same. The unit begins and ends with the same activities. In between are the actions that require courage from the person concerned. Even if the occupational therapist has the feeling that they are repeatedly performing the same activities, this repetition gives those affected a sense of security. As a result, the therapy is predictable, which is important for those affected.

On the basis of security and predictability, those affected can make gradual progress in therapy.

Personal Causation in Occupational Therapy Intervention

Personal causation is a key issue for the occupational therapist when working with the target group. The personal causation is often shaken by the illness and the experience of flight. The work that is done in the field of occupational therapy on the personal causation of those affected is very complex. It is often difficult for people with PTSD or, in particular, CPTSD to formulate goals for therapy but also for their own future. In these cases, it is necessary to work on their personal causation in advance in order to regain a sense of their own abilities.

By experiencing the ability to act, the personal causation is simultaneously promoted; see also 'Promotion of occupational performance'.

The Occupational Therapist's Attitude

Working on their personal causation constitutes a significant challenge for those affected. As measures must be repeated frequently, the therapist needs to possess a certain level of endurance. Genuine interest on the part of the occupational therapist is a prerequisite for finding out together who the person concerned is. This discovery already supports the person's personal causation.

Promotion of Personal Causation through Activity

Personal causation and occupational performance are closely intertwined. A person's sense of personal causation can be observed in the evaluation of their own actions; a negative evaluation entails a self-devaluation. The guilt and shame experienced by those affected often manifests itself in negative self-talk. This negative personal causation, which has been shaped by past experiences, causes a lack of confidence in one's own actions. The experience of having successfully performed an action and a subsequent positive response from the environment strengthens the personal causation. Performing actions creates an awareness of resources, which has a positive influence on the personal causation. If those affected have had the experience of being able to carry out actions and influence the environment through these actions, this conveys a certain degree of control over the situation. As a result of this experience, the feeling of being at the mercy of the environment is counteracted and a feeling of coherence is promoted.

Focus on Perception

Due to trauma, those affected are often strongly focused on their external environment. This heightened awareness of what is happening around them and the urge to adapt to the present environment were essential for survival during traumatic phases. As a result, their attention is directed outward, placing the value of the external world above their own. Therefore, it is necessary to strengthen their personal causation and support the establishment of boundaries to the environment. The affected individuals are guided to train their perception of feelings, bodily sensations, and thoughts. For this reason, the process-oriented approach is used in occupational therapy, often applied through craftwork. They need a protected space where they can act without being judged or observed. The craft itself does not need to have a deeper meaning, which is experienced as liberating. Even if a piece is created with guidance, it still holds personal expression and involves an internal process during its creation. In the follow-up discussion, the focus is on the process, specifically on the emergence of the piece. Feelings, thoughts, and bodily sensations experienced during the creation are discussed and thus communicated externally.

Promotion of Creativity

Open-ended tasks and new actions often pose a significant challenge for people with PTSD and CPTSD. These tasks involve a certain unpredictability and uncontrollability. In everyday life, we frequently encounter situations where we must find flexible and spontaneous solutions—for example, when the chosen train is cancelled or a bus is missed. Thus, creativity is required to respond effectively, combining environmental factors with an awareness of one's own capacities and trust in them. Therefore, therapy must create situations where those affected have to try something new or out of the ordinary. Patients are guided with minimal instruction to find their own way rather than following the therapists or other group members. Besides enhancing their perception, this approach fosters creativity and confidence in their own effectiveness, which positively shapes their personal causation.

Different Ways to Express Personal Causation

Using creative media enables individuals to express their self-image and make their feelings and needs transparent both to themselves and to the therapist. This approach is particularly valuable when working with people who have experienced displacement and have limited language abilities, providing a means of communication. While verbal language is often necessary when the occupational therapist wants to reflect on the product, the act of expression through activities such as painting can have a profound impact. Even when individuals are capable of verbal expression, they might still struggle to articulate their emotions. Therefore, expression with creative media offers a valuable way to communicate. As previously mentioned under the topic of narration, this method is essential not only for self-presentation to others but also for self-reflection, which ultimately influences one's personal causation.

Handling Emotions

The facial expressions of those affected are often blank. It is considered a success when tears flow, allowing the pain to find expression. Patients are encouraged to understand that expressing emotions is allowed. For example, screaming or crying can be a relief for them. In occupational therapy, various techniques such as throwing clay or boxing a punching bag are used to help mobilize emotions.

When dealing with the emotions of those affected, the therapist needs to have knowledge and a heightened awareness of the patient's socialisation. The intensity of emotional expression must be manageable for the individual to prevent the feeling of being overwhelmed.

Narratives: Verbal and Nonverbal Communication in Occupational Therapy Intervention

Narratives, whether verbal or nonverbal, are essential for identity work.

Narratives at the Beginning of the Intervention

At the start of occupational therapy interventions with individuals who have experienced forced migration and suffer from PTSD or CPTSD, communication is often nonverbal. It is conveyed that they are here to engage in action. Speaking is not required; the actions themselves can be viewed as a form of language. This allows for communication as well as therapy. The assessment of occupational performance can be conducted by observing the person's actions. However, language is necessary for a more detailed diagnosis.

Narratives in Later Phases of the Intervention

In later stages of therapy, verbal communication becomes increasingly important. Professional interpretation services are highly recommended and can be repeatedly utilized in occupational therapy interventions. Although the application of these services is straightforward, their implementation within an institution often poses challenges. Unfortunately, it is often the case that family members or friends act as translators. For example, a child may have to translate a diagnosis for his or her mother. Apart from possible translation errors, this is emotionally stressful for the child. Trust in the relationship may be violated. It is therefore clear that family members and friends should be avoided as translators if professional work is to be carried out.

Individuals affected may be highly distrustful due to their condition. Therefore, it is crucial to be very careful with expressions, gestures, and facial expressions in communication to avoid, in extreme cases, the risk of therapy being discontinued due to misunderstandings. A key part of therapy is taking responsibility and asking clarifying questions to understand what a statement meant. High transparency in documentation and reporting is essential. The individuals must feel involved to maintain trust.

Social, Physical, Economic and Cultural Environment in Occupational Therapy Intervention

Understanding the immediate environment of the individuals is a prerequisite for effective intervention.

The Occupational Therapist as a Health Advocate

Occupational therapy has the potential to more frequently incorporate methods from environmental therapy. This does not mean integrating the affected individuals but rather adapting the environment. There is a significant lack of environmental adjustments for individuals with mental health conditions. For example, a person with early childhood trauma who frequently dissociates may not be able to consistently arrive at work on time. This is an environmental issue, not a problem with the individual. Often, these individuals are highly intelligent but unable to work in a typical job setting due to their mental health conditions.

There is a need for greater awareness and education regarding psychiatric conditions. Stigmatisation is widespread. It is little known that people with refugee experiences often suffer from PTSD or CPTSD and the limitations these conditions impose on all areas of life. Advocacy is needed to regulate the workplace for these individuals, including managing breaks, work hours, noise reduction, and so on.

When occupational therapists work with this target group, networking becomes increasingly important. For example, communication with refugee shelters or employers where the affected individuals are involved is essential. Occupational therapists can inform the environment about the needs and challenges of individuals regarding their occupational performance. The goal is to discuss and implement possible adaptations to the environment with employers, educators, social workers, associations, etc. Refugee shelters can be conflict-laden without offering a perspective for the affected individuals to escape this situation. Developing future perspectives may require occupational therapy support over several years. Language skills are crucial for individuals' future opportunities.

Changes to the environment have a direct impact on the roles of the affected individuals. Therefore, when the roles of these individuals are addressed in therapy, work is indirectly being done on or with the environment.

Occupational Performance in Occupational Therapy Intervention

People with refugee experiences and PTSD or CPTSD often have a very low sense of self-efficacy. They need to regain their occupational performance, which in turn supports their personal causation. Occupational therapy and its methods promote self-efficacy and consequently promote the identity of the affected individuals. Expanding their ability to act is a central theme in working with traumatized refugees in occupational therapy. Occupational performance is not something that is achieved once and for all. Even different life phases demand that individuals acquire new skills or perform them differently. It is important to maintain the ability to act and to adapt to changing environmental conditions. Actions taken also affect the environment.

Fostering Self-Efficacy

The impact of self-initiated action on the environment strengthens the belief in one's effectiveness. The stronger the belief in one's self-efficacy, the greater the ability to adapt one's actions to everyday situations. Self-efficacy is consciously enhanced through reflection after performing an action. Self-efficacy, which occupational therapy is well-equipped to foster, is the key to improve well-being. Dissociation significantly reduces the sense of self-efficacy. Dissociations cause unpredictable memory gaps, leading to uncertainty about one's own effectiveness. Therefore, at the beginning of therapy, the most crucial approach is to enhance the sense of self-efficacy through action.

Taking Action as Soon as Possible

For those affected, the immediate priority is to engage in action. This helps individuals start to re-experience themselves, laying the foundation for rediscovering what they can do, what they enjoy or dislike, and which actions are important and meaningful to them. This process not only strengthens occupational performance but also reinforces values, personal causation, and interests.

Execution of Action

People with flight experience and PTSD or CPTSD may struggle with concentration difficulties, leading them to perform actions in a rushed and careless manner. This often results in dissatisfaction with the outcome. The discrepancy between the expected and actual result can be frustrating for those affected. Some may also exhibit perfectionism in their actions, yet still feel unsatisfied with the outcome. In such cases, feedback from a group about the action can be very effective. Additionally, addressing perfectionism in the execution of actions can gradually lead to changes in personal causation over time. Group activities that promote occupational performance and social skills (e.g., the ability to handle criticism and communication skills) are particularly beneficial.

In occupational therapy, individuals with flight experience and PTSD or CPTSD are supported in discovering more about their own abilities and skills. This discovery process is facilitated through action and is implemented throughout the course of therapy, from beginning to end.

The Personal Causation and External Perception Do Not Match

Individuals often underestimate their abilities, which leads to self-imposed limitations in their actions. For a person, the external perception of their abilities serves as an important mirror. The environment must recognize successful actions to help the individual become aware of their own resources. In occupational therapy, reflection on actions occurs both during and after the performance. The occupational therapist observes and analyses each step and the necessary skills and functions involved. These are then reflected upon with the individual, focusing on the resources and deficits within the different components of an action. This process helps to identify why an action may not have been carried out satisfactorily. More importantly, it makes resources transparent by identifying the parts of the intervention that are working well.

The experiences during the action must be reflected upon through discussion and further exploration. This reflection is crucial for reinforcing the experience of the action. Reflecting after the completion of an action is especially effective in a group setting led by the occupational therapist. It is essential that the individuals understand the reasoning behind the interventions. This understanding is vital for their motivation and comprehension of the therapy process. In this phase, it is advisable to use professional interpretation services. The impact of the final product on the environment can also be perceived nonverbally. The occupational therapist considers this and creates situations in which the completed product is put to use.

Finding Trust in One's Own Ability to Act without Pressure

People with PTSD and CPTSD often struggle with the action sequence of 'initiating an action'. They may experience fear when starting a task. To help them overcome this, it is important that they first participate in the group without any pressure. Initially, it is essential for them to feel like part of the group simply by being present. Once this sense of belonging is established, external prompts at the right moment can gently encourage the initiation of independent action. This approach can also work nonverbally. The more trust the individuals have in the occupational therapist, and the more frequently they experience self-efficacy, the easier it becomes for them to begin an action independently.

Relaxation Techniques

Relaxation techniques allow people with PTSD and KTPBS to calm the stress system and distance themselves from survival mode. One consequence of traumatisation is a strong focus on the environment, which constantly stimulates the person's stress system. This reduces the ability to act (Kubny 2020).

Goals in Occupational Therapy Intervention

In occupational therapy, goals are usually set at the beginning of therapy. These are client-centred, which means they are adapted to the client's needs. Progress can be made visible through goals.

Overwhelming the Affected Individuals with Goal Setting

At the beginning of therapy, individuals with flight experience and PTSD or CPTSD often find it challenging to articulate goals. Before they can do so, their personal causation needs to be strengthened—in other words, they need to build trust in their ability to influence their environment through their actions. Setting goals at the start of therapy can be overwhelming for them, meaning that a client-centred approach may not be possible from the outset. However, this should not be a reason to exclude them from occupational therapy interventions. The occupational therapist must be able to justify to the team why the goals they have formulated are not client-centred.

Possible Approach to Goal Setting

Initially, it is helpful to allow the individuals to create identity drafts and fictional goals. They are encouraged to dream. For example, the first goals of people with refugee experiences might often be to leave the refugee shelter, enrol in a language course, or find work. As they move into a phase where they recognize the difficulty of achieving these goals, they will need support. During this process of discovery, individuals learn to accurately assess their current situation and become familiar with the opportunities and limitations offered by their environment. Support during this phase is crucial to help them ultimately set realistic identity goals.

Trust in their own ability to act fuels intrinsic motivation and broadens their perspective. Consequently, a goal can eventually be formulated in a truly client-centred manner.

Conclusion

Experiences in the home country, during flight and the challenges in the country of arrival very often lead to mental illness, most frequently post-traumatic stress disorder (PTSD). Moreover, the suicide rate among male refugees while waiting for asylum is higher than that among the host society. At the same time, it is evident that access to psychiatric care is difficult or impossible, although there is an increased need for it.

The degree of traumatisation is influenced by the extent of personal resilience and, in contrast, the cause of the situation or who caused it, as well as its duration and frequency. A person can also process a traumatic experience independently. Whether this is successful cannot be predicted. If the symptoms persist for a period of six months, we can speak of PTSD, which can become chronic and result in personality changes.

People who have experienced flight and post-traumatic stress disorder (PTSD) are affected by occupation deprivation and occupation injustice, which has a negative impact on their occupation identity. This group of people is up to ten times more affected by mental illness than the autochthonous population of Western countries due to their experiences in their country of origin and arrival as well as their flight. Socio-economic status and psychosocial stress in the country of arrival have a significant influence on their health. These factors have a negative impact on people's life satisfaction and put a strain on identity work. Identity work is a continuous process. People change roles, meaningful activities, interests, etc., throughout their lives. This aspect is intensified by illness and the experience of flight. Therefore, people should be supported in these phases to stabilize their identity. The following aspects of identity work need to be supported in occupational therapy: the areas of roles and routines, personal causation, narrative, environment, occupational performance, and goal setting.

Roles can be a sensitive issue and are addressed and worked on over a longer period of time. The loss of roles is associated with psychological pain and the fear of no longer being able to fulfil them. Self-efficacy conviction, personal causation, and occupational performance influence the resumption of and satisfaction with the respective role. At the same time, the revitalisation of past roles is very effective for the identity of those affected. Routines provide stability and support the energy balance of those affected.

Personal causation is a central issue in occupational therapy interventions for the target group. Dealing with this is a lengthy process. The personal causation is strengthened by reflecting on the performance of the activity. Process-oriented measures are also used to reflect on subjective perception. The feelings and needs of those affected are addressed. To do this, the occupational therapist uses the expression-centred method, among other things.

The expression-centred method promotes narratives or the telling of one's own emotional experience and needs, but action can also be used as a means of communication. In the later course of therapy, when trust in the therapist is established, it is advisable to use professional interpreters.

In their occupational therapy expertise as a health spokesperson, the occupational therapist represents those affected. People with mental illnesses need advocates who educate people about mental illnesses and point out stigmatisation. There is a need to adapt to environmental conditions for people with mental illnesses. Interprofessional networking should be sought.

Promoting the occupational performance, and reflecting on the execution and the end result of these actions, influences the personal causation and the conviction of self-efficacy. It helps those affected to (re)formulate (identity) goals. Working on occupational performance in occupational therapy promotes the personal causation and subsequently the identity of those affected.

At the beginning of therapy, those affected usually find it difficult to independently formulate goals for the therapy but also for the future. As the therapy progresses, the focus is on creating realistic goals in the current environment. The occupational therapist supports the process from a draft of identity to realistic identity goals.

Occupational therapy offers effective intervention options when working with people with PTSD. It can intervene at all stages of the therapy process. It works in a stabilising, resource-oriented and action-promoting way.

Occupational therapists have extensive knowledge of how they can support people who have experienced flight and PTSD in their identity work.

References

Bennett, Kayla Marie, et al. 2012. 'Immigration and Its Impact on Daily Occupations: A Scoping Review', *Occupational Therapy International*, 19.4: 185–203, https://doi.org/10.1002/oti.1336

Bering, Robert. 2011. *Verlauf der Posttraumatischen Belastungsstörung* (Aachen: Shaker Verlag).

Blaser, Marlys, and István Csontos. 2014. *Ergotherapie in der Psychiatrie. Handlungsfähigkeit und Psychodynamik in der Erwachsenen-, Kinder- und Jugendpsychiatrie* (Bern: Hans Huber Verlag).

Brandt, Benigna, et al. 2020. 'Ergotherapeutische Interventionsverfahren in der Psychiatrie', in *Ergotherapie in der Psychiatrie*, Vol. 4, ed. by Kubny Beate (Stuttgart: Georg Thieme Verlag), pp. 192–234.

Crumlish, Niall, and Killian O'Rourke. 2010. 'A Systematic Review of Treatments for Post-Traumatic Stress Disorder among Refugees and Asylum-Seekers', *The Journal of Nervous and Mental Disease*, 198.4: 237–51, https://doi.org/10.1097/nmd.0b013e3181d61258

DACHS. 2007. *Ergotherapie. Was bietet sie heute und in Zukunft?* (Bozen: CAUDIANA-Landesfachhochschule für Gesundheitsberufe).

de las Heras de Pablo, Carmen-Gloria, Chia-Wei Fan, and Gary Kielhofner. 2017. 'Dimensions of Doing', in *Kielhofner's Model of Human Occupation*, Vol. 5, ed. by Renée Taylor (Philadelphia: Lippincott Williams & Wilkins), pp. 107–122.

Dilling, Horst, et al. 1991. *Internationale Klassifikation psychischer Störungen: ICD-10, Kapitel V (F, klinisch-diagnostische Leitlinien*, http://www.who.int/iris/handle/10665/38221

Döring, A., Hülsewiesche, D., Flotho, W., Gläser, A., Koeser, P., Lorenz, C. P., Timmer, A. 2008. Ergotherapie bei Posttraumatischer Belastungsstörung. Update der AWMF-Leitlinie 051/010 ('Posttraumaitsche Belastungsstörung; ICD-10: F43.1') durch die DeGPT, Karlsbad-Ittersbach: Deutscher Verband der Ergotherapie e. V.

Fazel, Mina, Jeremy Wheeler, and John Danesh. 2005. 'Prevalence of Serious Mental Disorder in 7000 Refugees Resettled in Western Countries: A Systematic Review', *The Lancet*, 365.9467: 1309–14, https://doi.org/10.1016/s0140-6736(05)61027-6

Fischer, Gottfried, and Peter Riedesser. 2009. *Lehrbuch der Psychotraumatologie* (München: Ernst Reinhardt Verlag).

Flatten, Guido. et al. 2011. 'S3 - Leitlinie Posttraumatische Belastungsstörung', *Trauma & Gewalt*, 3: 202–210.

Flotho, Wiebke. 2009. 'Psychosomatik', in *Ergotherapie im Arbeitsfeld Psychiatrie*, Vol. 2, ed. by Kubny-Lüke, Beate (Stuttgart: Georg Thieme Verlag), pp. 363–389.

Gerritsen, Annette A., et al. 2006. 'Use of Health Care Services by Afghan, Iranian, and Somali Refugees and Asylum Seekers Living in The Netherlands', *European Journal of Public Health*, 16.4: 394–99, https://doi.org/10.1093/eurpub/ckl046

Goosen, Simone, et al. 2011. 'Suicide Death and Hospital-Treated Suicidal Behaviour in Asylum Seekers in the Netherlands: A National Registry-Based Study', *BMC Public Health*, 11.1, https://doi.org/10.1186/1471-2458-11-484

Grinberg, León, and Rebeca Grinberg. 2010. *Psychoanalyse der Migration und des Exils* (Klett-Cotta).

Heeren, Martina, et al. 2014. 'Psychopathology and Resident Status – Comparing Asylum Seekers, Refugees, Illegal Migrants, Labor Migrants, and Residents', *Comprehensive Psychiatry*, 55.4: 818–25, https://doi.org/10.1016/j.comppsych.2014.02.003

Herzig, J., Foka, C., & Fischer, D (2001). 'Fallgruppen traumatisierter Flüchtlinge im Asylverfahren', in *Asylpraxis. Traumatisierte Flüchtlinge, Band 7(Bundesamtes für die Anerkennung ausländischer Flüchtlinge)*, pp. 39–58.

Keupp, Heiner, et al. 2002. *Identitätskonstruktionen. Das Patchwork der Identitäten in der Spätmoderne*, 2nd edn (Reinbek bei Hamburg: Rowohlt).

Klingberg, Insa. 2011. *Psychische Folgen von Kriegen bei ZivilistInnen* (Belm-Vehrte/Osnabrück: Sozio-Publishing).

Kubny, Beate. 2020. 'Besondere Methoden', in *Ergotherapie in der Psychiatrie*, Vol. 4, ed. by Kubny, Beate (Stuttgart: Georg Thieme Verlag), pp. 366–382.

Lindert, Jutta. 2016. 'Traumatische Ereignisse bei Migranten und ihre Auswirkungen', in *Handbuch Transkulturelle Psychiatrie*, Vol. 2, ed. by Hegemann, Thomas, and Ramazan Salman (Köln: Psychiatrie Verlag).

Moser, Catherine. 2021. 'Traumatisierungen', in *Transkulturelle und transkategoriale Kompetenz*, 3rd edn., ed. by Dagmar, Domenig (Bern: hogrefe Verlag), pp. 332–359.

O'Brien, Jane C., and Gary Kielhofner (2017). The Interaction between the Person and the Environment', in *Kielhofner's Model of Human Occupation*, Vol. 5, ed. by Taylor, Renée (Philadelphia: Wolters Kluwer Health), pp. 24–37.

Reddemann, Luise. 2006. 'Was ist eine traumatische Erfahrung?', in *Psychotraumata*, ed. by Reddemann, Luise (Köln: Deutscher Ärzte-Verlag), pp. 3–10.

Reddemann, Luise, and Cornelia Dehner-Rau. 2006. 'Wenn die Traumaverarbeitung misslingt', in *Psychotraumata*, ed. by Reddemann, Luise (Köln: Deutscher Ärzte-Verlag), pp. 23–38.

Richter, Kneginja, Hartmut Lehfeld, and Günter Niklewski. 2015. 'Warten Auf Asyl: Psychiatrische Diagnosen in Der Zentralen Aufnahmeeinrichtung in Bayern', *Das Gesundheitswesen*, 77.11: 834–38, https://doi.org/10.1055/s-0035-1564075

Schreiner, Anke. 2016. 'Aus der Ohnmacht zur Handlung. Wege zur unterstützenden Heilung von komplex traumatisierten Patientinnen in der Ergotherapie', *ergotherapie*, 1: 20–26.

Sluzki, Carlos E. 2016. 'Psychologische Phasen der Migration und ihre Auswirkungen', in *Handbuch Transkulturelle Psychiatrie*, Vol. 2, ed. by Hegemann, Thomas, and Ramazan Salman (Köln: Psychiatrie Verlag), pp. 108–123.

Spevak, Christine. 2022a. 'Identitätsarbeit in der Ergotherapie: Vergleichende Analyse des sozialpsychologischen Ansatzes zur Identitätsarbeit von Heiner Keupp mit dem ergotherapeutisch-handlungswissenschaftlichen Model of Human Occupation' (Master of Science Master: Medical University Vienna, Vienna).

Spevak, Christine. 2022b. 'Stabilization of Identity through Occupational Therapy for Refugees with PTSD', *Journal of Occupational Science*, 29.1: 1–116, https://doi.org/10.1080/14427591.2022.2111001

Stock-Gissendanner, Scott, et al. 2013. 'Migrantinnen und Migranten zwischen Trauma und Traumabewältigung Implikationen aus Migrationssoziologie und interkultureller Psychotherapie für die psychiatrische, psychosomatische und psychotherapeutische Behandlungspraxis', in *Traum(a) Migration, Aktuelle Konzepte zur Therapie traumatisierter Flüchtlinge und Folteropfer*, ed. by Feldmann, Robert E. J., and Günter H. Seidler (Gießen: Psychosozial-Verlag).

World Federation of Occupational Therapists. 2019. 'Position Statement: Occupational Therapy and Human Rights', https://www.wfot.org/resources/occupational-therapy-and-human-rights

Whiteford, Gail. 2010. 'Occupational Deprivation: Understanding Limited Participation', in *Introduction to Occupation: The Art and Science of Living*, ed. by Christiansen, Charles, and Elizabeth Townsend, 2nd edn (Upper Saddle River, NJ: Pearson Education), pp. 303–328.

Wilcock, Ann, A., and Clare Hocking. 2015. *An Occupational Perspective of Health* (SLACK Incorporated).

Wintersperger, Sylvia. 2006. 'Wann ist das Trauma zu Ende', *Wege und Ziele in der Traumatherapie. Imagination*, 28.2: 39–48.

Wook Lee, Sun, and Gary Kielhofner. 2017a. 'Habituation: Patterns of Daily Occupation', in *Kielhofner's Model of Human Occupation*, Vol. 5, ed. by Taylor, Renée (Philadelphia: Wolters Kluwer Health), pp. 57–73.

Wook Lee, Sun, and Gary Kielhofner. 2017b. 'Volition', in *Kielhofner's Model of Human Occupation*, Vol. 5, ed. by Taylor, Renée (Philadelphia: Wolters Kluwer Health), pp. 38–56.

Index

About the Team

Alessandra Tosi was the managing editor for this book.

Lucy Barnes proof-read this manuscript. Sophia Bursey compiled the index.

Jeevanjot Kaur Nagpal designed the cover. The cover was produced in InDesign using the Fontin font.

Annie Hine typeset the book in InDesign and produced the paperback and hardback editions. The main text font is Tex Gyre Pagella and the heading font is Californian FB.

Jeremy Bowman produced the PDF and HTML editions. The conversion was performed with open-source software and other tools freely available on our GitHub page at https://github.com/OpenBookPublishers. Jeremy also created the EPUB.

Hannah Shakespeare was in charge of marketing.

This book was peer-reviewed by two anonymous referees. Experts in their field, these readers give their time freely to help ensure the academic rigour of our books. We are grateful for their generous and invaluable contributions.

This book need not end here...

Share

All our books — including the one you have just read — are free to access online so that students, researchers and members of the public who can't afford a printed edition will have access to the same ideas. This title will be accessed online by hundreds of readers each month across the globe: why not share the link so that someone you know is one of them?

This book and additional content is available at
https://doi.org/10.11647/OBP.0479

Donate

Open Book Publishers is an award-winning, scholar-led, not-for-profit press making knowledge freely available one book at a time. We don't charge authors to publish with us: instead, our work is supported by our library members and by donations from people who believe that research shouldn't be locked behind paywalls.

Join the effort to free knowledge by supporting us at
https://www.openbookpublishers.com/support-us

We invite you to connect with us on our socials!

BLUESKY
@openbookpublish
.bsky.social

MASTODON
@OpenBookPublish
@hcommons.social

LINKEDIN
open-book-publishers

Read more at the Open Book Publishers Blog
https://blogs.openbookpublishers.com

You may also be interested in:

Undocumented Migrants and Healthcare
Eight Stories from Switzerland
Marianne Jossen

https://doi.org/10.11647/OBP.0139

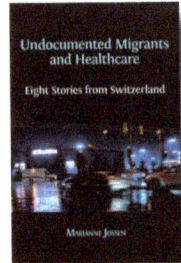

Non-communicable Disease Prevention
Best Buys, Wasted Buys and Contestable Buys
Edited by Wanrudee Isaranuwatchai, Rachel A. Archer, Yot Teerawattananon and Anthony J. Culyer

https://doi.org/10.11647/OBP.0195

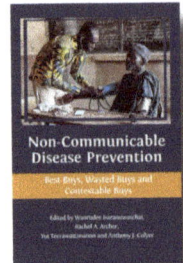

Intellectual Property and Public Health in the Developing World
Monirul Azam

https://doi.org/10.11647/OBP.0093

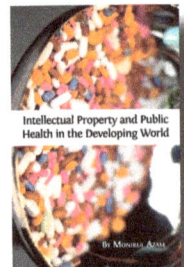

www.ingramcontent.com/pod-product-compliance
Lightning Source LLC
Chambersburg PA
CBHW042312210326
41598CB00042B/7370